The
SECTIONAL ANATOMY
LEARNING SYSTEM:

CONCEPTS

The SECTIONAL ANATOMY LEARNING SYSTEM:

CONCEPTS

Edith J. Applegate, M.S.
Professor of Science and Mathematics
Kettering College of Medical Arts
Kettering, Ohio

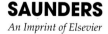
SAUNDERS
An Imprint of Elsevier

SAUNDERS
An Imprint of Elsevier
The Curtis Center
Independence Square West
Philadelphia, PA 19106

Library of Congress Cataloging in Publication Data

Applegate, Edith J.
  The sectional anatomy learning system / Edith J. Applegate.—2nd ed.
    p. ; cm.
  Includes bibliographical references and index.
  Contents: v. 1. Concepts—v. 2. Applications.
  ISBN 0-7216-8443-2 (v.1)—ISBN 0-7216-8443-2 (v.2)
  1. Anatomy, Surgical and topographical. 2. Diagnostic imaging. I. Title.
  [DNLM: 1. Anatomy, Cross-Sectional. 2. Magnetic Resonance Imaging.
  3. Tomography. 4. Ultrasonography. QS 4 A648s 2001]
  QM531 .A65 2001
  611—dc21
                                                                2001040049

Executive Editor: Jeanne Wilke
Developmental Editor: Jennifer Moorhead
Project Manager: John Rogers
Senior Production Editors: Mary Turner and Helen Hudlin
Designer: Julia Ramirez
Art: Julia Ramirez

THE SECTIONAL ANATOMY LEARNING SYSTEM: CONCEPTS   ISBN 0–7216–8443–2
                                                         Volume 1: 9997633717

Printed in the United States of America

Last digit is the print number: 9   8   7   6   5   4   TG/MVY

Dedicated to the three favorite men in my life: Stan, Dave, and Doug

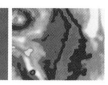

The *Sectional Anatomy Learning System* was created to provide teachers and students in the diagnostic imaging sciences with a tool for understanding anatomy in three dimensions. A thorough comprehension of anatomy from a sectional perspective greatly enhances the understanding of gross anatomy. Students should be able to observe a transverse, sagittal, or coronal section and mentally reconstruct the three-dimensional relationships of that area. Conversely, given a gross dissection of a region, students should be able to visualize the appearance and the relationships in the planar sections.

The Sectional Anatomy Learning System: Concepts is designed for radiography students and for those involved with the technologies of sonography, computed tomography, and magnetic resonance imaging. It is also valuable to practicing clinicians who want to improve their skills and expertise through continuing education. Basic anatomy and physiology—at least one semester and preferably two—is necessary for background information and terminology.

ORGANIZATION

The text is designed for use with its companion workbook, *Applications*. *Applications* is a collection of drawings of transverse, sagittal, and coronal sections for students to label. Coloring exercises are included to help readers see the relationships of important structures and follow them through several levels. Each line drawing is accompanied by questions, and there is a post test at the end of each chapter.

The common focus of both books is "anatomical relationships." In other words, the emphasis is on the relationship of one organ to another, one blood vessel to another, a blood vessel to a nerve, or one body part to another. Understanding these relationships is essential if one is to truly understand sectional anatomy rather than engage in a rote memorization process.

Both *Concepts*, the textbook, and *Applications*, the workbook, are divided into nine chapters. Chapter 1 introduces basic concepts and terminology. This introductory chapter is followed by eight chapters, each of which deals with a specific region of the body: the head, the neck, the thorax, the abdomen, the male and female pelves, the vertebral column and spinal cord, the upper extremity, and the lower extremity. Each chapter may be used as a self-contained unit for a series of minicourses, or the books may be used in their entirety for a complete semester course. Instructors can choose topics as the allotted class time permits.

Organization Within Chapters

Each chapter begins with an outline and a list of learning objectives that represent student goals. The first part of each chapter is an overview of the anatomy of the region being discussed, providing a common starting point for all the students in the class. It reviews and refreshes the terminology appropriate to the region so students can concentrate on the anatomical relationships of structures rather than becoming bogged down in the anatomy and terminology.

The sectional anatomy of the region is presented after the review of gross anatomy and terminology. Sectional anatomy is discussed first in the transverse plane and then in the sagittal and coronal planes. Each level of section that is presented is illustrated by a labeled line drawing.

Each chapter concludes with a series of review questions and a chapter quiz that students may use for self-testing. In general, there is at least one question pertaining to each of the objectives that is listed at the beginning of the chapter. Instructors may wish to assign them for homework or use them as test questions.

NEW TO THIS EDITION

The revised edition contains 60 brand-new halftones from various modalities, including radiographs, angiograms, computed tomography and magnetic resonance images, and sonograms. All the line drawings are new. Each chapter of the *Concepts* volume now includes a chapter quiz. Case studies with images and pathology sections have been added to selected chapters.

ANCILLARIES

An Instructor's Electronic Resource and an Electronic Image Collection are available as part of this comprehensive learning system. The Instructor's Electronic Resource contains a test bank and an instructor's manual. The test bank includes questions and answers different from those in either volume of the learning system. Instructors may use these questions for homework, in-class review, quizzes, or tests. The instructor's manual remains a multifaceted teaching aid for the instructor. It contains suggestions for teaching methods, lists of structures to be identified, and techniques for testing. The instructor's manual also contains a description of each image in the electronic image collection with notes on the important structures and the anatomical relationships that are evident on the images. The instructor's manual also contains the correct responses for all the labeling exercises in *Applications* and for all of the questions in both the *Concepts* textbook and the *Applications* workbook.

The Electronic Image Collection includes radiographs, sonograms, computed tomography and magnetic resonance images, and photographs of cadaver specimens that are sectioned in the transverse plane. These photographs correspond to the line drawings of transverse sections in *Applications*. Both a labeled and an unlabeled version of each of the line drawings in *Concepts* and all of the line drawings in *Applications* are included. These may be used at the instructor's discretion for teaching or for testing.

AUTHOR'S FINAL NOTE

I have used these materials in a variety of ways over the last 20 years–in collegiate courses for radiography, ultrasono-graphy, computed tomography, and magnetic resonance imaging. When conducting in-service programs for technologists in a hospital department, I usually concentrate on one region and use only one chapter. Because each chapter is self-contained, *The Sectional Anatomy Learning System* is a flexible teaching mechanism for a continuing education series.

It is my intent and hope that *The Sectional Anatomy Learning System* will serve as a comprehensive and effective teaching and learning package. There is always more to learn and many different teaching methods. You can help improve this package with your comments. I welcome any suggestions you have to offer.

Edith J. Applegate

ACKNOWLEDGMENTS

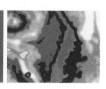

Writing a textbook requires the expertise, cooperation, collaboration, and encouragement of many people. This second edition of *The Sectional Anatomy Learning System* is no exception.

Four presidents of Kettering College of Medical Arts (KCMA), Kettering, Ohio, have had a role in the evolution of this publication. In the spring of 1980 Winton Beaven asked me to develop a course in cross-sectional anatomy for the then-new ultrasonography curriculum. Thus began this project. Early in 1989 Robert W. Williams encouraged me (maybe "nagged" is a better word) to put the material that I had developed into a publishable form. This was the second step. In 1991 Peter Bath rejoiced with me when the first edition of *The Sectional Anatomy Learning System* was published. Now in 2001 Charles Scriven shares with me the excitement of the second edition.

Larry Beneke and Rob Hoover from the Department of Radiologic Sciences and Imaging at KCMA provided the radiographs, angiograms, and the CT and MR images. Joyce Grube, Beth Maxwell, and Susan Price from the Department of Medical Sonography at KCMA and Margo Miller from Kettering Memorial Hospital provided the sonograms used in this book. Joyce Grube and Rob Hoover provided the case studies. The assistance of these individuals add a great deal to the learning experience provided by the second edition of *The Sectional Anatomy Learning System*.

My students, with their probing quest for knowledge, have been a driving force behind my efforts. Numerous colleagues and other friends, including Norman Wendth, the Dean of Academic Affairs at KCMA, have prodded me with their interest. Although many miles away, Doug, Dave, and Barb—my two sons and daughter-in-law—have encouraged me with their phone calls and enthusiasm. My husband and best friend for more than 40 years has been a constant source of love, encouragement, reassurance, strength, and patience.

To all I say a big *thank you!*

CONTENTS

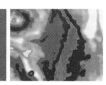

CHAPTER ONE

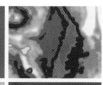

Introduction to Sectional Anatomy

1

BODY PLANES
DIRECTIONAL TERMS

BODY CAVITIES
  Membranes of the Ventral Cavity
REGIONAL TERMINOLOGY

OBJECTIVES

Upon completion of this chapter, the student should be able to do the following:

- Identify transverse, sagittal, midsagittal, parasagittal, and frontal planes.
- Describe the anatomical position.
- Use correct directional terms to describe the relative position of one body part to another.
- Describe the location, subdivisions, and contents of the dorsal body cavity and the ventral body cavity.
- Name and identify the nine abdominopelvic regions.
- Distinguish between the visceral and the parietal layers of serous membranes.
- State the specific locations of the parietal and visceral layers of pleura, pericardium, and peritoneum.
- Use correct regional terms to refer to specific areas of the body.

Before starting the study of sectional anatomy, it may be profitable to review some of the terminology and concepts you learned in gross anatomy or anatomy and physiology. This will help get you back into the "anatomy" mode and provide a common foundation for the class. The introductory material will include body planes, directional terms, body cavities, membranes, and regional terminology.

BODY PLANES

To aid in visualizing the spatial relationships of internal body parts, the body is sectioned, or cut, along a flat surface or plane. The ability to interpret sections in various planes is becoming increasingly important in the clinical sciences, especially in the imaging sciences. The three most commonly used planes are the transverse, sagittal, and frontal planes, which are at right angles to each other. These are illustrated in Fig. 1-1.

Transverse planes, or horizontal planes, cut across the body horizontally from right to left and divide the body into superior and inferior portions. Sections cut along transverse planes are sometimes called cross sections. These are the most frequently used sections in imaging modalities.

Sagittal planes are vertical planes that cut through the body from top to bottom and divide the body into right and left portions. The specific sagittal plane that passes through the midline is the **midsagittal plane,** or median plane, and

divides the body into right and left halves. All other sagittal planes are **parasagittal planes.**

Frontal planes, like sagittal planes, are vertical planes. They are at right angles to the sagittal and transverse planes and divide the body into anterior and posterior portions. Frontal planes are also called coronal planes.

DIRECTIONAL TERMS

If directional terms are to be meaningful, there must be some point of reference with which to start. In the body, the point of reference is the anatomical position. In this position, the body is standing erect, the face is forward, and the arms are at the sides with the palms and toes directed forward. Fig. 1-2 illustrates the body in anatomical position.

The following directional terms are used to describe the relative position of one part to another. Note that the two items in each pair of terms are opposites.

Superior means that a part is above another portion, or closer to the head.
Inferior means that a part is below another part, or closer to the feet.
Anterior (or ventral) means toward the front surface.
Posterior (or dorsal) means that a part is toward the back.
Medial means toward, or nearer, the midline of the body.

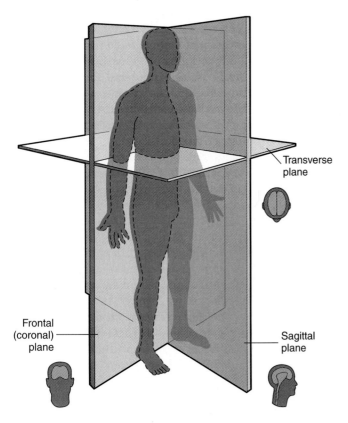

FIG. 1-1 Transverse, sagittal, and frontal planes of the body.

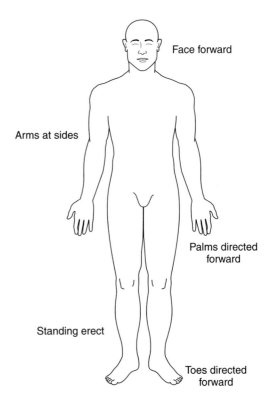

FIG. 1-2 Anatomical position.

Lateral means toward, or nearer, the side, away from the midline.

Proximal means that a part is closer to a point of attachment, or closer to the trunk of the body, than another part.

Distal is the opposite of proximal. It means that a part is farther away from a point of attachment than is another part.

Superficial means that a part is located on or near the surface.

Deep is the opposite of superficial. It means that a part is away from the surface.

BODY CAVITIES

The two large enclosed spaces within the axial portion of the body that contain the internal organs are called **body cavities.** In addition to the two closed body cavities, there are several smaller cavities such as the oral cavity, nasal cavity, and orbital cavity. Most of these open to the exterior of the body.

The smaller of the two closed cavities is the **dorsal body cavity.** This is subdivided into the **cranial cavity,** which contains the brain, and the **spinal cavity,** which contains the spinal cord. The cranial and spinal cavities are continuous with each other at the foramen magnum.

The larger and more anterior of the two closed body cavities is the **ventral body cavity.** This cavity contains the group of internal organs that are commonly called the viscera or visceral organs. The ventral body cavity is subdivided by the diaphragm into a smaller superior **thoracic cavity** and a larger inferior **abdominopelvic cavity.** The thoracic cavity is further subdivided into the right and left **pleural cavities** and the mediastinum. The pleural cavities contain the lungs, and the mediastinum, which is between the two pleural cavities, contains the **pericardial cavity,** which encloses the heart. The mediastinum also contains the esophagus and trachea.

Although there is no partition to separate it, the abdominopelvic cavity is often subdivided into the **abdominal cavity** and the **pelvic cavity.** The abdominal cavity is more superior and contains the stomach, liver, spleen, intestines, and other organs. The inferior part, the pelvic cavity, contains the urinary bladder, rectum, and reproductive organs. The closed body cavities are illustrated in Fig. 1-3.

To help describe the location of body parts or pain, health care professionals frequently divide the abdominopelvic cavity into regions by using imaginary lines. One method uses a vertical plane through the midline and a horizontal plane that passes through the umbilicus. This divides the abdominopelvic cavity into four quadrants, illustrated in Fig. 1-4. Another method uses two parasagittal planes to divide the cavity into nine regions, illustrated in Fig. 1-5. The three central regions are, from superior to inferior, the epigastric, umbilical, and hypogastric. To the right and left of these central regions, from superior to inferior, are the hypochondriac, lumbar, and inguinal, or iliac, regions.

Membranes of the Ventral Cavity

Very thin, double-layered **serous membranes** line the ventral cavity and cover the organs within the cavities. The portion of the membrane that lines the cavity wall is the **parietal layer,** or **parietal serosa.** It folds in on itself to form the **visceral serosa,** which covers the organs within the cavity. Serous membranes secrete a serous fluid that lubricates the surfaces of the membranes to allow the organs to move without friction.

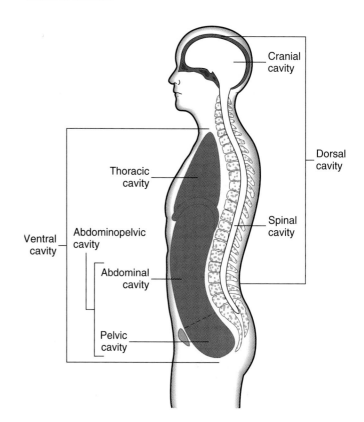

FIG. 1-3 The two major cavities in the body.

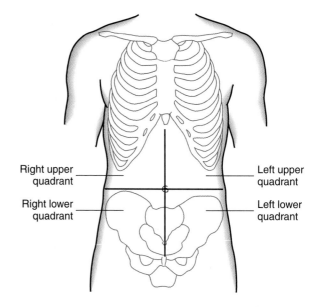

FIG. 1-4 Abdominopelvic quadrants.

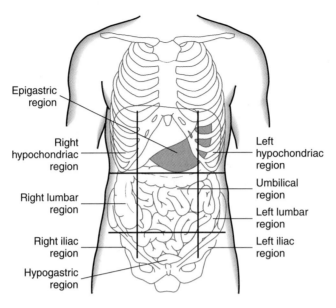

FIG. 1-5 Nine abdominopelvic regions.

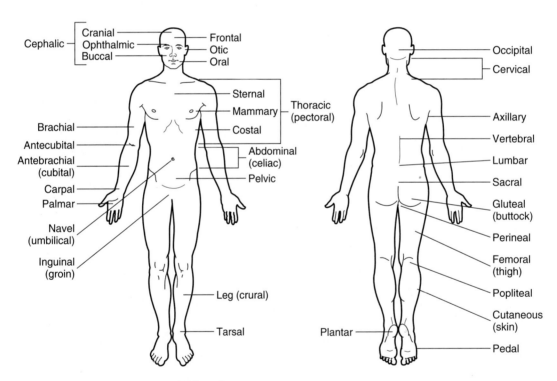

FIG. 1-6 Terms for the regions of the body.

Serous membranes have specific names according to their location. The membrane that lines the walls of the thoracic cavity is the **parietal pleura,** and that covering the lungs is the **visceral pleura.** The **parietal pericardium** lines the pericardial cavity, and the **visceral pericardium** covers the heart. In the abdominopelvic cavity, the serous membrane is called peritoneum, with the **parietal peritoneum** lining the wall of the cavity and the **visceral peritoneum** covering the organs.

REGIONAL TERMINOLOGY

The body may be divided into **axial** and **appendicular** portions. The axial part makes up the main axis of the body and consists of the head, neck, and trunk. The appendicular portion consists of the appendages, or limbs, that are attached to the main axis. Regional terms that refer to specific parts or areas of the body are listed in Table 1-1 and illustrated in Fig. 1-6.

TABLE 1-1 *Terms for Specific Body Regions*

Term	Body Region	Term	Body Region
Abdominal	Portion of the trunk below the diaphragm; between the thorax and pelvis	Lumbar	Region of the lower back and side between the lowest rib and the pelvis
Antebrachial	Region between the elbow and the wrist; forearm; cubital region	Mammary	Breast
Antecubital	Space in front of the elbow	Occipital	Lower portion of the back of the head
Axillary	Armpit area	Ophthalmic	Eyes
Brachial	Arm; proximal portion of the upper limb	Oral	Mouth
Buccal	Region of the cheek	Otic	Ears
Carpal	Wrist	Pectoral	Chest region
Cephalic	Head	Pelvic	Inferior region of the abdominopelvic cavity; lower portion of the trunk
Cervical	Neck region	Perineal	Region between the anus and pubic symphysis; includes the region of the external reproductive organs
Costal	Ribs		
Cranial	Skull		
Cubital	Antebrachial	Plantar	Sole of the foot
Femoral	Thigh; the part of the lower extremity between the hip and the knee	Popliteal	Area behind the knee
		Sacral	Posterior region between the hipbones
Gluteal	Buttock region	Sternal	Anterior midline of the thorax
Inguinal	Depressed region between the abdomen and the thigh; groin	Thoracic	Chest; part of the trunk inferior to the neck and superior to the diaphragm
Leg	Portion of the lower extremity between the knee and the foot; also called the crural region	Umbilical	Navel; middle region of the abdomen
		Vertebral	Pertaining to the spinal column; backbone

· REVIEW QUESTIONS ·

1. Define the following terms: transverse plane, sagittal plane, and frontal plane.
2. What is the difference between a sagittal plane, a midsagittal plane, and a parasagittal plane?
3. What are the five conditions of a body in anatomical position?
4. Define each of the following pairs of directional terms and use each term in a sentence that describes the relative position of two body parts:
   a. Superior/inferior
   b. Anterior/posterior
   c. Medial/lateral
   d. Proximal/distal
   e. Superficial/deep
5. Indicate whether each of the following is a part of the dorsal body cavity or a part of the ventral body cavity:
   a. Thoracic cavity
   b. Spinal cavity
   c. Abdominal cavity
   d. Cranial cavity
   e. Mediastinum
6. Name the three abdominopelvic regions in the middle, horizontal row of the nine regions.
7. Name the three abdominopelvic regions in the middle, vertical row of the nine regions.
8. What type of membrane lines the cavities and covers the organs in the ventral body cavity?
9. What specific layer of serous membrane covers the organs in the abdominopelvic cavity?
10. What regional term refers to each of the following?
    a. Armpit area
    b. Neck region
    c. Ears
    d. Sole of the foot
    e. Area behind the knee

· CHAPTER QUIZ ·

Name the Following:

1. The specific plane that divides the body into right and left halves
2. The vertical plane that is not a sagittal plane
3. The directional term that means toward, or nearer, the midline of the body
4. The dorsal body cavity that contains the brain
5. The most central of the nine abdominopelvic regions
6. The abdominopelvic region that contains most of the stomach
7. The serous membrane that lines the abdominopelvic cavity
8. The specific layer of serous membrane that covers the heart
9. The regional term that refers to the ribs
10. The regional term that refers to the wrist

True/False:

1. The plane that divides the body into anterior and posterior portions is a horizontal plane.
2. A frontal plane is the same as a coronal plane.
3. The brachial region is proximal to the carpal region.
4. The oral region is inferior to the ophthalmic region.
5. The mediastinum is a part of the dorsal body cavity.
6. Two divisions of the ventral body cavity are the thoracic cavity and the abdominopelvic cavity.
7. Parietal pleura covers the lungs.
8. The right hypochondriac region contains most of the liver.
9. The leg is also called the crural region.
10. The cephalic region refers to the lower portion of the back of the head.

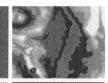

The Head 2

OBJECTIVES

Upon completion of this chapter, the student should be able to do the following:

- Name the bones of the cranium and face.
- Identify the four paranasal sinuses.
- Name five muscles of facial expression, describe the location of each, and state the insertion and innervation of this group.
- Name four muscles of mastication, describe the location of each muscle, and state the insertion and innervation of this muscle group.
- Compare the location and relationships of the three salivary glands.
- Identify the five lobes of the cerebrum.
- Describe the relationships of the basal ganglia.
- Describe the location and structure of the diencephalon.
- Locate the components of the brainstem.
- Compare the cerebrum and cerebellum with respect to size, appearance, location, and structure.
- Trace the flow of cerebrospinal fluid through the ventricles in the brain.
- Describe the three layers of meninges.
- Identify six subarachnoid cisterns by describing their location and significance.
- Describe the arterial blood supply to the brain.
- Identify the major venous sinuses that return blood from the brain to the internal jugular vein.
- Name the 12 cranial nerves and the foramen that serves as a passageway for each; state functions of each nerve.
- Describe the structure of the eye, including the bulbus oculi, musculature, vascular supply, and protective features.
- Discuss the relationships of the internal jugular vein, external jugular vein, internal carotid artery, and external carotid artery to each other and to other surrounding structures such as the parotid gland and the sternocleidomastoid muscle.

General Anatomy of the Head

The principal bony structure of the head is the skull, which is especially adapted to house and protect the brain and pituitary gland, the two organs that integrate body activities. The head is the location of the special sensory organs of vision, hearing, equilibrium, taste, and smell, which provide information concerning our surroundings. The digestive and respiratory systems begin with openings in the head and continue as passageways in the neck. The intricate structure of the head is an appropriate complement to the functional complexity of this region.

OSSEOUS COMPONENTS

The bony framework of the head is called the skull. This is the most complex osseous structure of the body, and it consists of 22 bones connected by immovable joints called sutures. For descriptive purposes, these bones are divided into the cranium and the facial skeleton, although there is no distinct line of demarcation between the two parts. Some of the bones surround a large cranial cavity that contains the brain. The superior surface of this region is covered by the scalp. Some skull bones adjacent to the nasal cavity contain air-filled spaces called paranasal sinuses. Many of the bones in the skull have holes or openings called foramina that serve as passageways for nerves and blood vessels. In addition to the skull, there are seven other bones associated with the head. These are the auditory ossicles and the hyoid bone. The osseous components of the head are summarized in Table 2-1.

Cranium

The eight bones of the cranium surround the cranial cavity, which houses the brain. The single **frontal bone** forms the forehead and superior part of the orbit of the eye. It contains frontal sinuses, which communicate with the nasal cavity. Two **parietal bones** form most of the top of the cranium. Two **temporal bones** form a portion of the sides and base, or floor, of the cranium. Each temporal bone has a thin, flat, squamous portion that forms the inferior lateral part of the cranium. The posterior portion of the temporal bone is the **mastoid process.** The **external auditory canal** (meatus), the tympanic membrane, the middle ear, and the inner ear are located in the **petrous portion,** which extends medially to form part of the base of the cranium. The single **ethmoid bone** is located between the eyes and forms most of the medial wall of each orbit. The superior surface of the ethmoid bone forms a part of the base of the cranial cavity and the roof of the nasal cavities. A thin, perpendicular plate of the ethmoid bone extends inferiorly to form part of the **nasal septum.** The superior and middle conchae (turbinates) in the nasal cavity are part of the ethmoid bone. The single **sphenoid bone** lies at the base of the skull anterior to the temporal bones. Often described as bat shaped, the sphenoid bone has "wings" that form the ante-

TABLE 2-1   *Summary of Bones Associated With Head*

Bone	Number	Total
Bones of the Cranium		8
Frontal	1	
Parietal	2	
Occipital	1	
Temporal	2	
Sphenoid	1	
Ethmoid	1	
Bones of the Face		14
Maxillae	2	
Nasal	2	
Zygomatic	2	
Lacrimal	2	
Mandible	1	
Vomer	1	
Inferior nasal conchae	2	
Palatine	2	
Middle Ear Bones		6
Malleus	2	
Incus	2	
Stapes	2	
Hyoid Bone		1

rior lateral portion of the cranium and the lateral walls of the orbits. The sella turcica is found in the center of the bone and is the location of the pituitary gland. The single **occipital bone** forms the posterior portion and part of the base of the cranium. It has a large hole, the foramen magnum, for passage of the spinal cord and the vertebral vessels. The bones of the cranium are illustrated in Fig. 2-1.

The domelike superior portion of the cranium is the **calvaria,** or skullcap. It is composed of the superior portions of the frontal, parietal, and occipital bones. The calvaria is covered by the scalp, which extends from the eyebrows to the superior nuchal line on the occipital bone. Structurally, the scalp has five layers. The outer layer, the **skin,** covers the second layer, which is composed of highly vascularized **subcutaneous connective tissue.** The third layer, or epicranium, consists of two thin muscles that are connected by a broad, flat tendon, or aponeurosis. This musculoaponeurotic sheet has the frontalis muscle at the anterior end and the occipitalis muscle at the posterior end. The strong aponeurosis that connects the two muscles is known as the **epicranial aponeurosis,** or **galea aponeurotica.** These three layers of the scalp are bound tightly together and move as a unit. Collectively, they are often referred to as the scalp proper. A fourth layer that consists of **loose connective tissue** separates the scalp proper from the fifth layer, the **periosteum,** or pericranium. The loose connective tissue layer permits mobility of the scalp proper, but it is also considered a potentially dangerous area because it allows scalp infections to spread easily. Lacerations of the scalp typically bleed profusely because of the extensive vascularization of the subcutaneous

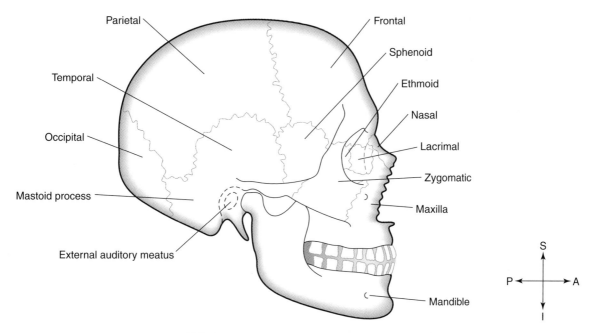

FIG. 2-1 Bones of the skull (cranium and face).

connective tissue. The letters SCALP serve as a useful mnemonic tool for remembering the five layers of the scalp.

S = Skin
C = Connective tissue
A = Aponeurosis
L = Loose connective tissue
P = Periosteum

The cranial cavity, a large space formed by the eight cranial bones, contains the brain. The floor of the cranial cavity is subdivided into anterior, middle, and posterior cranial fossae, as illustrated in Fig. 2-2. The **anterior cranial fossa** is formed by portions of the ethmoid, sphenoid, and frontal bones. This fossa houses the frontal lobes of the brain. The floor of the **middle cranial fossa** is composed of the body and greater wings of the sphenoid, and the squamosal and petrous portions of the temporal bones. This region contains the temporal lobes of the brain. The **posterior cranial fossa** comprises the remainder of the cranial cavity and is formed by parts of the sphenoid, temporal, and occipital bones. This region contains the cerebellum, the pons, and the medulla oblongata. The inferiormost portion of the posterior cranial fossa shows the large **foramen magnum** through which the spinal cord passes.

Face

The facial portion of the skull consists of 14 bones. Some of these bones are illustrated in Fig. 2-1. The two **maxillae** (singular, **maxilla**) unite in the midline to form the upper jaw. A horizontal piece of each maxilla, the **palatine process,** forms the anterior portion of the roof of the mouth, which is the hard palate. If the palatine processes of the two max-

illae fail to join during prenatal development, a cleft palate results. Each maxilla contains a maxillary sinus, which is a large air space that communicates with the nasal cavity. Two **palatine bones** form the posterior portion of the hard palate. Two **zygomatic bones,** one on each side, form the prominence of the cheek and the lateral margin of the orbit. A posteriorly extending process of the zygomatic bone unites with the temporal bone to form the **zygomatic arch.** Two small, rectangular **nasal bones** join in the midline to form the bridge of the nose. Fractures of these bones are common facial injuries. The anterior part of the medial wall of each orbital cavity consists of a small, thin **lacrimal bone.** Each bone has a groove that helps to form the nasolacrimal canal, which allows the tears of the eye to drain into the nasal cavity. The single **vomer** is a thin bone shaped like the blade of a plow. It forms the inferior portion of the nasal septum. The two **inferior nasal conchae** are scroll-like bones that project horizontally from the lateral walls of the nasal cavities. The **superior** and **middle conchae** are part of the ethmoid bone, but the inferior nasal conchae are separate bones. The conchae are covered by mucous membrane that warms and moistens the air that enters the nasal cavities. The single **mandible** forms the lower jaw. The posterior ends of the mandible extend vertically to form the **rami** (singular, **ramus**). Each ramus has a knoblike condyle and a pointed coronoid process. The mandibular condyle articulates with the temporal bone to form the temporomandibular joint, which is the only movable joint in the skull.

Paranasal Sinuses

The **paranasal sinuses** are air-filled spaces in some of the bones adjacent to the nasal cavity. There are four sets of

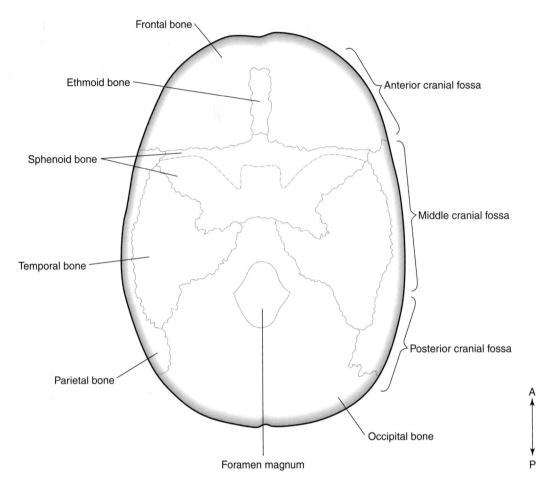

FIG. 2-2 Cranial fossae (floor of cranial cavity).

paranasal sinuses, and they are named according to the bone in which they are located: **frontal, ethmoidal, sphenoidal,** and **maxillary.** Usually developing after birth as outgrowths of the nasal cavity, the sinuses retain their original openings so that their secretions drain into the nasal cavity. The mucous membrane that lines the sinuses is continuous with the mucosa of the nasal cavity, but it is thinner and less vascular than the nasal mucosa.

The **frontal sinuses** are located in the frontal bone near the midline. They develop in the child and are usually visible on radiographs by the time the child is 7 years of age; however, the sinuses continue to enlarge throughout adolescence. The frontal sinuses drain into the **middle meatus** of the nasal cavity, between the middle and inferior nasal conchae, by way of a frontonasal duct.

The **ethmoidal sinuses** consist of numerous air spaces in the ethmoid bone between the orbit of the eye and the upper part of the nasal cavity. Although a few ethmoidal air cells are present in the neonate, they are not readily visible on radiographs until the infant is 2 years old and do not enlarge significantly until later in the childhood years—usually around 6 to 8 years of age. The ethmoidal sinuses have numerous openings into the **superior meatus** between the superior and middle conchae and into the **middle meatus** between the middle and inferior conchae.

The **sphenoidal sinuses** are located in the body of the sphenoid bone just posterior to the ethmoidal sinuses and nasal cavity. The sinuses occupy most of the volume of the sphenoid body so that only a thin plate of bone separates the sinuses from the pituitary gland, the optic nerve, the optic chiasma, the internal carotid artery, and the cavernous sinus. Tiny sphenoidal sinuses may be present in the newborn, but their development is more likely to occur in a child of about 2 years of age, with additional growth during late childhood and adolescence. The sphenoidal sinuses drain into the **sphenoethmoidal recess** above the superior nasal conchae.

Small **maxillary sinuses,** which are located in the bodies of the maxillae, are present in the newborn and grow slowly until the child reaches puberty. The accelerated development of the maxillary sinuses during adolescence contributes to the apparent change in facial features that typically occurs during this period. When fully developed, the maxillary sinuses are the largest of the paranasal sinuses. The maxillary sinus drains into the nasal cavity by way of a relatively long **hiatus semilunaris,** which opens into the **middle meatus.** A couple of factors hinder the drainage of this sinus: the hiatus traverses a superior direction when the body is erect, thus necessitating drainage "against gravity"; and the opening from the sinus into the hiatus is in a supe-

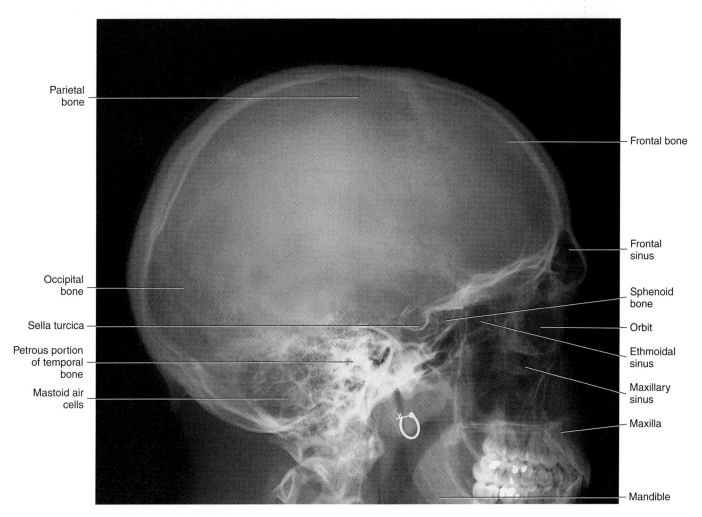

FIG. 2-3 Lateral skull radiograph.

rior location. The drainage problem is further complicated by the fact that the maxillary sinus is the most inferiorly located of the paranasal sinuses and communicating channels allow the other sinuses to drain into the maxillary sinus. These are the reasons why the maxillary sinus is the sinus that is most often involved in infections. The frontal, ethmoidal, and sphenoidal sinuses are innervated by branches of the ophthalmic division of the trigeminal nerve, which is the fifth cranial nerve. The maxillary sinus is innervated by branches of the maxillary division of the fifth cranial nerve. The cranial nerves will be discussed later in this chapter. Sinuses and other features of the skeleton of the head are illustrated by the radiographs in Figs. 2-3 and 2-4.

Foramina of the Skull

Foramina are openings in bones that serve as passageways for nerves and blood vessels. Because the vessels that transport blood and the nerves that carry impulses must pass through the sutured, helmetlike bones of the skull on their way to and from the brain, there are numerous foramina in these bones. Table 2-2 provides a summary of the foramina of the skull.

Additional Bones Associated With the Skull

There are six auditory ossicles (three pairs) and a single hyoid bone associated with the head, in addition to the eight bones of the cranium and the fourteen bones of the facial skeleton. There are three chambers in the ear: the inner ear, the middle ear, and the external ear. The ear ossicles, the **malleus, incus,** and **stapes,** are located within the middle ear chamber in the petrous portion of the temporal bone. The ossicles transmit and amplify sound waves through the middle ear. The single **hyoid bone** is located in the neck just superior to the larynx. The hyoid is unique because it does not attach directly to any other bone; instead, it is suspended by ligaments. Muscles associated with the hyoid bone are described in Chapter 3.

MUSCULAR COMPONENTS

There are numerous muscles located in the head, many of them small and difficult to separate from adjacent muscles. They are even more difficult to isolate by imaging techniques. These muscles have functional significance because they deal with facial expression and chewing food. Only the larger and more significant muscles are presented in this text (Table 2-3).

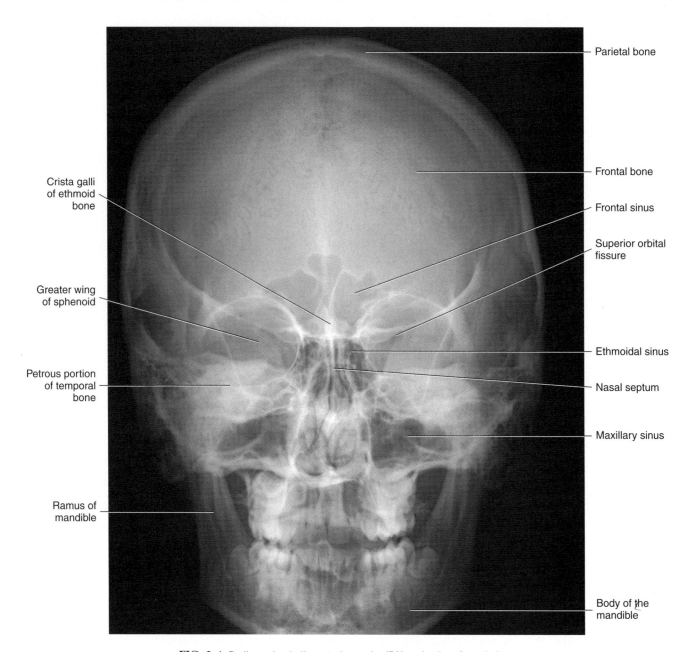

FIG. 2-4 Radiograph, skull, posterioanterior (PA) projection, frontal view.

TABLE 2-2   *Major Foramina of the Skull*

Foramen	Location	Structures Transmitted
Carotid canal	Temporal bone	Internal carotid artery; sympathetic nerves
Hypoglossal canal	Occipital bone	Hypoglossal nerve
Infraorbital	Maxilla	Maxillary branch of trigeminal nerve; infraorbital nerve and artery
Internal auditory meatus	Temporal bone	Vestibulocochlear nerve
Jugular	Temporal bone	Internal jugular vein; vagus, glossopharyngeal, and spinal accessory nerves
Magnum	Occipital bone	Medulla oblongata/spinal cord; accessory nerves; vertebral arteries
Nasolacrimal canal	Lacrimal bone	Nasolacrimal (tear) duct
Olfactory	Ethmoid bone	Olfactory nerves
Optic	Sphenoid bone	Optic nerve; central artery and vein of retina
Ovale	Sphenoid bone	Mandibular branch of trigeminal nerve
Rotundum	Sphenoid bone	Maxillary branch of trigeminal nerve
Stylomastoid	Temporal bone	Facial nerve

TABLE 2-3 *Muscles Associated With Facial Expression and Mastication*

Muscle	Origin	Insertion	Action	Innervation
Muscles of Facial Expression				
Frontalis	Aponeurosis of scalp	Skin of eyebrow and forehead	Elevates eyebrows; wrinkles forehead	Facial (cranial nerve VII)
Orbicularis oris	Maxillae and mandible	Lip mucosa and skin at corner of mouth	Closes mouth and puckers lips, as in whistling	Facial (cranial nerve VII)
Orbicularis oculi	Frontal bones and maxillae around orbit	Eyelid	Closes eye, as in winking and blinking	Facial (cranial nerve VII)
Buccinator	Buccinator ridge of mandible, alveolar processes of maxillae, pterygomandibular ligament	Orbicularis oris at angle of mouth	Compresses cheeks when blowing, as when playing a musical instrument	Facial (cranial nerve VII)
Platysma	Fascia of the cervical region	Mandible, the skin of the neck, and the orbicularis oris	Depresses lower jaw, forms ridges on neck	Facial (cranial nerve VII)
Muscles of Mastication				
Temporalis	Temporal bone	Mandible	Elevates mandible to close mouth	Trigeminal (cranial nerve V), mandibular division
Masseter	Zygomatic arch	Mandible	Elevates mandible	Trigeminal (cranial nerve V), mandibular division
Lateral pterygoid	Sphenoid	Mandible	Pulls mandible forward (protracts)	Trigeminal (cranial nerve V), mandibular division
Medial pterygoid	Sphenoid	Mandible	Protracts mandible and moves mandible laterally	Trigeminal (cranial nerve V), mandibular division

Muscles of Facial Expression

The muscles of facial expression are located in the subcutaneous tissue of the face. They originate in the fascia or on the underlying bone, and they insert on the skin of the face. All are innervated by cranial nerve VII, the facial nerve. Many of these muscles are small and thin and are difficult to dissect or to distinguish on sections. Actions of the facial muscles are easily observed, however, because they are used to express feelings. Five of the more prominent facial muscles are mentioned here. The **frontalis** muscle is a part of the scalp. Originating from the aponeurosis, which is located on the top of the head, the frontalis inserts on the skin of the eyebrow and forehead. When it contracts, this muscle elevates the eyebrows and produces transverse wrinkles in the skin of the forehead. The **orbicularis oris** muscle is an important sphincter that encircles the mouth and forms the muscular bulk of the lips. This muscle's function involves closing the mouth and puckering the lips, as in whistling. It plays an important role in the enunciation of words. A similar sphincter, the **orbicularis oculi** muscle, surrounds the eye. Contraction of these muscle fibers reduces the orbital opening, as in winking and blinking. The **bucci-**

nator muscle is an accessory muscle in mastication and compresses the cheeks when blowing, as in playing a musical wind instrument. It inserts on the orbicularis oris at the angle of the mouth. The **platysma** muscle is a broad, flat muscle in the subcutaneous tissue of the neck. It inserts on the mandible, the skin of the neck, and the orbicularis oris muscle. When it contracts, it depresses the lower jaw and forms ridges in the skin of the neck.

Muscles of Mastication

The four muscles of mastication provide chewing movements by acting on the temporomandibular joint to move the mandible (see Table 2-3). All insert on the mandible and are innervated by the mandibular division of the fifth cranial nerve. They are quite readily seen on transverse sections. The fan-shaped **temporalis** muscle covers the squamosal portion of the temporal bone and is a powerful muscle used to close the mouth by elevating the mandible. The **masseter,** or chewing muscle, is located on the lateral aspect of the ramus of the mandible. Both the **lateral** and **medial pterygoid** muscles originate on the lateral pterygoid plate of the sphenoid bone and insert on the medial surface of the mandible. When these muscles are observed in transverse sections, the temporalis is seen in the more superior sections. In lower sections, starting at the lateral surface, you see, in sequence, the masseter, the ramus of the mandible, the lateral pterygoid, and the medial pterygoid.

SALIVARY GLANDS

There are three pairs of salivary glands located in the region of the face. These glands are usually considered to be a part of the digestive system because they secrete a fluid to moisten food particles for taste and swallowing. They also secrete an enzyme, salivary amylase, which initiates digestion of carbohydrates. All of the salivary glands are easily seen in sectional views.

Parotid Gland

The largest of the glands is the **parotid gland,** wedged between the ramus of the mandible and the mastoid portion of the temporal bone. The parotid gland occupies the space just anterior and inferior to the auricle of the ear, and a portion of the gland overlies the masseter muscle in the cheek. The well-defined duct of the parotid gland, Stensen's duct, extends across the masseter muscle, then turns to penetrate the buccinator muscle and opens into the vestibule of the mouth near the upper second molar tooth.

Submandibular Gland

The **submandibular (submaxillary) gland** is located medial to the body and angle of the mandible. The gland can be felt as a small lump along the inferior border of the posterior half of the mandible. The secretions of this gland reach the oral cavity by means of the submandibular (Wharton's) duct, which opens near the midline beneath the tongue.

Sublingual Gland

The third salivary gland is the **sublingual gland.** It is the smallest and most deeply situated of the salivary glands. Located under the mucous membrane in the floor of the mouth, the two sublingual glands unite anteriorly to form a glandular mass around the lingual frenulum. These glands open into the floor of the mouth by means of a major sublingual duct (Bartholin's duct) and numerous small sublingual ducts (of Rivinus) along the midline. Sometimes ducts from the sublingual glands may open into the submandibular duct.

BRAIN

The predominant structure in the cranial cavity is the brain—a rather unimpressive looking mass of tissue that weighs approximately 3 pounds. It is composed of organized regions of white matter and gray matter. The **white matter** consists of nerve fibers that are covered with a white, fatty substance called myelin. The **gray matter** consists of nerve cell bodies and unmyelinated fibers. Some of the gray matter is grouped together to form regions called **basal ganglia.** Generally, the gray areas are regions of synapse—electrical communication between neurons. Spaces called **ventricles** are located within the brain and are surrounded by brain tissue. The brain is separated from the cranial bones by layers of connective tissue called **meninges** that help protect the surface of the brain. Further protection is provided by cerebrospinal fluid, which circulates through the ventricles and around the brain. Although the brain accounts for only about 2% of body weight, it is metabolically very active; consequently, it receives 15% to 20% of the cardiac output through its arterial blood supply. After the blood circulates through the capillaries to provide oxygen for the brain tissue, it is returned to the heart by veins. Another feature of the brain involves the 12 pairs of cranial nerves that emerge from the inferior surface. These nerves provide pathways for incoming sensory impulses, which are processed and interpreted by the brain, and for outgoing motor impulses, which travel from the brain to a muscle or gland and effectuate an action.

Regions of the Brain

For descriptive purposes the brain may be divided into the **cerebrum, diencephalon, brainstem,** and **cerebellum.**

Cerebrum.   The largest portion of the brain is the **cerebrum,** which consists of two cerebral hemispheres connected by a mass of white matter called the **corpus callosum.** The anterior end of the corpus callosum is called the **genu,** and the posterior end is called the **splenium.** The deep cleft between the two cerebral hemispheres is the **longitudinal fissure.** The surface of the cerebrum exhibits numerous convolutions, which greatly increase the surface area of the cerebral cortex. The ridges are called **gyri** (singular, **gyrus**), whereas the furrows between them are designated as **sulci** (singular, **sulcus**).

Superficially, the cerebrum is divided into lobes. A **central sulcus** separates the **frontal lobe** from the **parietal lobe.** Posteriorly, the **parieto-occipital sulcus** separates the parietal lobe from the **occipital lobe.** Laterally, the **temporal lobe** is situated below the **lateral fissure.** A fifth lobe that is called the **insula,** or island of Reil, is located deep within the lateral fissure. The lobes and fissures of the brain are illustrated in Fig. 2-5.

The surface layer of the cerebrum is **gray matter,** which consists of nerve cell bodies and unmyelinated fibers. This is called the cerebral cortex and is 2 to 4 mm thick. Lying beneath the cerebral cortex is the lighter colored **white matter,** which is made up of myelinated nerve fibers.

Scattered throughout the white matter are distinct regions of gray matter called **basal ganglia.** Two of the larger

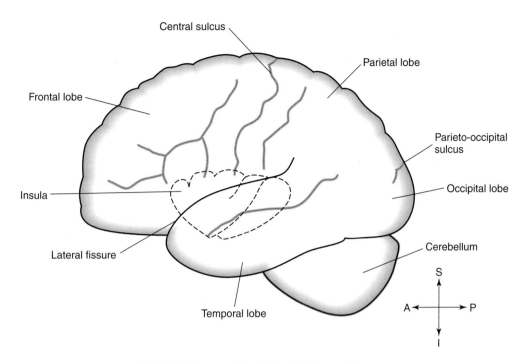

Central sulcus

Parietal lobe

Frontal lobe

Parieto-occipital
sulcus

Insula

Occipital lobe

Lateral fissure

Cerebellum

S

A ◄—— ——► P

I

Temporal lobe

FIG. 2-5 Surface of the brain with lobes and fissures.

basal ganglia are the **caudate nucleus** and the **lentiform** or **lenticular nucleus.** In sectional anatomy, the caudate nucleus is usually visualized in association with the lateral ventricle. The lentiform nucleus is rather centrally located in each cerebral hemisphere. It is subdivided into the lateral, or external, **putamen,** and the medial, or internal, **globus pallidus.** The **claustrum,** another of the basal ganglia, is a thin layer of gray matter just lateral to the lentiform nucleus and deep to the cortex of the insula. A band of white matter that is medial to the lentiform nucleus is called the **internal capsule.** The white matter that is present between the lentiform nucleus and the claustrum is the **external capsule.** The claustrum is separated from the insula by the **extreme capsule.** Because of their appearance, the caudate nucleus, the internal capsule, and the lentiform nucleus are sometimes referred to as the **corpus striatum.** Fig. 2-6 illustrates the arrangement of the basal ganglia in a transverse section.

Diencephalon. The diencephalon is centrally located and is nearly hidden from view by the large cerebral hemispheres. It surrounds the midline third ventricle and consists of the **epithalamus, thalamus,** and **hypothalamus.** The largest portion, the thalamus, is a mass of gray matter that lies on either side of the third ventricle and forms its lateral walls. This is a major relay station of the afferent, or sensory, pathway that carries impulses to the cerebral cortex. The epithalamus forms the roof of the third ventricle. A midline projection of the epithalamus forms the **pineal gland.** The hypothalamus forms the floor of the third ventricle. The following structures are located on the inferior aspect of the hypothalamus: the **infundibulum** or **pituitary**

stalk; the **optic chiasma,** where the optic nerves cross over and then emerge as optic tracts; and the **mammillary bodies,** which are two spherical masses of gray matter surrounded by a layer of white matter. The mammillary bodies function in some swallowing reflexes.

Brainstem. The brainstem is subdivided into the midbrain, the pons, and the medulla oblongata. The smallest division is the **midbrain,** which is located between the diencephalon and the pons. The midbrain surrounds the **cerebral aqueduct,** a long, slender channel for cerebrospinal fluid. Four rounded protuberances, the **corpora quadrigemina,** are visible on the dorsal aspect of the midbrain. The upper pair, **superior colliculi,** functions in the visual pathway, whereas the lower pair, the **inferior colliculi,** functions in the auditory pathway. Just above the corpora quadrigemina is a small glandular structure projecting from the diencephalon. This is the **pineal body,** or **pineal gland.** On the ventral aspect of the midbrain there are two ropelike bundles called **cerebral peduncles.** These are composed of motor fibers that extend from the cerebral cortex to the spinal cord. A narrow band of darkly pigmented cells crosses each cerebral peduncle. This is the **substantia nigra.** The dark color is due to the presence of melanin in the cells. The substantia nigra seems to be involved in the production of dopamine in the brain and also functions in muscle tone reflexes.

The **pons** appears as a prominent band of fibers located between the midbrain and medulla oblongata. Most of the fibers in the pons connect to the cerebellum, but some of the fibers extend from the cerebellum to other parts of the brain.

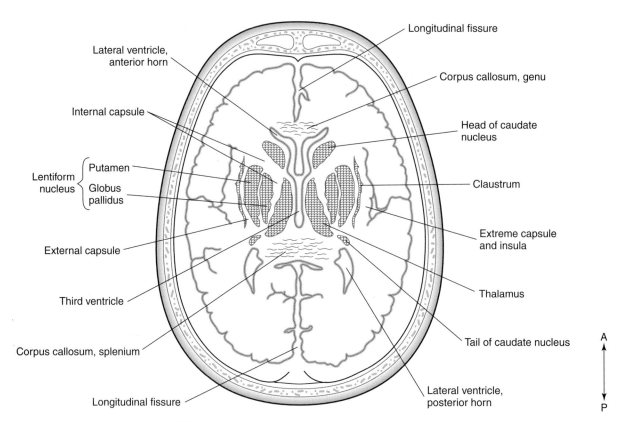

FIG. 2-6 Transverse section of cerebrum with basal ganglia.

The **medulla oblongata** looks somewhat conical and extends from the pons to the foramen magnum, where it is continuous with the spinal cord. A **median fissure** is located on the anterior surface of the medulla, and on either side of this fissure there is a small swelling called a **pyramid.** The **cerebral aqueduct** widens about halfway along the medulla to form the fourth ventricle.

Cerebellum.   Situated posterior to the pons and the medulla oblongata, the **cerebellum** occupies the posterior cranial fossa. It consists of two **cerebellar hemispheres** connected by a central **vermis,** which resembles a coiled-up worm. The word *vermis* is derived from the Latin word *verm,* which means worm. The surface of the cerebellum is covered by a layer of gray matter, the **cerebellar cortex.** Deep to the cortex is the white matter. Because the gray matter and white matter are laminated or foliated in appearance, the arrangement is sometimes called **arbor vitae.** **Cerebellar peduncles** connect the cerebellum with other portions of the brain. There are three pairs of cerebellar peduncles. The **superior cerebellar peduncles** connect the cerebellum to the midbrain. Fibers of the **middle cerebellar peduncles** connect the cerebellum and pons. The **inferior cerebellar peduncles** consist of fibers passing between the cerebellum and medulla oblongata. The cerebellum plays an important role in the control of muscle tone and coordinating muscular activity of the body. Some of the structures and regions of the brain are illustrated by the line drawing

in Fig. 2-7. The magnetic resonance image (MRI) in Fig. 2-8 also shows features of the brain in a midsagittal plane.

Ventricles of the Brain

Ventricles are fluid-filled cavities within the brain. These ventricles include the two lateral ventricles, the third ventricle, and the fourth ventricle. The ventricles and their communicating channels are illustrated in Fig. 2-9.

Lateral Ventricles.   There is a large **lateral ventricle** within each cerebral hemisphere. The major portion of each lateral ventricle is located in the parietal lobe. These ventricles extend into the frontal lobes as the anterior horns, into the occipital lobes as the posterior horns, and into the temporal lobes as the inferior horns. The lateral ventricles are separated from each other medially by a thin vertical partition called the **septum pellucidum.** Each lateral ventricle communicates with the third ventricle by a small opening called the **interventricular foramen,** or the foramen of Monro.

Third Ventricle.   The **third ventricle** is a narrow midline chamber that is enclosed by the diencephalon. The lateral walls of the third ventricle are formed by the right and left masses of the thalamus. The epithalamus and hypothalamus form the ventricle's roof and floor, respectively. A small band of white fibers, called the **intermediate mass,** passes through

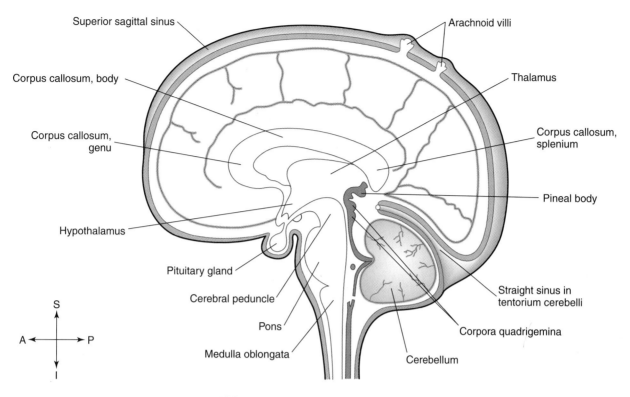

Superior sagittal sinus

Corpus callosum, body

Corpus callosum, genu

Hypothalamus

Pituitary gland

Cerebral peduncle

Pons

Medulla oblongata

Arachnoid villi

Thalamus

Corpus callosum, splenium

Pineal body

Straight sinus in tentorium cerebelli

Corpora quadrigemina

Cerebellum

S

A ← → P

I

FIG. 2-7 Midsagittal section of the brain.

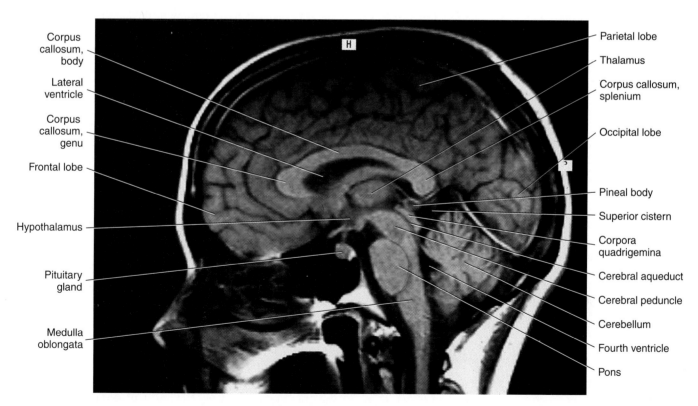

Corpus callosum, body

Lateral ventricle

Corpus callosum, genu

Frontal lobe

Hypothalamus

Pituitary gland

Medulla oblongata

Parietal lobe

Thalamus

Corpus callosum, splenium

Occipital lobe

Pineal body

Superior cistern

Corpora quadrigemina

Cerebral aqueduct

Cerebral peduncle

Cerebellum

Fourth ventricle

Pons

FIG. 2-8 Midsagittal MRI of the brain.

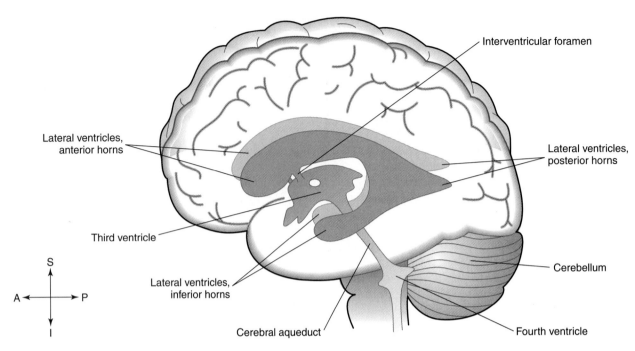

Interventricular foramen

Lateral ventricles,
anterior horns

Lateral ventricles,
posterior horns

Third ventricle

Cerebellum

Lateral ventricles,
inferior horns

S

A ← → P

I

Cerebral aqueduct

Fourth ventricle

FIG. 2-9 Ventricles of the brain.

the ventricle between the right and left thalami. The third ventricle communicates with the fourth ventricle by means of a relatively long **cerebral aqueduct,** also called the **aqueduct of Sylvius,** which passes through the midbrain.

Fourth Ventricle.   The **fourth ventricle** lies internal to the pons and the medulla oblongata at the level of the cerebellum. There are two openings called the **foramina of Luschka** in the lateral walls of the fourth ventricle. In the medial aspect of the dorsal wall there is a single opening called the **foramen of Magendie.** The ventricles communicate with the subarachnoid space through these three openings. The fourth ventricle is continuous with the narrow central canal that extends throughout the length of the spinal cord.

Choroid Plexus.   The **choroid plexus** is a group of specialized vascular structures that are located in the lateral, third, and fourth ventricles. The choroid plexus produces the **cerebrospinal fluid** by filtration and secretion. Originating in ventricles, the fluid circulates outward through the foramina in the fourth ventricle into the subarachnoid space around the brain and spinal cord. From there the fluid is reabsorbed into the venous system and returned to the heart as part of the blood.

Meninges

Three distinct connective tissue membranes called meninges cover the brain. These meninges are the dura mater, the arachnoid, and the pia mater. Cerebrospinal fluid circulates in the subarachnoid space between the arachnoid and the pia mater. In certain areas the arachnoid and the pia mater are widely separated, which creates spaces called cisterns.

Dura Mater.   The outermost layer of the meninges is the **dura mater,** which is composed of tough fibrous connective tissue. This forms a strong outer covering that serves as a supportive and protective structure for the brain. Although the dura mater is sometimes described as consisting of two layers, it is important to realize that what is called the outer layer of the dura is actually the endosteum (internal periosteum) of the calvaria. This outer layer is continuous with the external periosteum at the sutures and foramina. The inner, or meningeal, layer is the true dura mater, and it is continuous with the spinal dura at the foramen magnum. It also provides tubular sheaths for the cranial nerves as they pass through the foramina in the floor of the cranial fossa. The endosteum and true meningeal dura are closely adherent, except where there are venous sinuses.

The meningeal, or true, dura mater forms four inward-projecting folds that partially divide the cranial cavities into compartments. These four extensions of the dura mater are the **falx cerebri,** which is located between the cerebral hemispheres; the **falx cerebelli,** which is found between the cerebellar hemispheres; the **tentorium cerebelli,** which is between the cerebrum and cerebellum; and the **diaphragma sellae,** which forms a bridge over the sella turcica and covers the hypophysis.

Arachnoid.   The middle layer of the meninges is an extremely thin and delicate **arachnoid.** This layer is separated from the dura mater by a small subdural space that contains just enough fluid to keep the adjacent surfaces moist. The arachnoid is separated from the innermost pia mater by the **subarachnoid space,** which contains the cerebrospinal fluid and the larger blood vessels of the brain. Samples of cerebrospinal fluid may be withdrawn from the subarachnoid

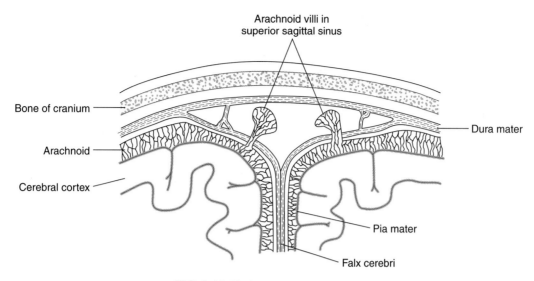

FIG. 2-10 Meninges and arachnoid villi.

Arachnoid villi in superior sagittal sinus

Bone of cranium

Arachnoid

Cerebral cortex

Dura mater

Pia mater

Falx cerebri

space and examined for evidence of infections or subarachnoid bleeding. This is usually done in the lumbar region of the vertebral column to minimize danger to the brain or spinal cord. From the inner surface of the arachnoid, minute trabeculae extend across the subarachnoid space to become continuous with the pia mater. This presents a cobweblike appearance and is the basis of the name arachnoid. In the vicinity of the venous sinuses there are numerous outgrowths, or diverticula, of the arachnoid that penetrate the dura and project into the venous sinuses. The interior of these **arachnoid villi** is continuous with the subarachnoid space and contains cerebrospinal fluid. This permits reabsorption of the fluid into the venous system. Arachnoid villi are illustrated in Fig. 2-10.

Pia Mater. The **pia mater** is the innermost layer of the meninges. It is a thin, highly vascular layer intimately adherent to the cortical tissue of the brain surface and closely follows the contours of the brain. The arachnoid and pia mater together are frequently referred to as the **leptomeninges.** These two layers of meninges are in close contact at the crests of the gyri, but as the pia mater follows the dips of the sulci and the arachnoid bridges over the top of the gyri, they become separated and triangular subarachnoid spaces are formed.

Subarachnoid Cisterns. In addition to the subarachnoid spaces described previously, there are certain other areas around the base of the brain where the arachnoid and pia mater are widely separated. This creates spaces called **cisterns,** which contain relatively large amounts of cerebrospinal fluid. Some of the cisterns are illustrated in Fig. 2-11. The **cerebellomedullary cistern,** or cisterna magna, is formed by the arachnoid as it bridges the interval between the medulla oblongata and the inferior surface of the cerebellum. The foramen of Magendie (median aperture) from the fourth ventricle opens into this cistern. When it is es-

pecially difficult or dangerous to perform a lumbar puncture to obtain samples of cerebrospinal fluid, the fluid may be taken from the cerebellomedullary cistern by a cisternal puncture. The **pontine cistern** is a space on the ventral surface of the pons. This cistern contains the basilar artery and receives cerebrospinal fluid from the fourth ventricle through the foramina of Luschka (lateral apertures). As the arachnoid bridges the gap from the temporal lobe to the frontal lobe, it forms the **cistern of the lateral sulcus,** which contains the middle cerebral artery. Between the two temporal lobes, the arachnoid is separated from the cerebral peduncles by an **interpeduncular cistern,** which contains the circle of Willis. Anteriorly and superiorly, the interpeduncular cistern continues as the **chiasmatic cistern. The cisterna ambiens** occupies the interval between the splenium of the corpus callosum and the superior surface of the cerebellum. It contains the great cerebral vein and the pineal gland. The cisterna ambiens is also called the cistern of the great cerebral vein, superior cistern, or quadrigeminal cistern. The pineal gland, which is located in this cistern, usually becomes calcified after adolescence and can be visualized on normal radiographs. This characteristic makes it an important landmark in neuroradiography and neurosurgery.

Arterial Blood Supply

The blood is supplied to the brain by two pairs of arteries, the **internal carotid** and the **vertebral arteries.** The **circulus arteriosus cerebri** is also discussed in this section.

Internal Carotid Artery. The cerebral portion of the internal carotid artery extends to the medial end of the lateral cerebral fissure, where it divides into the anterior cerebral and middle cerebral arteries. The two **anterior cerebral arteries** pass forward and medially toward the longitudinal fissure, where they are connected by a small **anterior commu-**

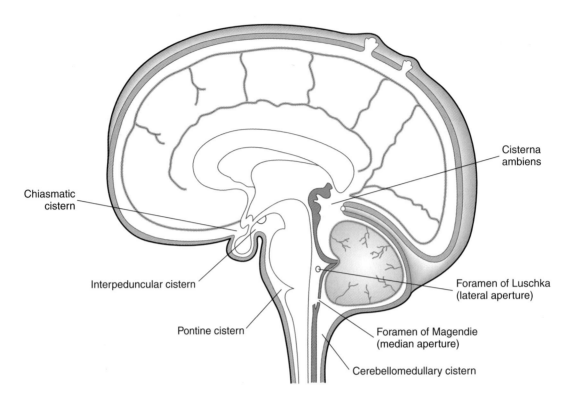

FIG. 2-11 Midsagittal section of the brain showing cisterns.

nicating artery. The two arteries then run parallel in the longitudinal fissure and give off numerous branches to supply much of the frontal and parietal lobes. The **middle cerebral artery** passes through the lateral fissure to spread out over the lateral surface of the brain. A third branch of the internal carotid artery, the **posterior communicating artery,** runs posteriorly to anastomose with posterior cerebral arteries.

Vertebral Arteries.   The right and left vertebral arteries, which are branches of the subclavian arteries, course superiorly through the transverse foramina of the cervical vertebrae beginning at C6. As they pass through the foramen magnum, they pierce the dura mater to enter the cerebellomedullary cistern of the subarachnoid space. The right and left vertebral arteries join to form the **basilar artery,** which passes over the surface of the pons. The basilar then divides to form two **posterior cerebral arteries,** which supply the occipital lobes.

Circulus Arteriosus Cerebri.   The typical configuration at the base of the brain shows the vessels anastomosing to form a "circle" called the **circulus arteriosus cerebri,** or **circle of Willis.** This circle, illustrated in Fig. 2-12, is formed by the internal carotid arteries, the anterior cerebral arteries, the anterior communicating artery, the posterior cerebral arteries, and the posterior communicating artery. Berry aneurysms often occur in the vessels of the circle of Willis. The circle of Willis, which is located in the interpeduncular cistern, encloses the optic chiasma, infundibulum, and

mammillary bodies. The angiogram in Fig. 2-13 shows some of the vessels in the circle of Willis.

Venous Drainage

Venous channels that drain blood from the brain and meninges are called sinuses. They are generally located between the endosteum of the calvaria and the meningeal dura or between two layers of dura mater. Unlike other veins, venous sinuses contain no valves. The **superior sagittal sinus** is triangular in cross section, occupies the entire length of the superior portion of the falx cerebri, and increases in size as it passes posteriorly. At the internal occipital protuberance it usually continues as the right lateral sinus. The smaller **inferior sagittal sinus** occupies the free inferior edge of the falx cerebri. At the junction of the falx cerebri with the tentorium cerebelli, the inferior sagittal sinus receives the great cerebral vein and becomes the **straight sinus,** which courses along the tentorium cerebelli. At the internal occipital protuberance the straight sinus usually continues as the left lateral sinus. The **lateral sinuses** are continuations of either the superior sagittal sinus or the straight sinus, but at their origin they may form a common space called the confluence of sinuses. The lateral sinuses are subdivided into transverse and sigmoid portions. The **transverse sinus** passes from the internal occipital protuberance (confluence of sinuses) to the junction of the petrous and mastoid portions of the temporal bone. The **sigmoid sinus,** which is a continuation of the transverse,

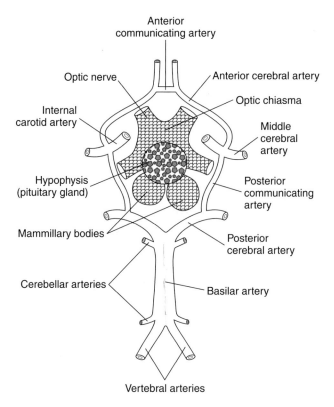

FIG. 2-12 Circulus arteriosus cerebri.

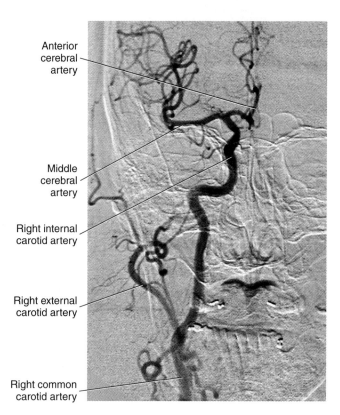

FIG. 2-13 Angiogram of portions of circle of Willis.

follows an **S**-shaped path that loops over the petrous and mastoid portions to the jugular foramen, where it becomes the **internal jugular vein.** The venous sinuses are illustrated in Fig. 2-14. In addition to these main sinuses, there are numerous smaller ones that drain specific portions of the brain and empty into one of the larger sinuses.

A rather large **cavernous sinus** is located on each side of the body and sella turcica of the sphenoid bone (see Fig. 2-14). These sinuses receive venous blood from the ophthalmic and middle cerebral veins and are drained by small petrosal sinuses that empty into the sigmoid sinus or into the internal jugular vein. The internal carotid artery enters the cavernous sinus through the foramen lacerum, makes a hairpin turn at the end of the sinus, and leaves the sinus to enter the subarachnoid space. The angiogram in Fig. 2-15 shows the internal carotid artery in the cavernous sinus. The abducens nerve is closely related to the internal carotid artery as it traverses the cavernous sinus. Associated with the lateral wall of the cavernous sinus, superior to inferior, are the oculomotor (III), trochlear (IV), and the ophthalmic and maxillary divisions of the trigeminal (V) nerves. The relationships of the vessels and nerves in the cavernous sinus are illustrated in Fig. 2-16. Injuries in the region of the cavernous sinus exhibit a variety of signs because there is an intimate relationship between the vessels and the nerves within the sinus. Some of these signs may be detected in the orbit of the eye. The proximity of the cavernous sinus with the sphenoidal paranasal sinus contributes to the development of meningitis as a sequela to sinusitis.

Cranial Nerves

Twelve pairs of cranial nerves emerge from the inferior surface of the brain. These nerves pass through foramina of the skull to innervate structures in the head and neck and in the viscera in the body. The cranial nerves are designated by name and by Roman numerals, according to the order in which they appear on the inferior surface of the brain.

Cranial Nerve I (Olfactory). The olfactory nerves provide the body with the sense of smell. They begin in the mucous membrane of the olfactory region of the nasal cavity and continue through the olfactory foramina in the cribriform plate of the ethmoid bone to enter the olfactory bulb on the inferior surface of the brain. From the olfactory bulb, the olfactory tract proceeds posteriorly to the olfactory cortex on the medial side of the temporal lobe of the brain.

Cranial Nerve II (Optic). Mediating visual function, the optic nerve originates in the nerve cells of the retina. From here, the two nerves, one for each eye, are directed posteriorly and medially through the optic foramen of the sphenoid bone into the cranial cavity, where they meet at the optic chiasma on the inferior surface of the hypothalamus. In the optic chiasma, the fibers from the medial part of the retina of each eye cross to the opposite side, whereas the fibers from the lateral portions of the retinas remain on the same side. After this partial decussation, or crossing over, in the chiasma, the fibers continue as the optic tract to the visual area of the occipital lobe.

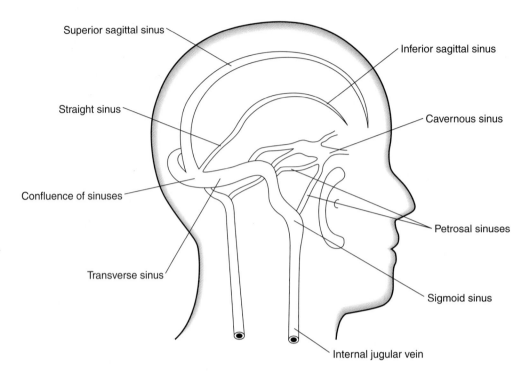

FIG. 2-14 Venous sinuses.

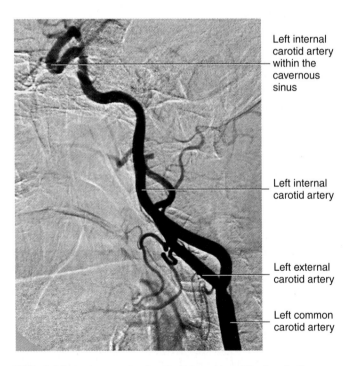

FIG. 2-15 Angiogram showing the internal carotid artery in the cavernous sinus, lateral projection.

Cranial Nerve III (Oculomotor). Cranial nerve III is a motor nerve to the superior, inferior, and medial rectus muscles and to the inferior oblique muscle of the eye. These muscles are responsible for a variety of eye movements. In addition to these four extrinsic muscles, the nerve also has fibers innervating the levator palpebrae superioris muscle,

which elevates the upper eyelid to open the eye. Some parasympathetic fibers supply the ciliary muscle, which changes the shape of the lens in accommodation, and the sphincter muscle of the iris, which changes the size of the pupil. In passing from the cranial cavity to the orbital cavity, the oculomotor nerve passes through the superior orbital fissure.

Cranial Nerve IV (Trochlear). The trochlear nerve is motor in function and supplies the superior oblique muscle of the eye. In passing from the cranial cavity to the orbital cavity, the trochlear nerve passes through the superior orbital fissure with the oculomotor nerve.

Cranial Nerve V (Trigeminal). The largest of the cranial nerves is the trigeminal, which contains motor fibers for the muscles of mastication and sensory fibers from the head. After emerging from the lateral side of the pons, the nerve divides into three branches. The ophthalmic branch passes through the superior orbital fissure to receive sensory impulses from the conjunctiva and cornea of the eye, the upper eyelid, the forehead, the nose, and the scalp. The maxillary branch first passes through the foramen rotundum, then curves around to enter the orbital cavity through the inferior orbital fissure. It leaves the cavity through the infraorbital foramen to receive sensory impulses from the skin of the cheek, the lateral nose, the upper lip, and the teeth. The mandibular branch emerges through the foramen ovale. It receives sensory impulses from the skin over the mandible and temporal region, the tongue, the floor of the mouth, the lower teeth and gingivae, and the buccal surface of the cheek. It also has motor fibers that stimulate the muscles of mastication.

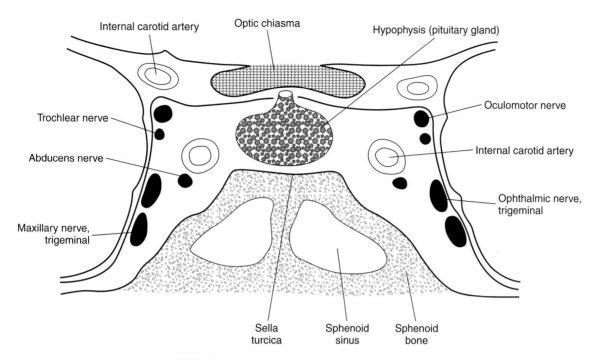

Internal carotid artery

Optic chiasma

Hypophysis (pituitary gland)

Trochlear nerve

Oculomotor nerve

Abducens nerve

Internal carotid artery

Ophthalmic nerve, trigeminal

Maxillary nerve, trigeminal

Sella turcica

Sphenoid sinus

Sphenoid bone

FIG. 2-16 Relationships within the cavernous sinus.

Cranial Nerve VI (Abducens). The abducens nerve emerges from the inferior surface of the brain at the junction of the pons and the medulla. It enters the orbital cavity through the superior orbital fissure to supply motor impulses to the lateral rectus muscle of the eye.

Cranial Nerve VII (Facial). The seventh cranial nerve, the facial nerve, contains both sensory and motor fibers. After leaving the skull through the stylomastoid foramen, it passes through the substance of the parotid gland, where it branches to supply motor impulses to the muscles of facial expression. The sensory component receives impulses from the taste buds on the anterior two thirds of the tongue. The nerve also stimulates the sublingual and submaxillary salivary glands and the lacrimal glands associated with the eye.

Cranial Nerve VIII (Vestibulocochlear). The eighth cranial nerve is a special sensory nerve with two distinct components. The vestibular branch functions in equilibrium by receiving sensory impulses from the semicircular canals, the utricle, and the saccule. These structures of the inner ear detect the position and movement of the head. The cochlear branch functions in hearing by receiving impulses from the organ of Corti in the cochlear duct, also in the inner ear. Both branches enter the cranial cavity through the internal auditory meatus. The vestibulocochlear nerve is sometimes referred to as the acoustic, or auditory, nerve.

Cranial Nerve IX (Glossopharyngeal). As the name implies, the chief distribution of the glossopharyngeal nerve is to the tongue and pharynx. It is a mixed nerve, with both sensory and motor functions. This nerve supplies motor impulses to muscles that aid in swallowing and to the parotid salivary gland. The sensory component may be divided into three functional groups. Some of the fibers convey the sensation of taste from the posterior one third of the tongue. Others transmit the general sensations of pain, temperature, and touch from the pharynx and middle ear. The third group is concerned with the regulation of respiration and blood pressure by receiving impulses from the chemoreceptors and pressure receptors associated with the carotid arteries in the neck. The ninth cranial nerve exits the cranial cavity through the jugular foramen.

Cranial Nerve X (Vagus). The word vagus is derived from the Latin word meaning "wandering." This is an appropriate name for the tenth cranial nerve, which has the most extensive distribution of all the nerves. It leaves the cranial cavity through the jugular foramen. The fibers of this mixed nerve may be divided into four groups: (1) somatic motor fibers supply the skeletal muscles of the pharynx and larynx; (2) visceral motor fibers carry impulses to the thoracic and abdominal viscera; (3) somatic sensory fibers convey impulses concerned with pain, temperature, and touch from the external ear; and (4) visceral sensory fibers function in the regulation of heart rate, blood pressure, and respiration by transmitting impulses from the stretch receptors in the heart, aorta, superior vena cava, and lungs. This component also receives sensory impulses from the abdominal viscera.

Cranial Nerve XI (Accessory). The accessory nerve, the eleventh cranial nerve, is entirely motor in function. It leaves the cranial cavity through the jugular foramen and stimulates the trapezius and sternocleidomastoid muscles to contract.

Cranial Nerve XII (Hypoglossal).   The numerous roots of the twelfth cranial nerve emerge through the hypoglossal canal in the occipital bone. After passing through the canal, the roots unite to form the hypoglossal nerve. This nerve, which is motor in function, stimulates the muscles of the tongue to contract.

Summary of the Cranial Nerves.   The cranial nerves are summarized in Table 2-4. Most cranial nerves have both sensory and motor components. Three of the nerves (I, II, VIII) are associated with the special senses of smell, vision, hearing, and equilibrium and consist of sensory fibers only. Five other nerves (III, IV, VI, XI, XII) are primarily motor in function but have some sensory fibers for proprioception. The remaining four nerves (V, VII, IX, X) consist of significant amounts of both sensory and motor fibers.

ORBITAL CAVITY AND CONTENTS

Cavity Walls

The orbital cavity is a pyramid-shaped structure with an apex, base, and four triangular walls. The **optic foramen** is at the apex in the posterior part of the orbit. The base, which is the anterior part that opens onto the face, is formed by the zygomatic, maxilla, and frontal bones. The medial walls of the two orbits are nearly parallel and have portions of the ethmoid and sphenoid sinuses between them. Each medial wall is formed by the lacrimal bone and the fragile orbital plates of the ethmoid and palatine bones. The superior wall, or roof, of the cavity is formed by the orbital plate of the frontal bone. The maxilla and a small portion of the zygomatic make up the inferior wall, or floor. The lateral walls of the two orbits are positioned at right angles (90 degrees) to each other and, if extended, would intersect in the region of the pituitary gland. The sturdy lateral wall is formed by the zygomatic bone and the greater wing of the

TABLE 2-4   *Summary of Cranial Nerves*

Number	Name	Associated Foramen	Type	Function
I	Olfactory	Olfactory foramina in cribriform plate of ethmoid bone	Sensory	Sense of smell
II	Optic	Optic foramen of sphenoid bone	Sensory	Vision
III	Oculomotor	Superior orbital fissure of sphenoid bone	Motor	Movement of eye and eyelid
IV	Trochlear	Superior orbital fissure of sphenoid bone	Motor	Movement of the eye
V	Trigeminal		Mixed	
	Ophthalmic branch	Superior orbital fissure of sphenoid bone	Sensory	Cornea, skin of nose, forehead, scalp
	Maxillary branch	Foramen rotundum of sphenoid bone	Sensory	Cheek, nose, upper lip, and teeth
	Mandibular branch	Foramen ovale of sphenoid bone	Mixed	Skin over mandible, tongue, lower lip, and teeth; contraction of muscles of mastication
VI	Abducens	Superior orbital fissure of sphenoid bone	Motor	Eye movement
VII	Facial	Stylomastoid foramen of temporal bone	Mixed	Contraction of muscles of facial expression; lacrimal and submaxillary gland secretion; taste from anterior two thirds of tongue
VIII	Vestibulocochlear	Internal auditory meatus of temporal bone	Sensory	Hearing and equilibrium
IX	Glossopharyngeal	Jugular foramen of temporal bone	Mixed	Taste from posterior one third of tongue; contraction of muscles used in swallowing; parotid gland secretion
X	Vagus	Jugular foramen of temporal bone	Mixed	Contraction of muscles of pharynx and larynx; gastric motility; general visceral sensation; alters heart rate, respiration, blood pressure
XI	Accessory	Jugular foramen of temporal bone	Motor	Contraction of trapezius and sternocleidomastoid muscles
XII	Hypoglossal	Hypoglossal canal of occipital bone	Motor	Contraction of muscles of tongue

sphenoid bone. A depression for the lacrimal gland is located in the superior portion of the lateral wall.

Bulbus Oculi

The primary structure located in the orbital cavity is, of course, the **bulbus oculi,** or **eyeball.** It is somewhat spherical, approximately 2 to 3 cm in diameter, and has an anterior bulge. The eyeball is surrounded by orbital fat within the orbital cavity.

The wall of the bulbus oculi is made up of three concentric coats, or tunics. The **external,** or **fibrous, tunic** is the supporting layer. It consists of the white opaque **sclera,** which covers the posterior five sixths of the eyeball, and the transparent **cornea,** which covers the anterior one sixth.

The **middle vascular tunic** consists of the **choroid, ciliary body,** and **iris.** The **choroid** is a highly vascular, brown-pigmented layer that is located between the sclera and the retina. It is the largest part of the middle tunic, and it lines most of the sclera, although it is only loosely connected to the fibrous coat and can easily be stripped away. The choroid is, however, firmly attached to the retina. Anteriorly, the choroid is continuous with the **ciliary body. Suspensory ligaments** connect the ciliary body to the lens of the eye. Numerous fingerlike ciliary processes that secrete the aqueous humor are within the ciliary body. Externally, the ciliary body contains ciliary muscle. When this muscle contracts, the suspensory ligaments relax and the lens bulges to allow focusing for close vision. The **iris** is the conspicuous, colored portion of the eye. It is a doughnut-shaped diaphragm with a central aperture, the **pupil.** The muscles of the iris are continually contracting and relaxing to change the size of the pupil, which regulates the amount of light entering the eye.

The **innermost nervous tunic** is the **retina,** which has several layers. The outer layer of the retina is deeply pigmented and firmly attached to the choroid. The rods and cones, which are the light receptor cells, are adjacent to the pigmented layer. Other layers consist of bipolar neurons and ganglion cells. The axons of the ganglion cells converge to form the optic nerve, which penetrates the tunics at the optic disc, then passes through the apex of the orbital cavity to reach the brain. The slight depression in the retina is the fovea centralis.

A transparent, biconvex **lens** is located just posterior to the iris. The curvature of the lens surface changes by action of the ciliary muscles and suspensory ligaments to permit focusing on objects at different distances. The space anterior to the lens is the anterior cavity, which is filled with **aqueous humor.** The posterior cavity, between the lens and the retina, is filled with a colorless, transparent, gellike **vitreous humor.** Unlike the aqueous humor, which is continually being replaced, the vitreous humor is formed during embryonic development and is not exchanged. Fig. 2-17 illustrates the structure of the bulbus oculi.

Six extrinsic ocular muscles, which insert on the sclera, are associated with movements of the eye. These muscles are summarized in Table 2-5.

Vascular Supply to the Orbital Contents

Most of the vascular supply to the orbital contents is by way of the **ophthalmic artery,** a branch of the internal carotid artery. Ciliary branches of the ophthalmic artery provide the blood supply to the sclera, choroid, ciliary body, and iris. One of the smallest, but most important, branches of the ophthalmic artery is the **central artery of the retina.** This vessel enters the bulbus oculi through the optic disc, then it branches over the surface of the retina to provide the blood supply. If the central artery is blocked by a tumor, thrombus, or massive edema, the result is sudden blindness.

Venous drainage of the orbital cavity is furnished by the **superior** and **inferior ophthalmic veins,** which pass through the orbit to enter the cavernous sinus located adjacent to the pituitary gland. The **central vein of the retina** follows the pathway of the central artery along the optic nerve. The central vein drains into the cavernous sinus along with the ophthalmic veins. Increased intracranial pressure restricts the blood flow in the central vein as it passes through the subarachnoid space. This restricted venous drainage results in edema at the optic disc, which is directly observable with an ophthalmoscope. Papilledema, swelling at the optic disc, is one of the earliest indications of increased intracranial pressure.

Protective Features of the Eye

The eyes are protected by the **eyelids,** or **palpebrae.** The upper eyelid consists of the **levator palpebrae superioris** muscle, which is covered by thin skin and lined by a highly vascular **conjunctiva.** The levator palpebrae superioris muscle elevates the upper eyelid to open the eye and is innervated by the oculomotor nerve.

TABLE 2-5 *Extrinsic Muscles Associated With Eye Movement*

Muscle	Function	Innervation
Superior rectus	Rotates eye upward and laterally	Oculomotor (cranial nerve III)
Inferior rectus	Rotates eye downward and medially	Oculomotor (cranial nerve III)
Lateral rectus	Rotates eye laterally	Abducens (cranial nerve VI)
Medial rectus	Rotates eye medially	Oculomotor (cranial nerve III)
Superior oblique	Rotates eye downward and laterally	Trochlear (cranial nerve IV)
Inferior oblique	Rotates eye upward and laterally	Oculomotor (cranial nerve III)

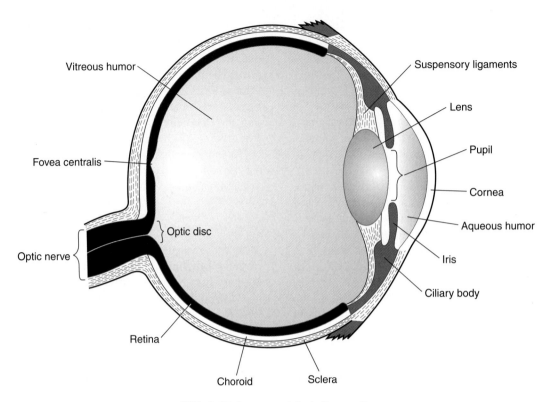

FIG. 2-17 Structure of the bulbus oculi.

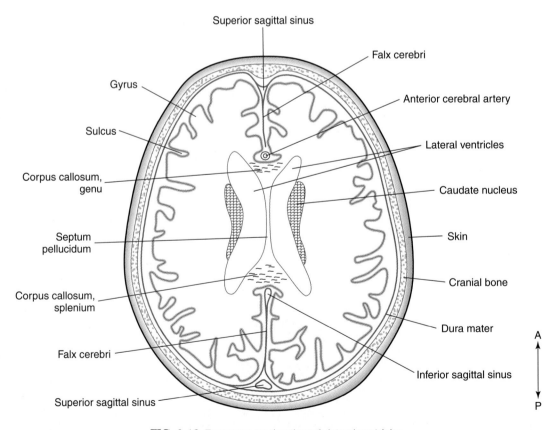

FIG. 2-18 Transverse section through lateral ventricles.

The **lacrimal apparatus** is another protective structure associated with the eye. The **lacrimal gland,** located in the upper and lateral part of the orbit, produces the lacrimal fluid, or tears. The lacrimal fluid moistens the surface of the eye, lubricates the eyelids, and washes away foreign particles. It also contains an enzyme that destroys certain bacteria. After spreading across the surface of the eye, the fluid drains through the nasolacrimal duct into the inferior meatus of the nasal cavity.

Sectional Anatomy of the Head

TRANSVERSE SECTIONS

Sections Through the Lateral Ventricles

Sections superior to the lateral ventricles will demonstrate the **cerebral gyri** and **sulci** with cortical gray matter and underlying white matter. The **longitudinal fissure** containing the **falx cerebri** and **superior sagittal sinus** is readily identifiable. In cadaveric specimens the **dura mater** and **arachnoid** may be seen; however, the **subdural space** is frequently exaggerated because of shrinkage of tissue.

Sections taken a little more inferiorly, 6 to 7 cm from the top of the head, show the roof or upper portion of the **lateral ventricles** (Fig. 2-18). Just inferior to this, the lateral ventricles are separated by a thin partition, the **septum pellucidum.** The **genu** of the corpus callosum is between the anterior horns, and the **splenium** is between the posterior horns of the lateral ventricles. The body of the **caudate nucleus** is lateral to the lateral ventricles. Depending on the angle of the plane, the **inferior sagittal sinus** may be present.

Section Through the Basal Ganglia

Proceeding inferiorly from the upper portions of the lateral ventricles, numerous internal brain structures are noted (Fig. 2-19). This plane passes just above the tentorium cerebelli. The **genu** and the **splenium** of the **corpus callosum** are readily identified as bands of white fibers passing from one hemisphere to the other. Both the anterior and the posterior horns of the **lateral ventricles** are present at this level. Just posterior and lateral to the anterior horns, in fact forming the floor of the anterior horns, are regions of gray matter, the head of the **caudate nucleus.** The **septum pellucidum** is seen as a thin midline partition between the two lateral ventricles. A slight enlargement of the septum pellucidum is the **fornix.** Posterior to the fornix, in a midline position, is a narrow slit representing the **third ventricle.** The **interventricular foramen,** sometimes called the foramen of Monro, is an opening between each of the lateral ventricles and the single midline third ventricle. Two regions of gray matter, the **thalami,** which make up a significant portion of the diencephalon, form the lateral walls of the third ventricle. The posterior horns of the lateral ventricles are posterior to the thalamic areas. **Choroid plexus,** a capillary network that produces cerebrospinal fluid, is evi-

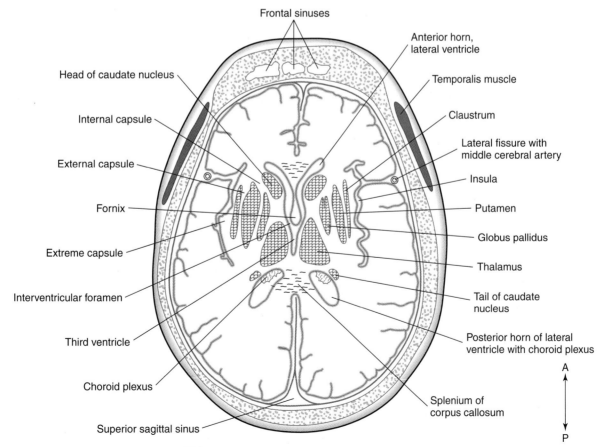

FIG. 2-19 Transverse section through basal ganglia.

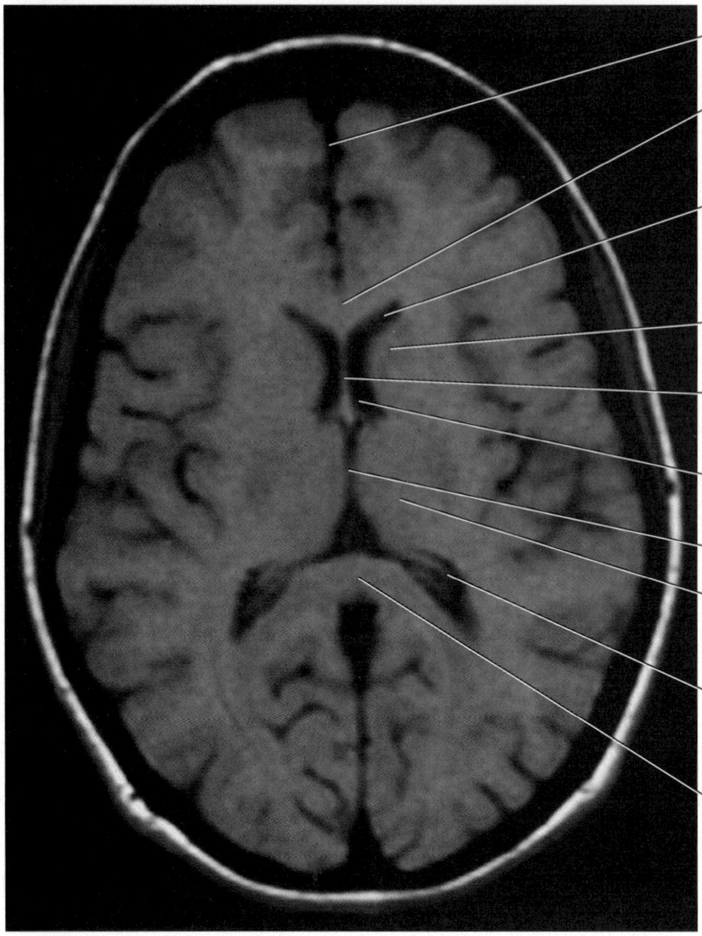

Longitudinal fissure

Corpus callosum

Lateral ventricle, anterior horn

Caudate nucleus

Septum pellucidum

Lateral ventricle, body

Third ventricle

Thalamus

Lateral ventricle, posterior horn, with choroid plexus

Corpus callosum

FIG. 2-20 Axial MRI showing lateral ventricles.

dent in the wall of the ventricles. A small area of gray matter, the **tail of the caudate nucleus,** may be seen in the roof of the posterior horns. The posterior horns are separated by the splenium of the corpus callosum. The MRI in Fig. 2-20 shows horns of the lateral ventricles and the choroid plexus.

The **insula,** or island of Reil, which is buried deep within the lateral fissure, usually is evident at this level. Branches of the **middle cerebral artery** are within the lateral fissure and around the insula. Deep to the insula, there is a mass of gray matter, which is the **lentiform nucleus.** The lentiform nucleus is made up of two parts, an outer darker segment, which is the **putamen,** and an inner paler segment, which is the **globus pallidus.** The lentiform nucleus is separated from the caudate nucleus by a band of white fibers constituting the **anterior limb of the internal capsule.** Between the thalamus and the lentiform nucleus the internal capsule continues as the **posterior limb.** A thin strip of gray matter, the **claustrum,** is located between the insula and the putamen of the lentiform nucleus. A portion of the **frontal sinus** may be seen in some specimens at this level.

Section Through the Superior Cistern

If the posterior portion of a section through the basal ganglia is at a slightly lower level, such as that which is ob-

tained parallel to the orbital-meatal line, then some additional structures may be noted. The splenium of the corpus callosum may be absent, and the top portion of the **tentorium cerebelli** may be seen. Along with this will be the **superior cistern,** which is located between the splenium of the corpus callosum and the tentorium cerebelli (Fig. 2-21). The **great cerebral vein** and the **pineal gland** are located in the superior cistern, and the corpora quadrigemina project into this space. The **straight sinus,** which runs along the junction between the falx cerebri and the tentorium cerebelli, is present in sections showing the tentorium cerebelli. The straight sinus is continuous with the inferior sagittal sinus and also receives the great cerebral vein.

Section Through the Midbrain

The next few paragraphs deal with sections at the level of the midbrain. If the plane of section is parallel to the orbital-meatal line, sections at this level pass through the superior part of the orbit anteriorly, and pass through the cerebellum posteriorly. If the plane of section is more oblique, say a 15- to 20-degree angle to the orbital-meatal line, then anterior views are above the orbit and more of the cerebellum is shown posteriorly.

Fig. 2-22 illustrates the area surrounding the **midbrain.** The two anteriorly projecting **cerebral peduncles** are partic-

DATE: 04/30/07
TS2R0006 - P0020

INSTRUCTOR: DAVID WHIPPLE
SCORING METHOD USED: PERCENTAGE SCORE

STUDENT ANSWER SHEET
DEPT CRS SEC
2760-288:001

TEST #: 01
TEST FORM: A

SOC. SEC. #	STUDENT NAME		# RIGHT	# WRONG	# OMITTED	# NOT GRADED	SCORE
279-02-3793	MANIVONG	SUNGKOM	41	9	0	0	82.00

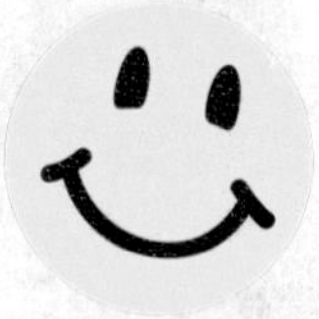

```
QUESTION #            1 1 1 1 1 1 1 1 1 1 2 2 2 2 2 2 2 2 2 2 3 3 3 3 3 3 3 3 3 3 4 4 4 4 4 4 4 4 4 4 5
            1 2 3 4 5 6 7 8 9 0 1 2 3 4 5 6 7 8 9 0 1 2 3 4 5 6 7 8 9 0 1 2 3 4 5 6 7 8 9 0 1 2 3 4 5 6 7 8 9 0

STUDENT     B D B C A D E C D B A D A C C D E A D A A C D A A E B C A B E D E B B A C E A D D E C C A D C B A B
ANSWER KEY  A A D                               C   B   B                   D                   B                   E
ALTERNATE
```

****
*** ANSWER KEY RESPONSES ARE ONLY PRINTED IF THE CORRECT ANSWER DIFFERS FROM THE STUDENT'S ***
*** ANSWER.   ALTERNATE ANSWERS WILL BE PRINTED WHENEVER THEY EXIST.   ***
****

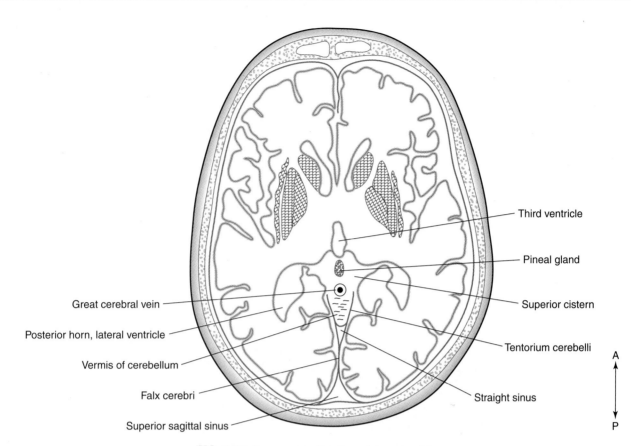

Third ventricle

Pineal gland

Superior cistern

Great cerebral vein

Tentorium cerebelli

Posterior horn, lateral ventricle

Vermis of cerebellum

Falx cerebri

Straight sinus

Superior sagittal sinus

A
P

FIG. 2-21 Transverse section through superior cistern.

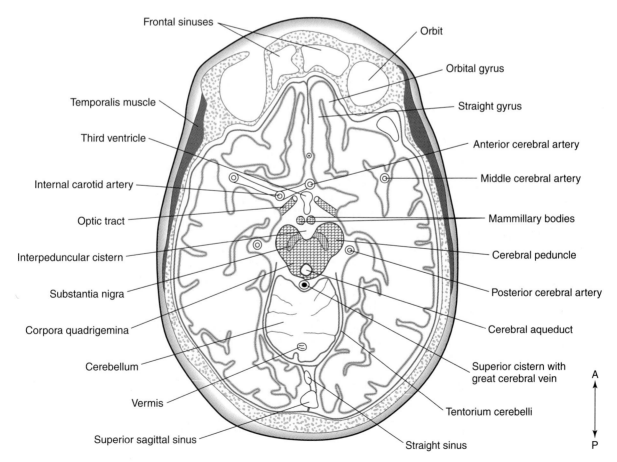

Frontal sinuses

Orbit

Orbital gyrus

Temporalis muscle

Straight gyrus

Third ventricle

Anterior cerebral artery

Internal carotid artery

Middle cerebral artery

Optic tract

Mammillary bodies

Interpeduncular cistern

Cerebral peduncle

Substantia nigra

Posterior cerebral artery

Corpora quadrigemina

Cerebral aqueduct

Cerebellum

Superior cistern with
great cerebral vein

Vermis

Tentorium cerebelli

Superior sagittal sinus

Straight sinus

A
P

FIG. 2-22 Transverse section through midbrain.

ularly noticeable because of the presence of a very dark substance called **substantia nigra.** The **interpeduncular cistern** is between the two cerebral peduncles. Two **mammillary bodies,** which form a portion of the floor of the **third ventricle,** project into the interpeduncular cistern. The narrow space that is anterior to the mammillary bodies is the third ventricle. **Optic tracts** project posteriorly and laterally from the third ventricle. The aqueduct of Sylvius, or **cerebral aqueduct,** forms a small opening near the **superior colliculi of the corpora quadrigemina.** The space between the corpora quadrigemina and the cerebellum is the **superior cistern,** or cistern of the great cerebral vein. Compare the line drawing in Fig. 2-22 with the axial MRI in Fig. 2-23.

In sections that are nearly parallel to the orbital-meatal line, the frontal bone exhibits a large **frontal sinus.** The **orbits,** on either side, contain some **orbital fat,** or possibly some of the superior muscles such as the **levator palpebrae superioris,** or superior rectus. Laterally, the **temporalis muscle** is superficial to the temporal bone. Posteriorly, the **cerebellum** is sectioned so that it shows the centrally located **vermis.** The **tentorium cerebelli** separates the cerebellum from the cerebrum. The **anterior cerebral arteries** are present in the longitudinal fissure, the **middle cerebral arteries** are in the lateral fissure, and the **posterior cerebral arteries** are in the superior cistern with the great cerebral vein.

In more oblique sections through the midbrain, say at 15 or 20 degrees to the orbital-meatal line, the plane will pass superior to the orbit and frontal sinus anteriorly and will pass through the cerebellum at a more inferior level than the section described above. Either a **sigmoid sinus** or a **transverse sinus** will probably be present instead of the superior sagittal sinus.

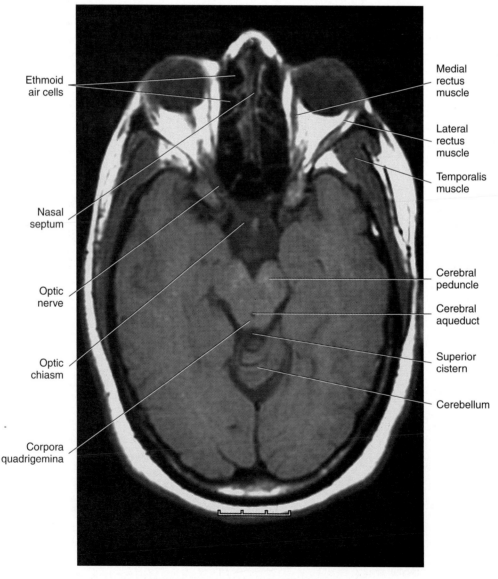

FIG. 2-23 Axial MRI through midbrain.

Section Through the Pons

Transverse sections through the pons, illustrated in Fig. 2-24, show the **pontine cistern** with the single **basilar artery.** The **fourth ventricle** is posterior to the pons, with the **superior cerebellar peduncles** forming the walls of the ventricle. Large **middle cerebellar peduncles** are lateral to the superior cerebellar peduncles. Two large **trigeminal nerves** emerge laterally from the pons. In sections that are cut more or less parallel to the orbital-meatal line, the **pituitary gland** is just anterior to the pontine cistern. Some sections may also pass through the body of the **sphenoid bone,** with a cavernous sinus located on either side. The **internal carotid arteries** and some nerves are in the cavernous sinus (see Fig. 2-16). Sections at this level also show the **sphenoid sinuses** and **ethmoid air cells.** Compare the line drawing in Fig. 2-24 with the axial MRI in Fig. 2-25.

Fig. 2-24 also shows that the **lateral walls** of the orbit are perpendicular to each other, whereas the **medial walls** are parallel. The **optic nerve** is centrally located within each orbit, between the **lateral rectus muscle** and the **medial rectus muscle.** The axial computed tomography image in Fig. 2-26 is at the level of the orbit and shows some of the features in this region.

In the posterior region, the dural venous sinuses are **transverse sinuses.** In the region of the pons, the **petrous** portions of the temporal bone project between the cerebellum and the temporal lobes of the cerebrum. The **temporalis muscle** is in the temporal fossa. In more oblique sections through the level of the pons, the anterior portion is cut above the level of the orbit and the nasal cavity and still shows the frontal lobes of the cerebrum.

Section Through the Medulla Oblongata

At the level of the medulla oblongata, the **right** and **left vertebral arteries** are present in the **cerebellomedullary cistern,** which is anterior to the medulla. The venous sinuses present in the **petrous portion of the temporal bone** are **sigmoid sinuses,** which are continuations of the transverse sinuses. In some cases, the **jugular foramen** is present at this level. The **internal carotid arteries** are lateral to the basilar portion of the occipital bone. In sections parallel to the orbital-meatal line (Fig. 2-27), the facial region shows the **nasal septum, middle nasal conchae,** and **maxillary sinuses.** The **zygomatic arch** is present in the cheek area, and the **temporalis muscle** is medial to the arch. This region is also illustrated by the axial MRI in Fig. 2-28.

The axial computed tomography image in Fig. 2-29 is at a slightly lower level and passes through the ramus of the mandible and mastoid process. Compare the features at this level with those at the level of the medulla oblongata.

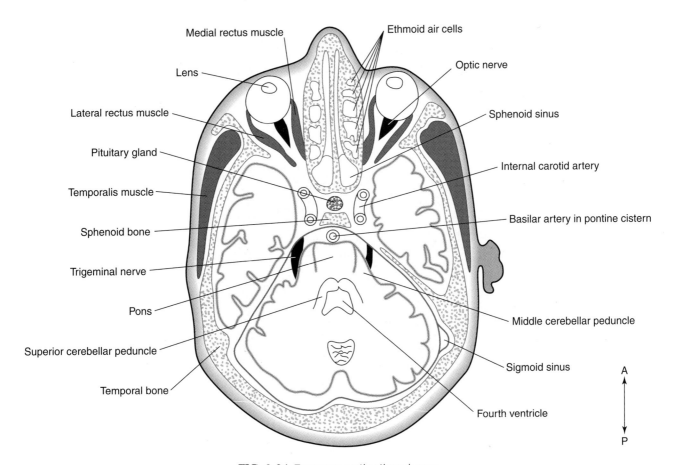

FIG. 2-24 Transverse section through pons.

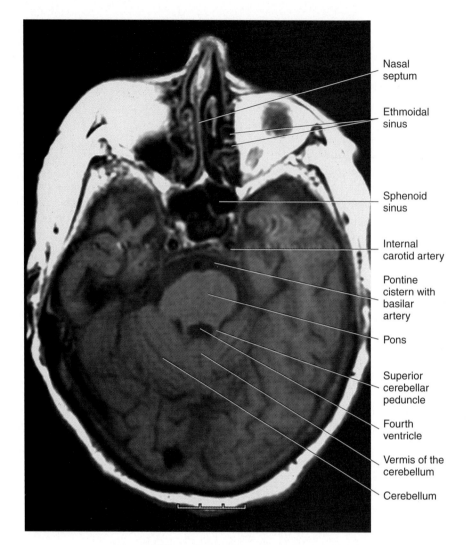

Nasal septum

Ethmoidal sinus

Sphenoid sinus

Internal carotid artery

Pontine cistern with basilar artery

Pons

Superior cerebellar peduncle

Fourth ventricle

Vermis of the cerebellum

Cerebellum

FIG. 2-25 Axial MRI through pons.

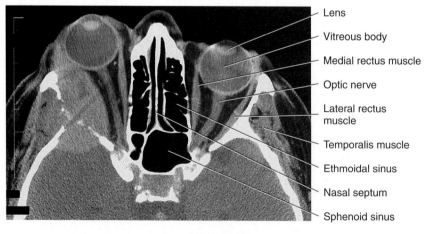

Lens

Vitreous body

Medial rectus muscle

Optic nerve

Lateral rectus muscle

Temporalis muscle

Ethmoidal sinus

Nasal septum

Sphenoid sinus

FIG. 2-26 Axial CT image through orbit.

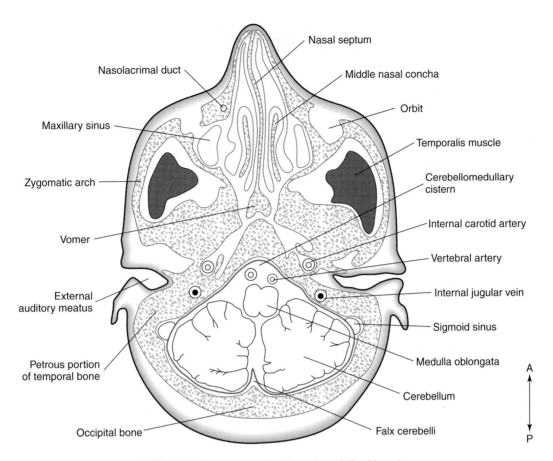

Nasal septum

Nasolacrimal duct

Middle nasal concha

Maxillary sinus

Orbit

Temporalis muscle

Zygomatic arch

Cerebellomedullary cistern

Internal carotid artery

Vomer

Vertebral artery

Internal jugular vein

External auditory meatus

Sigmoid sinus

Medulla oblongata

Petrous portion of temporal bone

Cerebellum

Occipital bone

Falx cerebelli

A
P

FIG. 2-27 Transverse section through medulla oblongata.

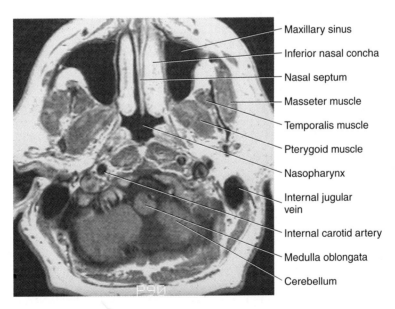

Maxillary sinus

Inferior nasal concha

Nasal septum

Masseter muscle

Temporalis muscle

Pterygoid muscle

Nasopharynx

Internal jugular vein

Internal carotid artery

Medulla oblongata

Cerebellum

FIG. 2-28 Axial MRI through base of skull.

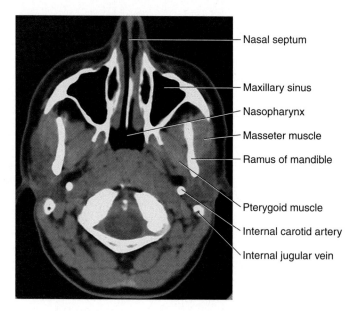

FIG. 2-29 Axial CT image through ramus of mandible.

SAGITTAL SECTIONS

Section Through the Temporomandibular Joint

Fig. 2-30 illustrates a parasagittal section through the lateral surface of the head and neck, particularly through the **temporomandibular joint.** The **condyle** of the mandible articulates in the **mandibular fossa** of the temporal bone. Using the joint as a reference, the **zygomatic process** of the temporal bone projects anteriorly, the **external auditory meatus** is immediately posterior to the joint, and this is followed by the **mastoid process.** The superficial cheek muscle is the **masseter,** followed posteriorly by the **parotid gland** and the **sternocleidomastoid** muscle. The sternocleidomastoid muscle, a landmark muscle in the neck, courses obliquely along the neck to insert on the mastoid process. The **temporalis** muscle overlying the temporal bone is superior to the masseter. Only the surface of the brain is visible inside the cranial cavity.

Section Through the Orbit

Sagittal sections through the orbit, as illustrated in Fig. 2-31, are too lateral to show many details of the brain; however, numerous other structures of the head are illustrated. This plane passes through the **frontal, parietal, occipital,** and **temporal** lobes of the cerebrum. The **tentorium cerebelli,** with the **transverse sinus** in its posterior margin, forms a partition between the cerebrum and cerebellum. Note that the tentorium cerebelli is anchored to the **petrous ridge** of the temporal bone and the **sigmoid venous sinus** is along the posterior margin of the ridge.

The **frontal** and **maxilla** bones form the superior and inferior portions of the orbit. Within the orbit, fat surrounds the **bulbus oculi** and **extrinsic eye muscles.** The **mandible** is a recognizable structure in the face. The **buccinator muscle,** one of the muscles of mastication, is in the cheek superior to the mandible, and the **submandibular gland** is inferior to the mandible. The sublingual gland is not present because it is nearer the midline. A portion of the **temporalis** and **pterygoid** muscles may be evident superior and posterior to the buccinator.

Midsagittal Section

Fig. 2-32 illustrates a midsagittal section through the head. Also refer to Fig. 2-8, which is a midsagittal MRI of the brain. Because many parts of the brain are midline or nearly so, they are evident on midsagittal sections. The **cerebrum** curves around the **thalamus** to enclose it, except inferiorly. The **lateral ventricle** is superior to the thalamus. Posteriorly, the **tentorium cerebelli** forms a partition between the cerebrum and cerebellum. The brainstem, consisting of the **midbrain, pons,** and **medulla oblongata,** extends inferiorly from the thalamus. A large **middle cerebellar peduncle** connects the cerebellum with the pons. The **hypophysis,** or **pituitary gland,** is located in the sella turcica of the sphenoid bone, and the **sphenoid sinuses** are anterior to the sella turcica. Midsagittal sections show the **nasal septum,** made up of the vomer and the perpendicular plate of the ethmoid bone.

In the region of the mouth, the **maxilla** forms the upper jaw, the **mandible** forms the lower jaw, and the **hard** and **soft palates** form the roof of the mouth. The **uvula** is the terminal portion of the soft palate. The largest structure present in the mouth is the **tongue.** Inferior to the tongue, between it and the mandible, the **sublingual gland** is visible as a midline structure.

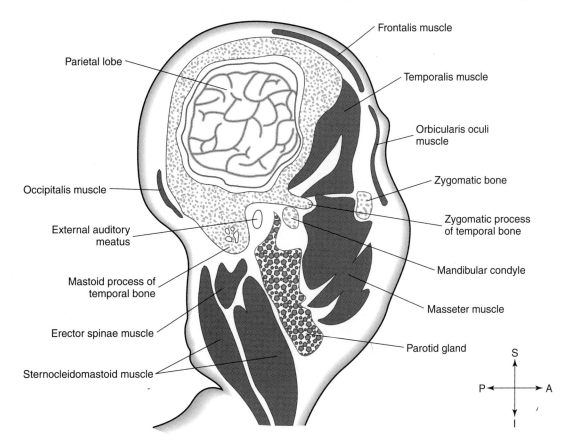

FIG. 2-30 Sagittal section through the temporomandibular joint.

Parietal lobe

Frontalis muscle

Temporalis muscle

Orbicularis oculi muscle

Zygomatic bone

Zygomatic process of temporal bone

Occipitalis muscle

Mandibular condyle

External auditory meatus

Masseter muscle

Mastoid process of temporal bone

Parotid gland

Erector spinae muscle

Sternocleidomastoid muscle

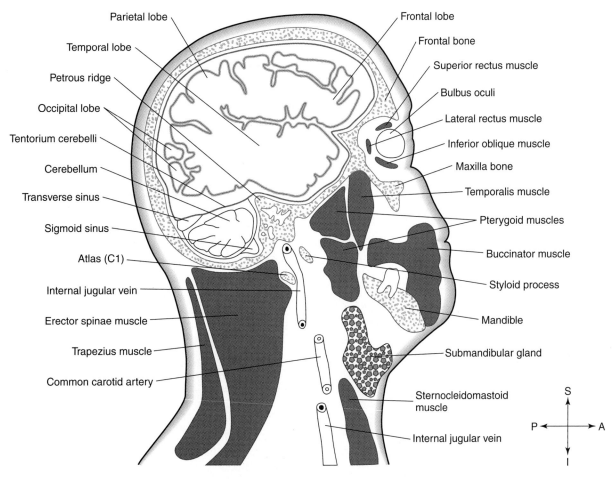

FIG. 2-31 Sagittal section through the orbit.

Parietal lobe

Frontal lobe

Temporal lobe

Frontal bone

Petrous ridge

Superior rectus muscle

Occipital lobe

Bulbus oculi

Tentorium cerebelli

Lateral rectus muscle

Cerebellum

Inferior oblique muscle

Transverse sinus

Maxilla bone

Sigmoid sinus

Temporalis muscle

Atlas (C1)

Pterygoid muscles

Internal jugular vein

Buccinator muscle

Erector spinae muscle

Styloid process

Trapezius muscle

Mandible

Common carotid artery

Submandibular gland

Sternocleidomastoid muscle

Internal jugular vein

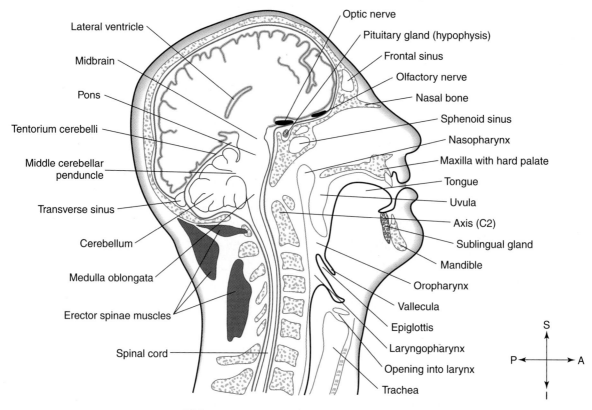

Lateral ventricle
Midbrain
Pons
Tentorium cerebelli
Middle cerebellar peduncle
Transverse sinus
Cerebellum
Medulla oblongata
Erector spinae muscles
Spinal cord

Optic nerve
Pituitary gland (hypophysis)
Frontal sinus
Olfactory nerve
Nasal bone
Sphenoid sinus
Nasopharynx
Maxilla with hard palate
Tongue
Uvula
Axis (C2)
Sublingual gland
Mandible
Oropharynx
Vallecula
Epiglottis
Laryngopharynx
Opening into larynx
Trachea

FIG. 2-32 Midsagittal section through the head.

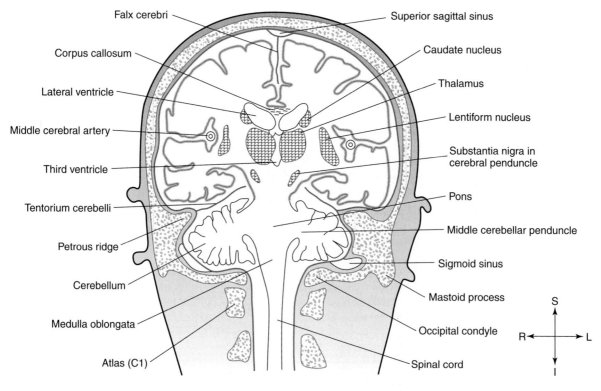

Falx cerebri
Corpus callosum
Lateral ventricle
Middle cerebral artery
Third ventricle
Tentorium cerebelli
Petrous ridge
Cerebellum
Medulla oblongata
Atlas (C1)

Superior sagittal sinus
Caudate nucleus
Thalamus
Lentiform nucleus
Substantia nigra in cerebral peduncle
Pons
Middle cerebellar peduncle
Sigmoid sinus
Mastoid process
Occipital condyle
Spinal cord

FIG. 2-33 Coronal section through third ventricle and brainstem.

CORONAL SECTIONS

Section Through the Third Ventricle and Brainstem

Fig. 2-33 illustrates a coronal section through the third ventricle and the brainstem. The two cerebral hemispheres are separated by the **longitudinal fissure,** which contains the **falx cerebri** and the **anterior cerebral arteries.** The **superior sagittal sinus** is in the superior margin of the falx cerebri. At the inferior margin of the falx cerebri, the **corpus callosum** forms a communicating band of white fibers between the two hemispheres. The two **lateral ventricles** are separated by a thin partition, the **septum pellucidum.** A region of gray matter, the **caudate nucleus,** forms the lateral portion of the floor of the lateral ventricle. Inferior to the lateral ventricles, in the midline, the **third ventricle** appears as a thin slitlike opening, with the **thalamus** forming the wall on each side. Another region of gray matter, the **lentiform nucleus,** is lateral to the thalamus, between the thalamus and the **lateral sulcus.** The **cerebral peduncles** of the midbrain, easily identified by the small dark band of **substantia nigra,** extend inferiorly from the thalamus and third ventricle. The brainstem is completed by the **pons** and **medulla oblongata.** At the **foramen magnum,** between the occipital condyles, the medulla oblongata continues as the **spinal cord.** Large **middle cerebellar peduncles** form a connection between the cerebellar hemispheres and the pons. Fig. 2-33 shows the petrous and mastoid portions of the temporal bone. The **tentorium cerebelli** extends medially from the petrous ridge to form the dural partition between the cerebrum and cerebellum. Sigmoid venous sinuses are associated with the petrous ridge. Fig. 2-34 is a coronal MRI

slightly anterior to the illustration in Fig. 2-33 and shows lateral ventricles, the internal carotid artery, optic chiasma, and other features in this region.

Section Through the Orbit and Nasal Cavity

Fig. 2-35 illustrates a coronal section through the posterior portion of the orbit and the nasal cavity. This plane intersects the frontal lobes of the cerebral hemispheres, with the longitudinal fissure and falx cerebri between them. Within the orbit, the **optic nerve** appears as a central structure with the extrinsic eye muscles and other nerves surrounding it. All are embedded in the orbital fat. The **bulbus oculi** is anterior to this plane and not visible. **Ethmoid sinuses** are medial to the orbits. Within the nasal cavity, the central structure is the thin **perpendicular plate of the ethmoid,** which forms the nasal septum. Three **nasal conchae** project medially from the lateral walls of the cavity. The superior and middle conchae are part of the ethmoid bone, but the inferior concha is a separate bone. A portion of the large **maxillary sinus** is lateral to the nasal cavity. The palate separates the nasal cavity from the oral cavity. Bones and muscle make up the framework of the sides of the face. Extending inferiorly from the temporal bone, the **temporalis muscle** inserts on the medial side of the mandible. The **masseter muscle,** lateral to the mandible, originates on the zygomatic arch and maxilla and inserts on the mandible. The **submandibular gland** is near the inferior margin of the mandible. Fig. 2-36 is a coronal computed tomography image through the nasal cavity. Compare this with the line drawing in Fig. 2-35.

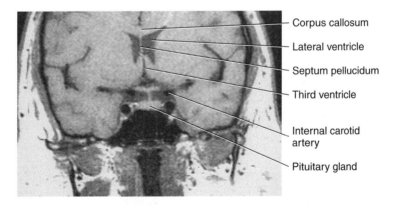

- Corpus callosum
- Lateral ventricle
- Septum pellucidum
- Third ventricle
- Internal carotid artery
- Pituitary gland

FIG. 2-34 Coronal MRI through ventricles.

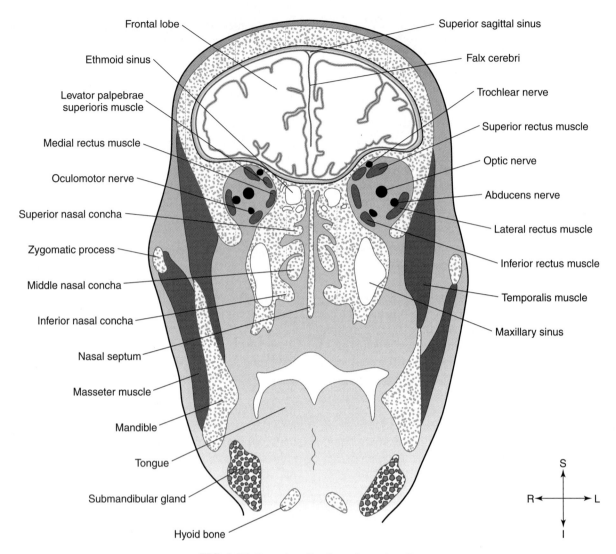

FIG. 2-35 Coronal section through nasal cavity.

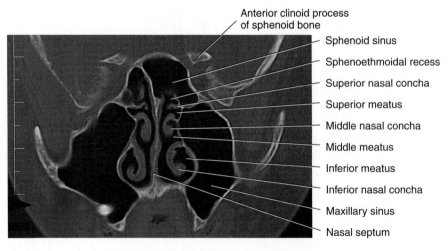

FIG. 2-36 Coronal CT image through nasal cavity.

Pathology

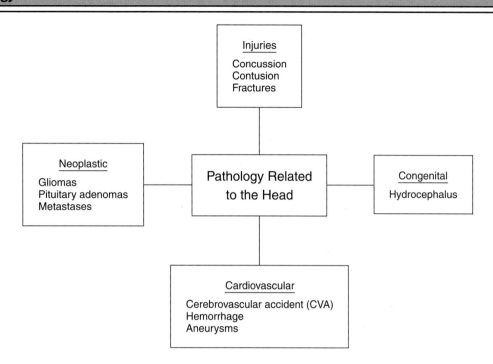

Concussion

A concussion results from a blow to the head that causes the brain to shift within the cranial vault and hit the cranial wall. Signs and symptoms include a short-term loss of consciousness following the injury, severe headache, nausea, and vertigo. This type of injury is common in automobile, motorcycle, and bicycle accidents, child abuse, and falls in the home.

Contusion

A contusion is injury to the brain tissue. It is a bruise of the brain, possibly accompanied by a collection of blood (hematoma) in the epidural or subdural space. This is more severe than a concussion and usually occurs as a result of direct impact by a blunt object, often in automobile accidents and violent acts.

Fractures

Fractures of the bones of the skull are often accompanied by damage to brain tissue, such as concussion or contusion. Skull fractures are of additional concern when they cross an artery because the vessel may tear, resulting in an epidural hematoma. Because bleeding from an artery is usually rapid, intracranial pressure increases quickly. If the fracture enters the mastoid air cells or a sinus, there is the danger that an infection from these areas may potentially spread throughout the cranial vault and possibly result in encephalitis or meningitis.

Hydrocephalus

Hydrocephalus is excessive accumulation of cerebrospinal fluid (CSF) in the ventricles of the brain (internal hydrocephalus), in the subarachnoid space (external hydrocephalus), or in both locations. Noncommunicating hydrocephalus is caused by an obstruction in the channels between the ven-

tricles. Communicating hydrocephalus results when there is diminished resorption of cerebrospinal fluid by the arachnoid villi. The accumulation of cerebrospinal fluid leads to ventricular enlargement, compression of brain tissue, and increased intracranial pressure.

Cerebrovascular Accident (CVA or Stroke)

A cerebrovascular accident is sudden interruption of cerebral circulation. The loss of cerebral circulation results in a diminished supply of oxygen (ischemia) and leads to an area of necrosis in brain tissue. This area is referred to as an infarct. There are two major causes of a cerebrovascular accident. The most common is the blockage of a blood vessel, either by a thrombus (more common) or an embolus. The second, more serious cause, is cerebral hemorrhage. The precipitating cause is usually chronic hypertension or an aneurysm that weakens the vessel wall. Symptoms depend on the arteries involved. The internal carotid, anterior cerebral, middle cerebral, vertebral, and basilar arteries are most commonly affected.

Hemorrhage

Hemorrhage is the escape of blood from a ruptured vessel. A ruptured or torn artery bleeds faster than a vein because of the higher pressure in the arterial system. There are four primary types of hemorrhage. **Epidural** hemorrhage is external to the dura mater and usually is in the temporal region as a result of rupture of the middle meningeal artery. **Subdural** hemorrhage is between the dura mater and arachnoid and usually is the result of slow venous leakage. **Subarachnoid** hemorrhage occurs between the arachnoid and pia mater, often as the result of a ruptured berry aneurysm. The intersections, or junctions, along the circle of Willis are vulnerable locations for berry aneurysms. **Intracerebral** hemorrhage occurs within the brain, often with the bleeding originating

Continued

Pathology—cont'd

Hemorrhage—cont'd

from a hemangioma that develops as a result of chronic hypertension. With all types of hemorrhage, the surrounding brain tissue is usually swollen and edematous.

Aneurysm

An aneurysm is a sac formed by a localized dilation of a vessel wall, usually an artery. It is caused by a weakness in the vessel wall. Most aneurysms enlarge with time and become increasingly susceptible to rupture with subsequent hemorrhage. Cerebral aneurysms are most often associated with the circle of Willis.

Glioma

A glioma is a primary tumor of the brain that is composed of neuroglia. Approximately one half of all primary brain tumors are gliomas of some type, such as glioblastomas (most common), astrocytomas, oligodendrogliomas, and ependymomas.

Often the location of the tumor is just as important as the malignancy of the tumor. Any tumor, whether benign or malignant, primary or metastatic, usually causes an increase in intracranial pressure resulting in headaches, vomiting, and blurred vision. Seizures may occur as a result of the presence of a tumor.

Pituitary Adenoma

Pituitary adenomas are tumors of the pituitary gland. These tumors grow out of the sella turcica and usually are benign, slow growing, and well encapsulated. These features contribute to a high rate of cure with surgery and irradiation. Symptoms of pituitary adenomas include headaches and, if the tumor compresses the optic chiasm, visual disturbances.

Metastatic Tumors

Metastases of tumors from other sites may invade any intracranial structure. Usually the metastases arise form lung carcinoma, adenocarcinoma of the breast, or malignant melanoma.

· REVIEW QUESTIONS ·

1. Indicate whether each of the following is a bone of the face or a bone of the cranium:
   a. Maxilla
   b. Frontal
   c. Ethmoid
   d. Temporal
   e. Zygomatic
2. What nerve innervates the muscles of facial expression?
3. On what bone do all of the muscles of mastication insert?
4. What salivary glands are medial to the angle of the mandible?
5. Where are the basal ganglia located?
6. What is the largest portion of the diencephalon?
7. Name the three parts of the brainstem.
8. Where are the ventricles located?
   a. Lateral ventricles
   b. Third ventricle
   c. Fourth ventricle
9. Between which layers of meninges are the subarachnoid cisterns located?
10. Name six subarachnoid cisterns.
11. What are the two pairs of arteries that supply blood to the brain?
12. What venous structures collect blood and cerebrospinal fluid from the brain and return it to the internal jugular vein?
13. Name the three cranial nerves that are primarily sensory in function.
14. Name the three tunics, or coats, in the wall of the bulbus oculi.
15. What is contained in the anterior cavity of the eye and in the posterior cavity, and what separates the two cavities?

· CHAPTER QUIZ ·

Name the Following:

1. The largest of the paranasal sinuses
2. The bone that has a mastoid process, spinous process, and external auditory meatus
3. The muscle of mastication that is superficial to the ramus of the mandible
4. The salivary gland that is between the ramus of the mandible and the mastoid process
5. The component of the basal ganglia that is closely associated with the lateral ventricles
6. The portion of the diencephalon that forms the lateral walls of the third ventricle
7. The passageway between the third and fourth ventricles
8. The largest of the subarachnoid cisterns
9. The venous sinus that empties into the internal jugular vein
10. The anterior portion of the fibrous tunic of the eye

True/False:

1. The sphenoid bone is a facial bone.
2. The falx cerebri is an extension of the arachnoid that is found in the longitudinal fissure.
3. The tentorium cerebelli is between the cerebrum and cerebellum.
4. The internal capsule is a band of white matter between the globus pallidus and putamen.
5. The cerebrospinal fluid is located in the subarachnoid space between the arachnoid and the dura mater.
6. The two vertebral arteries join to form the basilar artery, which passes over the midbrain.
7. The longitudinal sulcus (fissure) separates the frontal lobe from the parietal lobe.
8. The cavernous sinus contains the internal jugular vein.
9. The venous sinus that follows along the tentorium cerebelli from the inferior sagittal sinus to the confluence of sinuses is the straight sinus.
10. The lacrimal gland for the production of tears is located in the superior and medial margin of the orbit.

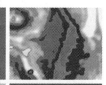

OBJECTIVES

Upon completion of this chapter, the student should be able to do the following:

- Identify the features of "typical" vertebrae and compare these with the features unique to cervical vertebrae.
- Describe the structure of intervertebral discs and state the functions of the discs.
- Identify the margins of the anterior and posterior triangles of the neck, and name the principal components in each triangle.
- Identify the regions of the pharynx by describing the location and features of each region.
- Describe the features of the larynx.
- Discuss the relationships of the esophagus and trachea as they descend through the neck.
- Describe the location of the thyroid and parathyroid glands relative to the trachea.
- Discuss the relationships of the internal jugular vein with other vessels and anatomic structures as it descends from the jugular foramen to the brachiocephalic vein.
- Describe the pathways and the relationships of the common carotid, external carotid, and internal carotid arteries.
- State the origin and pathway of the vertebral arteries.
- Explain what is meant by the term *sympathetic trunk* and describe its location.
- Name one cranial nerve located in the neck.
- Identify the nerve plexus located in the neck and name one nerve that emerges from this plexus.
- Describe the composition and location of the brachial plexus and name the region innervated by the nerves that emerge from this plexus.
- Identify the features of the neck, including vertebrae, muscles, viscera, and blood vessels, in transverse and midsagittal sections.

General Anatomy of the Neck

The principal bony structures in the neck are the cervical vertebrae. These bones and the muscles in the neck provide support for the head, yet they permit some degree of movement. The digestive and respiratory systems begin with openings in the head and continue as passageways in the neck. The thyroid and parathyroid glands, which are important endocrine organs, are located in the neck region. The neck also serves as a passageway for the spinal cord, blood vessels, and nerves. As you can see, there are many important structures located in the limited region of the neck and an understanding of the relationships of these structures is important for the imaging professional.

OSSEOUS COMPONENTS

The bony skeleton of the neck consists of seven cervical vertebrae. These vertebrae are similar to all the other vertebrae, but they have some features that are unique. In order to make comparisons, it is necessary to first describe the "typical" vertebra.

General Structure of Vertebrae

Vertebrae, in general, have a thick, disc-shaped body. Two small bridges of bone, called *pedicles*, project posteriorly from the vertebral body. The pedicles continue as flat plates of bone, called *laminae*, which unite with each other posteriorly. The body, pedicles, and laminae form a complete circle that encloses a large opening, called the **vertebral foramen,** which contains the spinal cord. Two **transverse processes** project laterally from the laminae, and a single **spinous process** projects posteriorly from the midline. Fig. 3-1 illustrates the features of a typical vertebra such as the one just described.

Features of Cervical Vertebrae

Cervical vertebrae, illustrated in Fig. 3-2, are distinguished from other types of vertebrae by the holes, or foramina, that are present in the transverse processes. These holes, called **transverse foramina,** are for the passage of the vertebral arteries. Another unique feature is the forked, or bifid, spinous processes on the first six cervical vertebrae. The spinous process of the seventh cervical vertebra may not be **bifid,** and is usually long and pointed, which makes it easily palpable. This is a good reference point for counting the vertebrae.

The first two cervical vertebrae are unique and have special names. The first cervical vertebra, C1, is called the **atlas.** It does not have a spinous process, and it has no vertebral body mass, but instead it is shaped like an oval ring. It has smooth facets on the superior surface that articulate with the occipital condyles. Inferior facets articulate with the second cervical vertebra. The second cervical vertebra, C2, is called the **axis.** It has a superiorly projecting process called the **dens** or **odontoid process.** The dens projects into the vertebral foramen of the atlas above to form a pivot around which the atlas and skull rotate. Fig. 3-3 illustrates the atlas and the axis.

Intervertebral Discs

The structures that join the vertebrae together to form a continuous column are the **intervertebral discs.** Each disc consists of a fibrocartilaginous outer ring called the **anulus fibrosus** and an inner soft core, the **nucleus pulposus.** The size and shape of each disc corresponds to the adjoining vertebrae. In the cervical region the discs are slightly thicker anteriorly than posteriorly. This forms a normal curve in the cervical region that is convex anteriorly. This is illustrated by the radiograph in Fig. 3-4. The cervical curvature develops within a few weeks after birth, when infants begin to hold their head erect. The discs form a tight joint between the vertebrae and yet, by their design, are able to absorb the high compression forces that are generated in walking and

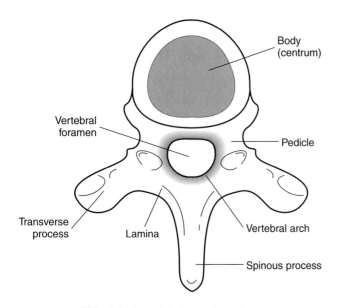

FIG. 3-1 General features of vertebrae.

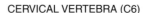
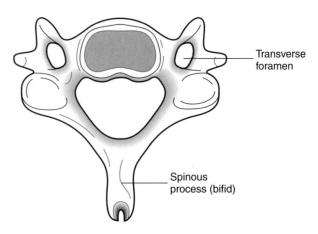

FIG. 3-2 Features of cervical vertebrae.

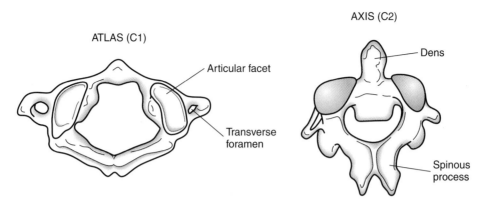

ATLAS (C1)

AXIS (C2)

Articular facet

Transverse foramen

Dens

Spinous process

FIG. 3-3 Atlas (C1) and axis (C2).

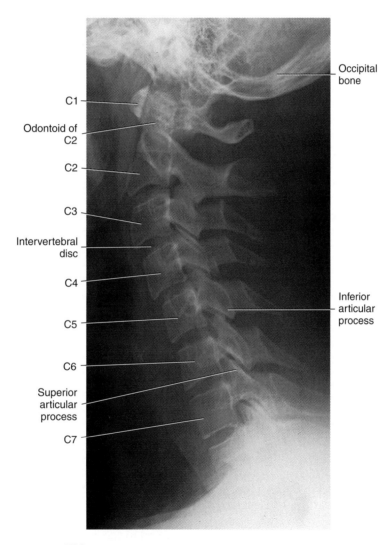

Occipital bone

C1

Odontoid of C2

C2

C3

Intervertebral disc

C4

C5

C6

Superior articular process

C7

Inferior articular process

FIG. 3-4 Radiograph showing normal cervical curvature.

other daily activities. As a result of disc degeneration or trauma, the soft nucleus pulposus may protrude through an opening or tear in the anulus fibrosus. This is called a **herniated disc.** Symptoms will depend on the location and severity of the herniation.

Muscular Components

There are numerous muscles located in the neck; however, many of them are small and difficult to separate from adjacent muscles. They may be even more difficult to isolate by imaging techniques. These muscles have functional significance because they deal with deglutition and with movements of the head, neck, and shoulder. The muscles of the neck are often described as being located within one of two triangles, which are separated by the sternocleidomastoid muscle. Fig. 3-5 illustrates the boundaries of the anterior and posterior triangles of the neck. Only the larger and more significant muscles are presented in this discussion.

Anterior Triangle of the Neck

The anterior triangle extends from the midline of the neck to the anterior margin of the sternocleidomastoid muscle. The lower border of the mandible forms the base, and the manubrium of the sternum forms the apex of the triangle.

The muscles of the anterior triangle, which are generally considered throat muscles, also help to form the floor of the oral cavity, and all are attached to the hyoid bone. They are involved with movements of the tongue and aid in swallowing. These muscles, summarized in Table 3-1, may be divided into two groups, the **suprahyoid muscles** and the **infrahyoid muscles.** As a group, the suprahyoid muscles are superior to the hyoid bone and raise the hyoid bone during swallowing, or open the jaw when the hyoid bone is fixed. These muscles are the digastric, stylohyoid, mylohyoid, and geniohyoid. The infrahyoid muscles are inferior to the hyoid bone and

pull down on the larynx and hyoid to return them to their normal positions after swallowing. These muscles are the sternohyoid, sternothyroid, thyrohyoid, and omohyoid.

In addition to the muscles, a significant structure located within the anterior triangle is the **carotid sheath,** which is a tubular arrangement of fascia that extends from the base of the skull to the inferior portion of the neck. The sheath encloses the common carotid artery, internal jugular vein, and the vagus nerve, as illustrated in Fig. 3-6. Superior to the bifurcation of the common carotid artery, the internal carotid artery is in the position previously occupied by the common carotid artery. Branches of the external carotid artery are within the anterior triangle but are not enclosed by the carotid sheath.

Other components within the anterior triangle include the carotid sinus, carotid body, lymph nodes, and the submandibular salivary gland. The carotid sinus and the carotid body are closely related to the common carotid artery near its point of bifurcation. The carotid sinus, which reacts to changes in arterial blood pressure, is an enlargement of the internal carotid artery as it branches from the common carotid artery. The carotid body, a small ovoid mass of tissue in the region of the carotid sinus, responds to changes in the chemical composition of the blood.

Posterior Triangle of the Neck

The posterior triangle of the neck extends from the posterior margin of the **sternocleidomastoid** muscle to the **trapezius** with the apex of the triangle at the junction of these two muscles. The base is formed by the clavicle. The muscular floor of the triangle is formed by the splenius capitis, the levator scapulae, and the middle and posterior scalene muscles. These muscles are summarized in Table 3-2. The external jugular vein, the phrenic and accessory nerves, and portions of the brachial plexus are located within the posterior triangle.

Viscera of the Neck

The neck region represents the connection between the head and the trunk of the body. Although the term *viscera* usually refers to the organs of the thoracic and abdominopelvic cavities, it is used here as a collective term for the miscellaneous structures of the neck that cannot be classified as nerves, muscles, or blood vessels. This includes the pharynx, larynx, trachea, and esophagus, which represent passageways for food and air, and the thyroid and parathyroid glands, which are important endocrine glands located in the neck.

Pharynx

The **pharynx** is a muscular tube about 12 cm long that extends from the base of the skull to the level of the sixth cervical vertebra and cricoid cartilage, where it becomes the **esophagus.** The wall of the pharynx consists of overlapping

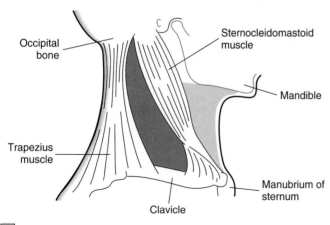

Anterior triangle

Posterior triangle

FIG. 3-5 Boundaries of the anterior and posterior triangles in the neck.

TABLE 3-1   *Muscles Associated With the Anterior Triangle of the Neck*

Muscle	Origin	Insertion	Action	Innervation
Sternocleidomastoid	Sternum and clavicle	Mastoid of temporal	Turn head side to side; flex neck	Spinal accessory (XI)
Suprahyoid Muscles				
Digastric	Mandible	Hyoid	Elevate hyoid; open mouth	Trigeminal (V)
Stylohyoid	Temporal	Hyoid	Elevate hyoid; retract tongue	Facial (VII)
Mylohyoid	Mandible	Hyoid	Elevate hyoid and floor of mouth	Trigeminal (V)
Geniohyoid	Mandible	Hyoid	Protracts hyoid	Hypoglossal (XII)
Infrahyoid Muscles				
Sternohyoid	Sternum	Hyoid	Depress hyoid	Hypoglossal (XII)
Sternothyroid	Sternum	Thyroid cartilage and hyoid	Depress thyroid cartilage and hyoid	Hypoglossal (XII)
Thyrohyoid	Thyroid cartilage	Hyoid	Depress hyoid	Hypoglossal (XII)
Omohyoid	Scapula	Hyoid and clavicle	Depress hyoid	Hypoglossal (XII)

TABLE 3-2   *Muscles Associated With the Posterior Triangle of the Neck*

Muscle	Origin	Insertion	Action	Innervation
Trapezius	Occipital bone and vertebral spines	Scapula	Elevates scapula	Spinal accessory (XI)
Splenius capitis	Cervical and thoracic vertebrae	Occipital bone	Extends head	Cervical nerves
Levator scapulae	Cervical vertebrae	Vertebral border of scapula	Elevates scapula	Dorsal scapular
Middle scalene	Cervical vertebrae	First rib	Elevates rib	Cervical plexus
Posterior scalene	Cervical vertebrae	Second rib	Elevates rib	Cervical plexus

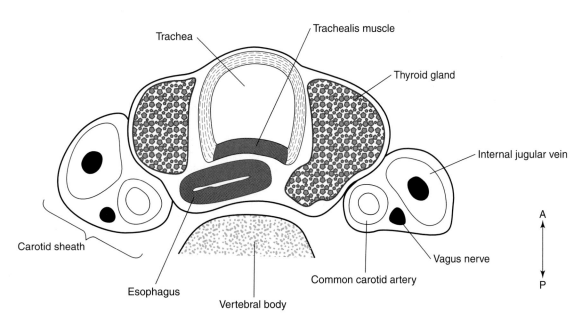

FIG. 3-6 Contents and location of the carotid sheath.

pharyngeal constrictor muscles lined with mucous membrane. For descriptive purposes it is divided into the nasal, oral, and laryngeal portions.

The **nasopharynx,** which is the region posterior to the nose, extends from the base of the skull to the soft palate. The anterior wall of the pharynx is somewhat lacking in structural elements but presents open space where the nasal cavity communicates with the pharynx through the **choanae** or internal nares. The **eustachian,** or auditory, tubes open into the lateral walls of the nasopharynx. The openings are recognized by the **torus tubarius,** a rounded protuberance of cartilage, which outlines the posterior wall of the opening. Posterior to the torus tubarius, the walls of the nasopharynx extend laterally to form the **pharyngeal recess.** Aggregations of lymphoid tissue, the pharyngeal tonsils, are found in the mucosa of the posterior wall of the nasopharynx. When enlarged, these tonsils are commonly called "adenoids."

The **oropharynx,** which is posterior to the oral cavity, extends from the soft palate to the tip of the epiglottis. The opening from the oral cavity into the pharynx is called the **fauces.** Collections of lymphoid tissue, the **palatine tonsils,** are in the wall of the oropharynx. These are commonly referred to as "the tonsils." The base of the tongue, with the associated lymphoid tissue called **lingual tonsils,** forms part of the anterior wall of the oropharynx. Between the tongue and the epiglottis are two valleys, called **valleculae,** which present a potential hazard since foreign objects may become lodged there.

The laryngeal portion of the pharynx, called the **laryngopharynx,** or hypopharynx, extends from the superior border of the epiglottis to the cricoid cartilage, which is located at the junction between the larynx and trachea at the level of the sixth cervical vertebra. The walls extend laterally around the opening of the larynx to form the **piriform recesses.** Foreign objects that enter the pharynx may become lodged in the recesses. Inferiorly the laryngopharynx is continuous with the esophagus.

The **retropharyngeal space** is a potential space between the fascia that surrounds the pharynx and the fascia that surrounds the vertebral column and its associated prevertebral muscles. The space contains loose connective tissue and permits the movement of the pharynx, larynx, trachea, and esophagus during swallowing. The retropharyngeal space is closed off by the skull superiorly, but it opens into the mediastinum of the thorax inferiorly. Laterally, the carotid sheath forms a barrier to the space. Infections in the region of the fascial layers may penetrate the fascia and enter the retropharyngeal space. Pus from infections may form abscesses that bulge into the pharynx and cause difficulty in speaking or swallowing. Once an infection enters the retropharyngeal space, it has a direct pathway into the mediastinum.

Larynx

Although the larynx is an essential part of the air passageway, it is especially modified for voice production. In the male the larynx typically extends from the level of the third cervical vertebra (C3) to the sixth cervical vertebra (C6). It is usually somewhat higher than this in females and children. The skeleton of the larynx is formed by nine cartilages joined by ligaments. The major cartilages are the single **thyroid, cricoid,** and **epiglottic cartilages** and the paired **arytenoids.** In addition, there are small **corniculate** and **cuneiform cartilages,** which are paired. The thyroid, cricoid, and arytenoids are hyaline cartilage. With age, the hyaline cartilage may calcify, making these cartilages visible on radiographs. The other cartilages (epiglottic, corniculate, and cuneiform) are elastic cartilage. The corniculate cartilages are attached to the tips of the arytenoids and are covered by a fold of tissue called the aryepiglottic fold. The cuneiform cartilages are enclosed within the aryepiglottic fold lateral to the arytenoids. The interior of the larynx is subdivided into three portions by folds of tissue that project from the lateral laryngeal wall. The upper folds are the **vestibular folds.** These form the inferior margin of the **vestibule,** which is the most superior chamber of the larynx. The opening between the two vestibular folds is called the **rima vestibuli.** Because the vestibular folds are frequently mistaken for the vocal cords, they are sometimes referred to as the false vocal cords, even though they play little or no part in voice production. The lower projections are the **vocal folds,** or true vocal cords, and the slit or opening between them is the **rima glottidis.** This aperture changes shape depending on the position of the folds during breathing and phonation. The space between the vestibular folds and the vocal folds is the **ventricle of the larynx.** Sometimes the ventricle is called the laryngeal sinus. This is the smallest and middle of the three regions. The remainder of the laryngeal cavity is the **infraglottic portion,** which extends from the vocal folds to the trachea. The term *glottis* refers to the true vocal folds and rima glottidis collectively.

If a foreign particle such as a bit of food enters the larynx, the musculature goes into a spasm and creates tension on the vocal folds, which closes the rima glottidis. This prevents air from reaching the trachea and lower air passageways, and the individual is in danger of asphyxiation.

Trachea

The **trachea** begins as a continuation of the larynx in the neck at vertebral level C6. It descends through the thorax, anterior to the esophagus, and enters the **superior mediastinum** of the thorax a little to the right of midline. It extends to vertebral level T5, where it bifurcates into the right and left bronchi. The walls of the trachea are supported by 16 to 20 incomplete rings of hyaline cartilage. The rings are deficient on the posterior side, where they are related to the esophagus; therefore the posterior margin of the trachea is flattened. The tracheal airway is kept open by the rings of cartilage; the soft tissue filling the posterior gap, between the tips of the rings, allows for expansion of the esophagus during swallowing. The **common carotid arteries** and lobes of the **thyroid gland** are lateral to the trachea in

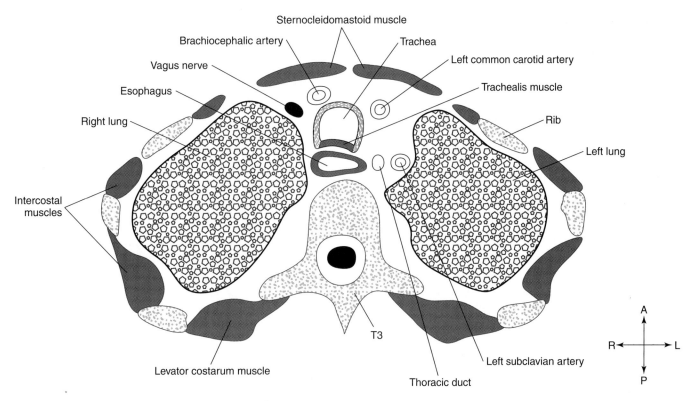

Sternocleidomastoid muscle

Brachiocephalic artery

Vagus nerve

Trachea

Left common carotid artery

Esophagus

Trachealis muscle

Right lung

Rib

Intercostal muscles

Left lung

A

R ← → L

P

T3

Levator costarum muscle

Thoracic duct

Left subclavian artery

FIG. 3-7 Relationships of the esophagus.

the neck (see Fig. 3-6). At lower levels, near the aortic arch, the **brachiocephalic artery** (trunk) is anterior and to the right of the trachea.

Esophagus

The **esophagus** is a thick, distensible, muscular tube that extends from the pharynx at the level of the cricoid cartilage (C6) in the neck to the stomach in the abdomen. As it descends through the neck, it is near the midline, between the trachea and the vertebral bodies. At the root of the neck, on the right side, the esophagus is related to the **parietal pleura** of the apex of the lung. On the left, the **thoracic duct** and **subclavian artery** are between the esophagus and the pleura. These relationships are illustrated in Fig. 3-7.

Thyroid and Parathyroid Glands

The **thyroid,** an important endocrine gland, consists of right and left lobes, usually connected by an **isthmus.** The lobes are lateral to the lower portion of the larynx and upper part of the trachea, and they may extend posteriorly enough to be related to the esophagus. The isthmus connecting the lobes passes over the second and third tracheal rings, and the lobes may extend inferiorly to the sixth tracheal ring. Four small **parathyroid glands** are usually embedded along the posterior margin of the thyroid, but these are difficult to visualize.

VASCULAR COMPONENTS

Internal Jugular Veins

The **internal jugular vein** begins as a continuation of the **sigmoid sinus** at the jugular foramen in the posterior cranial fossa. It is usually the largest vein in the neck, and it is generally larger on the right side than on the left. As the internal jugular vein descends toward the heart, it passes deep to the **sternocleidomastoid muscle,** then courses anteriorly to unite with the **subclavian vein.** Posterior to the sternal end of the clavicle, the internal jugular vein joins with the subclavian vein to form the **brachiocephalic vein.** The internal jugular vein is located within the carotid sheath with the common carotid artery (or internal carotid artery at higher levels) and vagus nerve. Within the sheath, the internal jugular vein is lateral to the common carotid artery and the vagus nerve is between the two vessels and slightly posterior to them. Figs. 3-6 and 3-8 illustrate these relationships. At higher levels the internal jugular vein is posterior to the internal carotid artery since the jugular foramen is posterior to the carotid canal. At lower levels the internal jugular vein is anterior to the common carotid artery because of the anteriorly positioned brachiocephalic veins.

Common Carotid Arteries

On the right side the **common carotid artery** begins posterior to the sternoclavicular joint as a branch of the

brachiocephalic artery. On the left it arises from the **aortic arch.** It ascends the neck, medial to internal jugular vein within the carotid sheath, to the level of the superior border of the thyroid cartilage, where it divides into the **external** and **internal carotid arteries.** This is at the level of the disc between the third and fourth cervical vertebrae. At the bifurcation the common carotid artery and the continuing internal carotid artery are dilated to form the **carotid sinus.** The carotid sinus contains receptors for the regulation of blood pressure.

The angiogram in Fig. 3-8, A and the sonogram in Fig. 3-8, B show the bifurcation of the common carotid artery into the internal and external carotid arteries.

Internal Carotid Arteries

Arising as a direct continuation of the common carotid artery, the **internal carotid artery** ascends almost vertically within the carotid sheath to enter the carotid canal in the petrous portion of the temporal bone. The right and left internal carotid arteries are two of the four major vessels supplying blood to the brain. Branches also supply the pituitary gland and orbit. The internal jugular vein is lateral to the internal carotid artery, and the vagus nerve is posterolateral (see Fig. 3-6).

External Carotid Arteries

The **external carotid artery** arises at the bifurcation of the common carotid artery. As the name implies, the external carotid artery and its numerous branches supply structures external to the skull. At low levels, near the bifurcation of the common carotid artery, the external carotid artery is anterior and medial to the internal carotid artery. At higher levels the external carotid artery becomes more superficial so that it is anterior and lateral to the internal carotid artery.

Vertebral Arteries

The right and left **vertebral arteries** begin as branches of the right and left **subclavian arteries.** The arteries ascend through the transverse foramina of the cervical vertebrae C6 through C1. The vessels then course along the superior portion of the atlas and enter the **foramen magnum.** As they pass through the foramen magnum, the arteries pierce the dura mater and arachnoid to enter the subarachnoid space of the **cerebellomedullary cistern.** Within the skull, at the base of the pons, the right and left vertebral arteries join to form a single basilar artery. The vertebral arteries are two of the four major arteries that supply the brain. The other two arteries are the right and left internal carotid arteries.

Major Nerves of the Neck

Sympathetic Trunks

The **sympathetic trunks** are strands of nerve fibers and ganglia that lie lateral to the vertebral column. They extend from the base of the skull to the coccyx. In the cervical region the trunks are posterior to the carotid sheath and are immediately anterior to the transverse processes of the ver-

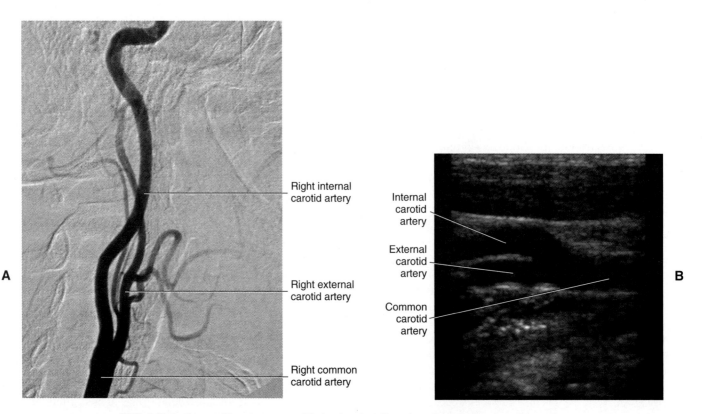

A

Right internal carotid artery

Right external carotid artery

Right common carotid artery

Internal carotid artery

External carotid artery

Common carotid artery

B

FIG. 3-8 Angiogram **(A)** and sonogram **(B)** showing the bifurcation of the common carotid artery.

tebrae. There are three ganglia in the cervical region of the sympathetic trunk. The superior cervical ganglion is located at the level of the axis, and because it is large, it serves as a good landmark for locating the trunk. The middle cervical ganglion is small and is located just anterior to the vertebral artery at the level of the transverse process of the sixth cervical vertebra. The inferior cervical ganglion is usually found posterior to the vertebral artery at the level of the superior border of the neck of the first rib.

Vagus Nerve

Cranial nerve X is named the **vagus** because of its wide distribution. The vagus nerve leaves the skull through the jugular foramen with the internal jugular vein. It descends in the anterior triangle of the neck, within the carotid sheath, and it is slightly posterior to and between the internal jugular vein and carotid artery, either common or internal depending on the level.

Cervical Plexus

The **cervical plexus** is a network of nerve fibers that are derived from the first four cervical nerves. It is located within the posterior triangle of the neck, lateral to the first four cervical vertebrae, and deep to the internal jugular vein and sternocleidomastoid muscle. Branches from this plexus innervate the skin and muscles of the neck and portions of the head and shoulders. The **phrenic nerve,** an important branch of the cervical plexus, is the only nerve that supplies motor impulses to stimulate contraction of the diaphragm. It descends the neck along the anterior surface of the anterior scalene muscle. At the root of the neck it enters the thorax between the subclavian artery and subclavian vein.

Brachial Plexus

The **brachial plexus** is a network of nerve fibers that are derived from the last four cervical nerves and the first thoracic nerve. Nerves from the brachial plexus innervate the upper extremity. The supraclavicular portion of this plexus is in the anterior and inferior portion of the posterior triangle of the neck, lying between the anterior and middle scalene muscles. The infraclavicular portion of the brachial plexus is located in the axilla. This plexus is discussed further with the thorax.

Sectional Anatomy of the Neck

TRANSVERSE SECTIONS

Section Through the Neck at Level of C1

Sections through the neck at the level of the first cervical vertebra, illustrated in Fig. 3-9, typically pass through the **hard** and **soft palate.** The **pharyngeal constrictor muscle** forms the wall of the **oropharynx** at the posterior edge of the soft palate. The dens, or odontoid process, of C2 projects upward, posterior to the arch of C1. The **ramus of the mandible** appears as a thin slice of bone, with the **masseter**

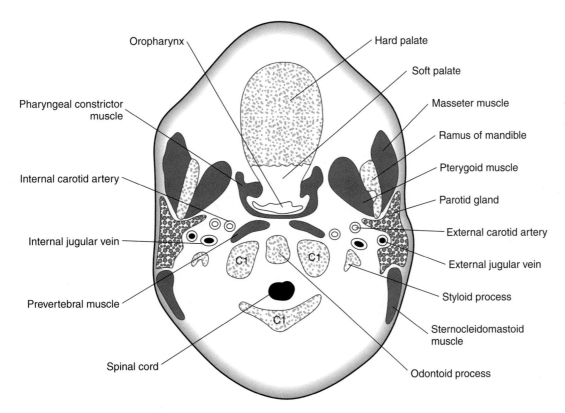

FIG. 3-9 Transverse section through the neck at level of C1.

muscle lateral to it and the **pterygoid muscle** medial to it. Another significant structure at this level is the **parotid gland.** The **sternocleidomastoid muscle** is posterior to the parotid gland, and the masseter muscle, the medial ptery-goid muscle, and the ramus of the mandible are anterior to the gland. Medially, the parotid gland is related to the **styloid process** of the temporal bone and the **internal jugular vein.** The tissue of the parotid gland may surround the **external jugular vein.**

Section Through the Neck at Level of C3

Sections through the third cervical vertebrae, illustrated in Fig. 3-10, will likely pass through the **mandible** and the **muscles of the tongue.** The **submandibular gland** is medial to the mandible, and a small portion of the **parotid gland** may still be present at this level. The arrangement of the vessels in the region is of particular significance. The **external** and **internal carotid arteries** are close together, which indicates that this is near their junction point. The external carotid artery is anterior to the internal carotid artery, and the **internal jugular vein** is lateral to both of these. The **external jugular vein** is lateral to the sternocleidomastoid muscle.

Section Through the Larynx

A representative transverse section through the larynx is illustrated in Fig. 3-11. The laminae of the laryngeal **thyroid**

cartilage are usually evident at vertebral levels of C3 or C4. Near the upper margin of the thyroid laminae, the **common carotid arteries** bifurcate into the external and **internal carotid arteries.** At this junction, the common carotid artery and the internal carotid artery that continues from it dilate to form the **carotid sinus,** which contains barorecep-tors to monitor blood pressure. The pharynx continues through this region as the **laryngopharynx.** Muscles forming the floor of the posterior triangle of the neck are lateral to the transverse processes of the vertebrae.

Section Through the Thoracic Inlet

Sections through the thoracic inlet, or superior thoracic aperture, are inferior to the larynx and show the structures that pass through the root of the neck into the thorax. Fig. 3-12 illustrates this region. At this level the **trachea** is present, with a lobe of the **thyroid gland** on each side. In some cases the isthmus of the thyroid will be present anterior to the trachea. The posterior soft tissue of the trachea, namely the **trachealis muscle,** allows for expansion of the **esophagus,** which is posterior to the trachea, during swallowing. At this level the **sternocleidomastoid muscles** are more anteriorly positioned than they are at higher levels. The **common carotid arteries** and **internal jugular veins** are lateral to the thyroid gland, with the artery medial to the vein.

Some of the components of the posterior triangle are evident in transverse sections at this level. The anterior scalene,

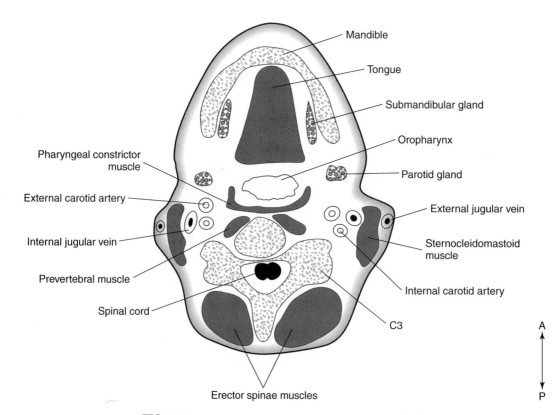

Mandible

Tongue

Submandibular gland

Oropharynx

Parotid gland

Pharyngeal constrictor muscle

External carotid artery

Internal jugular vein

Prevertebral muscle

Spinal cord

External jugular vein

Sternocleidomastoid muscle

Internal carotid artery

C3

A

P

Erector spinae muscles

FIG. 3-10 Transverse section through the neck at level of C3.

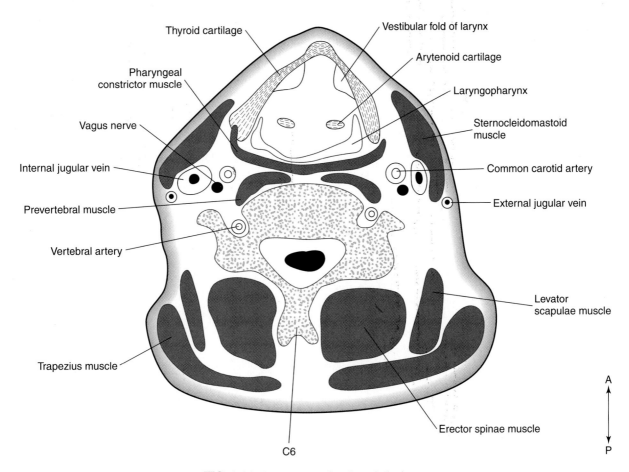

FIG. 3-11 Transverse section through the larynx.

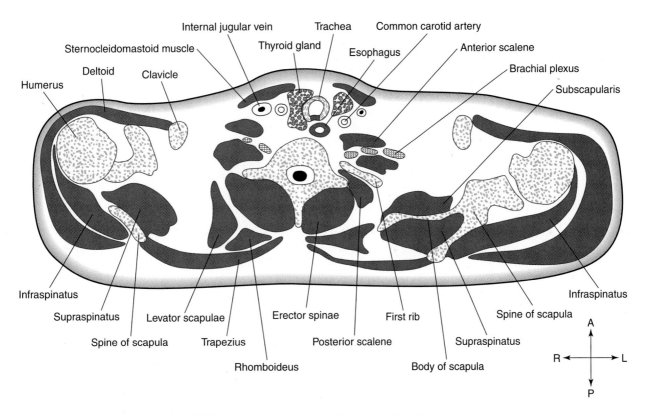

FIG. 3-12 Transverse section through the thoracic inlet.

middle scalene, and levator scapulae muscles are present, and the brachial plexus is visible between the anterior and middle scalene muscles. Sections at this level also show the shoulder region with the pectoral girdle and the upper extremity. The details of these regions will be discussed in Chapters 4 and 8.

MIDSAGITTAL SECTION

Fig. 3-13 illustrates a midsagittal section through the neck. This illustration shows features of the brain and oral cavity, but this discussion focuses on the neck region. The leaf-shaped epiglottis, one of the laryngeal cartilages, is quite ob-

vious. The trachea, with its cartilaginous rings, is inferior to the larynx.

The pharynx is immediately anterior to the vertebral column. The nasopharynx, which is located posterior to the nasal cavity, extends from the superior pharyngeal margin to the uvula. At the uvula the nasopharynx becomes the oropharynx, which continues inferiorly to the epiglottis. The laryngopharynx continues inferiorly from the epiglottis, posterior to the larynx. At the level of the first tracheal cartilage the laryngopharynx becomes the esophagus. Midsagittal sections provide nice views of the vertebral bodies, the intervertebral discs, and the spinal cord.

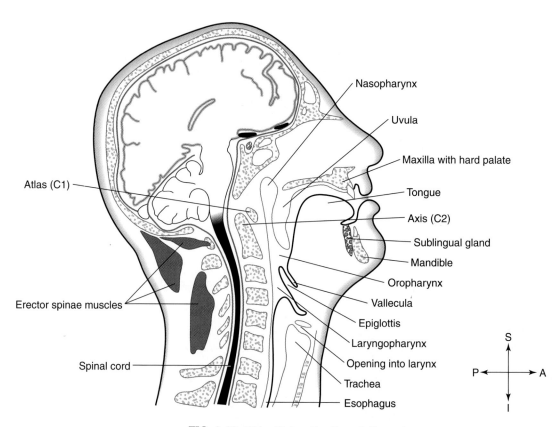

FIG. 3-13 Midsagittal section through the neck.

· REVIEW QUESTIONS ·

1. What two features are unique to cervical vertebrae?
2. What special names are given to C1 and C2?
3. What are the two parts of an intervertebral disc?
4. What muscle forms the dividing line between the anterior and posterior triangles of the neck?
5. In which triangle, anterior or posterior, is the carotid sheath located?
6. What are the three components located within the carotid sheath?
7. What three structures form the boundaries of the posterior triangle?
8. What are the three regions of the pharynx, and where are they located?
9. What are the three largest and unpaired cartilages of the larynx?
10. What two structures are immediately lateral to the trachea in the neck?
11. What distensible tube is between the trachea and the vertebral bodies in the neck?
12. What vein descends in the neck to join with the subclavian vein?
13. At what vertebral level does the common carotid artery divide into the external and internal carotid arteries?
14. What cranial nerve descends the neck within the carotid sheath?
15. What is the cervical plexus, and at what vertebral level is it located?

· CHAPTER QUIZ ·

Name the Following:

1. The superiorly projecting process on C2
2. The fibrocartilaginous outer ring of an intervertebral disc
3. The bone that forms the base of the anterior triangle of the neck
4. The most lateral component within the carotid sheath
5. The region of the pharynx that is the location of the pharyngeal tonsils
6. The most inferior cartilage of the larynx
7. The glandular structure immediately lateral to the trachea
8. The vessel that begins as a continuation of the sigmoid sinus in the posterior cranial fossa
9. The structure in the neck that contains receptors for the regulation of blood pressure
10. The nerve that emerges from the cervical plexus and innervates the diaphragm

True/False:

1. Cervical vertebrae are unique because they are the only ones that have laminae and pedicles.
2. The laryngopharynx is also called the hypopharynx.
3. The epiglottis is one of the unpaired laryngeal cartilages.
4. On the right side the esophagus is related to the pleura, and on the left side it is related to the thoracic duct and subclavian artery.
5. Within the carotid sheath the internal jugular vein is lateral to the common carotid artery and anterior to the vagus nerve.
6. At higher levels in the neck the internal carotid artery is posterior to the internal jugular vein.
7. The relationships of the external and internal carotid arteries change so that at higher levels the external carotid artery is medial to the internal carotid artery, but at lower levels it is lateral to the internal carotid artery.
8. The vertebral arteries ascend the neck within the transverse foramina of the cervical vertebrae and enter the skull through the foramen magnum.
9. The vagus nerve is the longest nerve in the body and, among other things, provides the primary innervation to the diaphragm.
10. In the cervical region the sympathetic trunk is posterior to the carotid sheath and anterior to the transverse processes of the cervical vertebrae.

CHAPTER FOUR

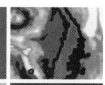

The Thorax   4

General Anatomy of the Thorax

OBJECTIVES

Upon completion of this chapter, the student should be able to do the following:
- Identify and describe the bones that form the thoracic cage.
- State the vertebral level of the jugular notch, sternal angle, and xiphisternal junction.
- State the boundaries of the superior and inferior thoracic apertures.
- List three muscles that form thoracic boundaries.
- Identify muscles associated with the pectoral, back, and shoulder regions.
- State the origin and location of the brachial plexus and name five nerves that emerge from the plexus.
- Describe the structure and hormonal control of the female breast.
- Name four groups of lymph nodes involved in lymphatic drainage of the breast.
- Describe the pleura and pleural cavities.
- Compare the features of the right and left lungs.
- List the divisions of the mediastinum and the contents of each region.
- Describe the pericardial sac, pericardium, and pericardial cavity.
- Describe the three layers of the heart wall.
- Define and state the location of the apex, base, surfaces, and borders of the heart.
- Discuss the features and relationships of the chambers and valves of the heart.

- Compare the right and left coronary arteries with respect to origin, branches, location, and regions they supply.
- Describe the venous drainage of the heart.
- Trace the pathway of a stimulus through the conduction system of the heart.
- Identify the great vessels associated with the heart by describing the location and relationships of each vessel.
- Trace the flow of blood through the heart from the right atrium to the ascending aorta.
- Discuss the location and relationships of the thymus, trachea, esophagus, azygos vein, and hemiazygos vein.
- Identify the skeletal components, muscles, blood vessels, and viscera of the thorax in transverse, sagittal, and coronal sections.

General Anatomy of the Thorax

The terms *thorax* and *chest* are used synonymously to refer to the region that is located between the neck and the abdomen. The **superior thoracic aperture,** or thoracic inlet, is rather small and oblique in position. It separates the thorax from the root of the neck. The most superior portion of the aperture is situated posteriorly, then it slopes inferiorly in the anterior direction. It is bounded posteriorly by the first thoracic vertebra, laterally by the first pair of ribs and costal cartilages, and anteriorly by the manubrium of the sternum. The **inferior thoracic aperture,** or thoracic outlet, is bounded posteriorly by the twelfth thoracic vertebra and anteriorly by the xiphisternal junction. The lateral margins of the thoracic outlet are formed by the twelfth rib and the sloping cartilage of the costal margin. The diaphragm covers the inferior thoracic aperture to separate the thoracic cavity from the abdominal cavity. The musculoskeletal wall of the thorax provides protection for the heart and lungs, contained in the thoracic cavity.

OSSEOUS COMPONENTS

The skeleton of the thorax is formed by the **sternum** anteriorly, the **twelve thoracic vertebrae** posteriorly, and the **ribs with their costal cartilages** laterally. These bones form a thoracic cage that serves as an attachment for muscles and provides protection for the vital viscera it encloses. The osseous components of the thorax are illustrated in Fig. 4-1.

Sternum

The **sternum** is an elongated, flat bone located in the anterior midline of the thorax. Anteriorly, it is covered only by skin, superficial fascia, and periosteum. It consists of three parts: the **manubrium,** the **body,** and the **xiphoid process.** The manubrium is the most superior of the three parts. Its upper border is indented by a midline **jugular notch,** sometimes called *suprasternal notch*, which is easily palpable. The jugular notch is at the level of the disc between the second and third thoracic vertebrae. **Clavicular notches,** located at the superolateral margins of the manubrium, on either side of the jugular notch, form articulating surfaces for the clavicle. Inferiorly, the manubrium is joined to the body of the sternum by fibrocartilage and ligaments. The manubrium and body of the sternum do not articulate in a straight line. Instead, their line of junction projects forward, forming the **sternal angle** (of Louis). This reliable landmark is generally 5 cm below the jugular notch and locates the sternal end of the second rib. This also marks the level of the intervertebral disc between the fourth and fifth thoracic vertebrae. The trachea bifurcates into the two bronchi and the aortic arch begins at the level of the sternal angle. The body, forming the bulk of the sternum, articulates with the second through seventh costal cartilages. The smallest and most inferior part of the sternum is the xiphoid process. It consists of hyaline cartilage in youth but gradually ossifies during adulthood so that by 40 years of age it is generally bony in nature and is fused with the body of the sternum at the xiphisternal junction. The xiphisternal junction is generally at the level of the ninth thoracic vertebra.

Ribs

The lateral boundaries of the chest are formed by the **12 pairs of ribs.** These flat, elongated, curved, and slightly twisted bones, along with their costal cartilages, extend from the thoracic vertebrae posteriorly to the sternum anteriorly. The ribs make up the major portion of the thoracic skeleton. The first seven ribs are considered **vertebrosternal ribs,** or true ribs, because they articulate directly with the sternum by way of their costal cartilages. The remaining five pairs are called false ribs. The costal cartilage of the eighth, ninth, and tenth ribs (the first three pairs of false ribs) is attached to the cartilage of the preceding rib rather than directly to the sternum. These are called **vertebrochondral ribs.** The last two pairs of false ribs are **vertebral ribs,** or floating, ribs, because they have no anterior attachment to the sternum. The costal cartilages of the vertebrochondral ribs join so that their inferior edges form a continuous **costal mar-**

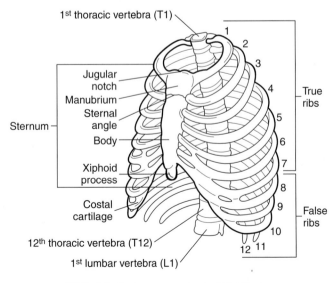

1st thoracic vertebra (T1)

Jugular notch
Manubrium
Sternal angle
Body

Sternum

Xiphoid process

Costal cartilage

12th thoracic vertebra (T12)

1st lumbar vertebra (L1)

1
2
3
4   True ribs
5
6
7
8
9   False ribs
10
12 11

FIG. 4-1 Osseous components of the thorax.

gin. As the costal margins diverge from the xiphisternal junction, they delineate the **infrasternal angle,** or **costal arch.**

Thoracic Vertebrae

The posterior median skeleton of the thoracic cage is formed by the **12 thoracic vertebrae.** Features of these vertebrae that are specifically related to the thorax include **facets** on the transverse processes and vertebral bodies for articulation with the ribs and **long spinous processes.** Features of the thoracic vertebrae are illustrated by Fig. 4-2. When the vertebral column is flexed, the most prominent spinous process is usually that of the seventh cervical vertebra, although sometimes the first thoracic spinous process may be just as evident. When the arms are at the sides, a

line drawn through the tip of the third thoracic spinous process indicates the level of the base of the scapular spine. The inferior angle of the scapula is at the same level as the middle of the seventh thoracic spinous process. The position of these landmarks changes when the arms are raised.

MUSCULAR COMPONENTS

Muscles of the Thoracic Wall

Numerous muscles are attached to the skeleton of the thorax. Most of these are muscles that move the pectoral girdle or are associated with the shoulder joint. In this section only those muscles that form a part of the thoracic boundary and are associated with changing the intrathoracic volume during breathing will be considered. Enlarging the volume of the cavity decreases the pressure and permits inspiration. Conversely, decreasing the volume increases the pressure and forces air out of the lungs during expiration. To increase intrathoracic volume, the boundaries of the cavity may increase in three different dimensions, vertically, transversely, and anteroposteriorly. Elastic recoil of the lungs and the weight of the thoracic wall primarily account for the decrease in each dimension during expiration. Muscles of the thoracic wall are illustrated in Fig. 4-3, and they are summarized in Table 4-1.

Diaphragm. The **diaphragm** covers the thoracic outlet, forming a muscular, movable partition between the thoracic and abdominal cavities. Contraction of the diaphragm enlarges the thoracic cavity in the vertical dimension during inspiration. Since the diaphragm is visualized to a greater extent in abdominal sections than in thoracic sections, it will be described in greater detail in the next chapter.

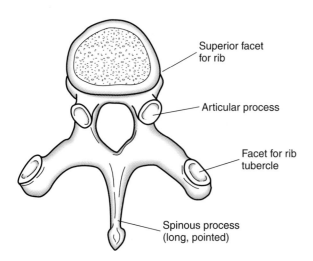

FIG. 4-2 Features of thoracic vertebrae.

Labels: Superior facet for rib; Articular process; Facet for rib tubercle; Spinous process (long, pointed)

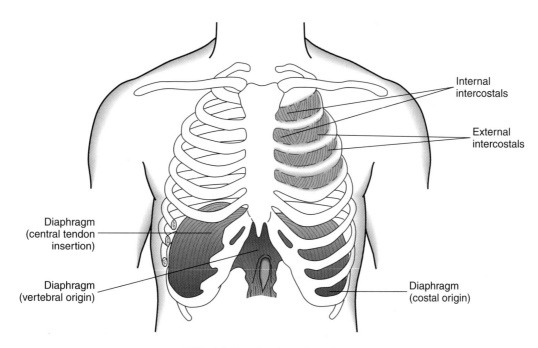

FIG. 4-3 Muscles of the thoracic wall.

Labels: Internal intercostals; External intercostals; Diaphragm (central tendon insertion); Diaphragm (vertebral origin); Diaphragm (costal origin)

TABLE 4-1   *Muscles of the Thoracic Wall*

Muscle	Origin	Insertion	Action	Innervation
Diaphragm	Interior body wall	Central tendon of diaphragm	Enlarges the thoracic cavity during inspiration	Phrenic nerve
External intercostal	Inferior border of rib above	Superior border of rib below	Assists in inspiration; synergists of diaphragm	Intercostal nerves
Internal intercostal	Inferior border of rib above	Superior border of rib below	Assists in expiration; antagonistic to external intercostals	Intercostal nerves
Innermost intercostal	Internal surface of rib above	Internal surface of rib below	Assists in expiration; antagonistic to external intercostals	Intercostal nerves
Levator costarum	Transverse processes of thoracic vertebrae	Ribs, close to the tubercle of rib below the vertebra from which it originates	Elevates the ribs	Dorsal branch of thoracic nerves

TABLE 4-2   *Muscles of the Pectoral Region*

Muscle	Origin	Insertion	Action	Innervation
Pectoralis major	Clavicle, sternum, and costal cartilages of ribs	Humerus	Adduct and medially rotate humerus	Pectoral nerves
Pectoralis minor	Third to fifth ribs	Coracoid process of the scapula	Pull scapula inferiorly	Pectoral nerves
Subclavius	First rib	Clavicle	Stabilize clavicle during shoulder movement	Subclavius nerve
Serratus anterior	First eight ribs	Scapula	Stabilize scapula; also rotate scapula	Thoracic nerve

Intercostals.   Three layers of intercostal muscles fill the spaces between the ribs. These are the external, internal, and innermost intercostal muscles, all of which receive motor impulses from the intercostal nerves. The **external intercostals** arise from the lower border of one rib and insert on the upper limit of the next rib below. The fibers are directed inferiorly and anteriorly. The **internal intercostals** occupy the intercostal spaces deep to the external intercostals. Also rising from the lower border of one rib and inserting on the upper limit of the next one below, the fibers are directed inferiorly and posteriorly, at right angles to the external intercostal fibers. The **innermost intercostals** appear similar to the internal intercostals but are separated from them by a neurovascular bundle containing an intercostal nerve, artery, and vein.

Levator Costarum.   Twelve fan-shaped **levator costarum** muscles originate on the transverse processes of the thoracic vertebrae and insert on the rib immediately below. These are visualized on transverse sections as extending from the vertebral column to a rib. Action of the levator costarum

muscles increases both the transverse and anteroposterior dimensions.

Muscles of the Pectoral Region

Numerous muscles span the back and pectoral regions of the thorax but are functionally associated with the upper extremity. Many of these muscles anchor the arm to the trunk, as well as function in movement. Sections of the thorax also show the humerus and bones of the pectoral girdle. The **pectoral girdle** consists of the **clavicle,** or collar bone, anteriorly and the **scapula,** or shoulder blade, posteriorly. Since these skeletal and muscle components are clearly evident on thoracic sections, they are included here. A more thorough discussion of the upper extremity and its associated articulations is presented in a later chapter.

The pectoral region is located on the anterior thoracic wall. Four muscles are associated with this region. These muscles help attach the upper limb to the thoracic skeleton. All are associated with movements of the arm either by acting directly on the humerus or by acting on the bones

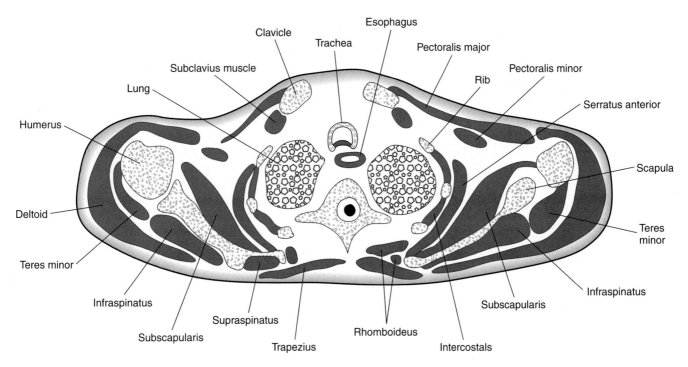

FIG. 4-4 Muscles of the pectoral region, the back, and the shoulder.

of the pectoral girdle. These muscles are summarized in Table 4-2 and are illustrated in Fig. 4-4.

Pectoralis Major. The **pectoralis major** is a large, fan-shaped muscle covering the anterior chest wall. From an extensive origin on the clavicle, sternum, and ribs, the muscle fibers converge to insert on the humerus. Near its insertion, this muscle forms the anterior wall of the axilla, the region of the armpit or junction of the arm and thorax.

Pectoralis Minor. The **pectoralis minor** is a smaller muscle lying deep to the pectoralis major. The origin of the pectoralis minor from ribs three, four, and five is much less extensive than the origin of the pectoralis major. The pectoralis minor inserts on the coracoid process of the scapula.

Subclavius. A small **subclavius** muscle lies deep to the clavicle. It extends from its origin on the first rib to the posterior surface of the middle portion of the clavicle. It appears to stabilize the clavicle during shoulder movement. It also affords some protection for the subclavian vessels when the clavicle is fractured. It is mentioned because it is usually seen in sections of this region.

Serratus Anterior. A fourth muscle, the **serratus anterior,** is associated with the pectoralis muscles in the axilla. The fan-shaped serratus anterior muscle originates from the first eight ribs then passes posteriorly to insert on the medial border of the scapula. As it runs its course from ribs to scapula, the muscle is closely applied to the wall of the thorax. The serratus anterior primarily acts with other muscles

to stabilize the scapula so it can be used as a fixed point in producing movement of the humerus.

Muscles of the Back and Shoulder Region

The muscles of the back and shoulder region may be divided into three groups: superficial back muscles, deep back muscles, and those muscles associated with the scapula. Several of these muscles are illustrated in Fig. 4-4, and they are summarized in Table 4-3.

Superficial Back Muscles. The **trapezius** and **latissimus dorsi** are the two superficial muscles of the back and shoulder region. The origin of the trapezius extends from the occipital bone to the spinous process of the twelfth thoracic vertebra. It inserts on both the clavicle and scapula. Weakness of the trapezius muscle or damage to the accessory nerve that innervates the muscle results in a drooping shoulder.

The latissimus dorsi is an extensive muscle that originates from the spinous processes of the vertebrae from the seventh thoracic down through the sacrum. Some fibers also arise from the crest of the ilium. From this broad origin, the muscle fibers converge into a tendon that inserts in the intertubercular groove of the humerus.

Deep Back Muscles. Three relatively thin straplike muscles lie deep to the trapezius. The **levator scapulae, rhomboideus minor,** and **rhomboideus major** all originate on the vertebral column and insert on the medial border of the scapula. These muscles act on the scapula to stabilize and control its position during active motion of the

TABLE 4-3 *Muscles of the Back and Shoulder Region*

Muscle	Origin	Insertion	Action	Innervation
Superficial back muscles				
Trapezius	Occipital bone to T12 vertebra	Clavicle and scapula	Adduct, elevate, and rotate scapula; also extend the head	Accessory nerve
Latissimus dorsi	Thoracic and lumbar vertebrae; crest of ilium	Humerus	Adduct and medially rotate humerus	Thoracodorsal
Deep back muscles				
Levator scapulae	Cervical vertebrae	Scapula	Elevate scapula	Dorsal scapular
Rhomboideus major and minor	Cervical and thoracic vertebrae	Scapula	Adduct scapula	Dorsal scapular
Serratus anterior	First eight ribs	Scapula	Stabilize scapula; also rotate scapula	Thoracic nerve
Muscles in scapular region				
Supraspinatus	Supraspinous fossa of scapula	Humerus	Abduct humerus	Suprascapular nerve
Infraspinatus	Infraspinous fossa of scapula	Humerus	Laterally rotate humerus	Suprascapular nerve
Subscapularis	Subscapular fossa	Humerus	Medially rotate humerus	Subscapular nerve
Deltoid	Clavicle and scapula	Humerus	Abduct humerus	Axillary nerve
Teres major	Margin of scapula	Humerus	Adduct arm	Subscapular nerve
Teres minor	Margin of scapula	Humerus	Laterally rotate arm	Axillary nerve

humerus. A fourth muscle, the **serratus anterior,** lies deep to the latissimus dorsi. This muscle has been described previously with the pectoralis muscles because of its association with them in the axilla.

Muscles in the Scapular Region. Six muscles are described in the scapular region. All of these muscles pass from the scapula to the humerus and act on the shoulder joint. The **supraspinatus** fills the supraspinous fossa of the scapula superior to the spine, whereas the **infraspinatus** lies in the infraspinous fossa inferior to the spine of the scapula. The **subscapularis** occupies the subscapular fossa on the costal surface of the scapula. The **deltoid** is a superficial muscle covering the shoulder. This muscle forms the lateral mass and rounded contour of the shoulder. In addition to origins on the spine and acromion of the scapula, the deltoid also has a portion originating on the clavicle. The insertion is on the humerus. The **teres major** is an oval muscle running from the inferior angle of the scapula to the intertubercular groove of the humerus, where it inserts with the tendon of the latissimus dorsi. It, along with the latissimus dorsi, forms a portion of the posterior wall of the axilla. Located superior to the teres major, the **teres minor** is frequently inseparable from the infraspinatus muscle. The supraspinatus, infraspinatus, subscapularis, and teres minor muscles all reinforce the fibrous capsule of the shoulder joint. These muscles, together with the fibrous capsule, are collectively referred to as the **rotator cuff** of the shoulder joint. The rotator cuff holds the head of the humerus in the glenoid cavity of the scapula, thus protecting and stabilizing the joint.

Several of the muscles associated with the back and shoulder are illustrated in Fig. 4-4. For further detail refer to Chapter 8.

BRACHIAL PLEXUS

The **brachial plexus** is a network of nerves formed by the ventral rami, or branches, of spinal nerves C5 to C8 and T1. It extends from the posterior triangle of the neck into the axilla and supplies innervation to the arm. Portions of the brachial plexus are clearly evident in transverse sections, between the anterior scalene and middle scalene muscles (see Fig. 3-13). Five nerves supplying innervation to the arm emerge from the brachial plexus. These are the **musculocutaneous, median, ulnar, axillary,** and **radial nerves.**

Injuries to the brachial plexus may occur by disease, trauma, or stretching. These injuries result in paralysis and/or anesthesia. The extent of the signs and symptoms depends on the part of the plexus that is injured.

BREAST

Both males and females have breasts. Mammary glands for the production of milk are located within the breast. Normally these become well developed and functional only in the female.

General Breast Anatomy

The breast is located in the superficial fascia of the pectoral region overlying the pectoralis major muscle. It normally extends from the lateral margin of the sternum to the anterior border of the axilla between the second and sixth ribs. Breast tissue is separated from the deep fascia of the underlying muscle by a retromammary layer of loose connective tissue. Some breast carcinomas may invade the loose connective tissue and deep fascia and become fixed to the underlying muscle. This restricts the movement of the breast.

At birth and throughout early childhood the male and female breasts are similar. Externally, near the center of the breast, a circular area of pigmented skin known as the **areola** surrounds an elevated nipple. Numerous sebaceous glands within the areola appear as small nodules under the skin and secrete an oily substance to keep the tissues soft. Internally there are a few rudimentary ducts radiating from the nipple. At puberty the mammary gland in the female undergoes developmental changes, but the male gland usually remains rudimentary.

In the adult male the breast consists of a few small ducts without any milk-secreting cells and some supporting adipose and fibrous tissue. The ducts in the male may become fibrous cords.

Female Breast Structure

In the female the breast includes glandular **parenchyma** and connective tissue **stroma.** The glandular parenchyma consists of 15 to 20 lobes of **alveoli,** or milk producing cells, arranged radially around the centrally located nipple. An excretory **lactiferous duct** extends from each lobe to the nipple, where it terminates in a tiny opening at the surface. The glandular lobes are embedded in the connective tissue stroma, which contains varying amounts of fat. Condensations of connective tissue, known as **suspensory** or **Cooper's ligaments,** extend from the underlying deep fascia through the breast to the skin. These ligaments provide support for the breasts. The components of the female breast are illustrated in Fig. 4-5.

Hormonal Control of the Female Breast

The development of the mammary gland in the female begins at puberty, when **estrogens** stimulate extensive growth of the lactiferous duct system, along with deposition of fat between the lobes. During pregnancy, the high level of **progesterone** stimulates the development of the milk-producing glands. However, no milk is actually produced until after parturition, when the sudden decrease in progesterone and estrogen signals the anterior pituitary gland to secrete **prolactin.** This hormone stimulates the production of the milk proteins and brings about the glandular secretion of milk. Stimulation by the suckling infant and the hormone **oxytocin** results in the ejection of the milk from the breast.

Lymphatic Drainage From the Breast

Although there are several routes of lymphatic drainage from the breast, about 75% of the drainage is by way of the **axillary lymph nodes.** In addition to the axillary nodes, other avenues of lymphatic drainage include the **paraster-**

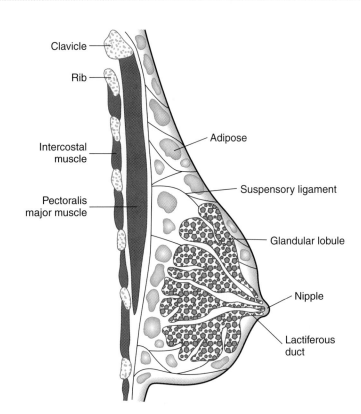

FIG. 4-5 Sagittal section of the female breast.

nal, supraclavicular, and **abdominal lymph nodes.** The drainage of one breast may also join the drainage of the opposite breast. The lymphatic drainage of the breast is of clinical significance in the diagnosis and treatment of breast cancer. As the cancer cells break loose, they travel through the lymphatic channels until they become trapped. Since 75% of the lymphatic drainage is through the axillary nodes, this is the most common site of metastases from breast carcinoma.

THORACIC CAVITY

The thoracic cavity, enclosed within the bones and muscles described in the previous paragraphs, is divided into three major divisions. The **right** and **left pleural cavities,** filled with the lungs, occupy the lateral regions. The **mediastinum** is the central region between the two pleural cavities. It contains the heart and other structures such as the trachea, esophagus, and thymus gland.

Pleural Cavities

The two pleural cavities are completely closed and separated and are lined by a serous membrane called the **pleura.** The pleura is essentially a continuous sheet in each cavity but, for descriptive purposes, it is divided into the **visceral** and **parietal layers.** You can picture this much as a balloon indented by your fist. The balloon is a single sheet of material, but when you stick your fist into it, you have two layers, the outside, or parietal, layer and the layer next to your

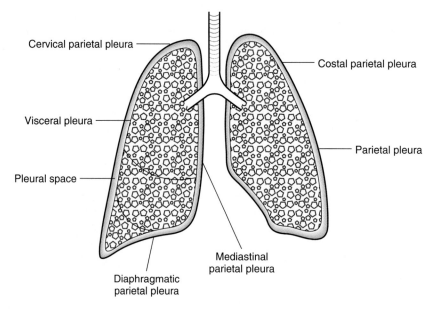

Cervical parietal pleura

Visceral pleura

Pleural space

Diaphragmatic
parietal pleura

Costal parietal pleura

Parietal pleura

Mediastinal
parietal pleura

FIG. 4-6 The pleura of the lung.

hand, the visceral layer. The **visceral pleura** is intimately adherent to the lung, covering its entire surface and continuing deeply into its fissures. The **parietal pleura** lines the thoracic wall and is divided into four regions, as illustrated in Fig. 4-6. The **costal parietal pleura** is applied to the ribs, costal cartilages, intercostal muscles, and sternum. The **diaphragmatic parietal pleura** is fused with the diaphragm and is continuous with the **mediastinal parietal pleura,** which is adjacent to the mediastinum. The **cervical parietal pleura** projects into the thoracic inlet to cover the apex of the lung.

The space between the two pleural layers, parietal and visceral, is the **pleural cavity** or **pleural space.** In reality, this is a **potential space** filled with only a capillary layer of serous lubricating fluid. This fluid reduces friction to allow the two surfaces to glide easily over each other during respiratory movements. The visceral pleura is insensitive to pain, but the parietal layer is very sensitive.

Lungs

Each lung is an elongated structure shaped roughly like a half cone. The apex, or cervical dome, lies posterior to the middle third of the clavicle. It extends slightly above the first rib to project through the superior thoracic aperture. On the slightly concave medial (mediastinal) surface, there is an opening called the **hilus,** where the bronchi, blood vessels, lymph vessels, and nerves enter and leave the lung. The structures that traverse the hilus are collectively called the **root** of the lung. Each lung is freely movable within its own pleural cavity except at the root or hilus, where it is attached. The right and left lungs are separated from each other by the mediastinum. The base of each lung is concave as it conforms to the dome of the diaphragm. Although shorter because of the volume of the liver on that side, the right lung is wider and has a greater volume than the left

lung. The heart makes an indentation, called the **cardiac notch,** in the left lung. Each lung is partially transected by an **oblique fissure** that separates the lung into **superior** and **inferior lobes.** The right lung is further subdivided by the **horizontal fissure** to form a wedge-shaped **middle lobe.** Within the lung each primary bronchus divides into secondary bronchi, two on the left side and three on the right side, providing a secondary bronchus for each lobe of the lung. Each secondary bronchus further divides into tertiary segmental bronchi that supply specific regions. A tertiary segmental bronchus with the specific sector of lung it supplies is called a **bronchopulmonary segment.**

Mediastinum

The lungs and pleura occupy the lateral portions of the thoracic cavity. All other thoracic structures are crowded into a central space called the **mediastinum.** This is divided into four regions, as illustrated in Fig. 4-7.

Superior Mediastinum.   The **superior mediastinum** is the area above the fibrous pericardium, and it is separated from the inferior mediastinum by a line passing from the sternal angle to the intervertebral disc between the fourth and fifth thoracic vertebrae. It contains all the structures passing between the neck and the thorax, the aortic arch with its branches, the brachiocephalic veins, the superior vena cava, the thymus, the trachea, the esophagus, and the vagus and phrenic nerves.

Inferior Mediastinum.   The **inferior mediastinum** is divided into the anterior, middle, and posterior mediastina.

Anterior Mediastinum.   The **anterior mediastinum** is a limited area anterior to the pericardium and posterior to the

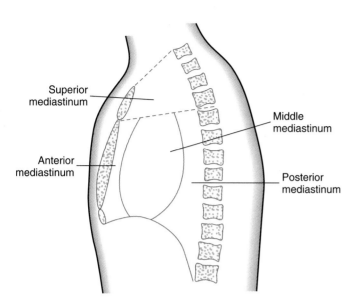

FIG. 4-7 The four regions of the mediastinum.

sternum, between the sternal angle and the diaphragm. At the sternal angle it is continuous with the superior mediastinum. It contains connective tissue with some fat, lymph nodes, and a portion of the thymus.

Middle Mediastinum.

The **middle mediastinum,** centrally located and limited by the fibrous pericardium, contains the heart and the roots of the ascending aorta, pulmonary artery, superior and inferior venae cavae, and the four pulmonary veins.

Posterior Mediastinum.

The **posterior mediastinum** is posterior to the pericardium and inferior to the fourth thoracic vertebra. The diaphragm limits the posterior mediastinum inferiorly. Between the two parietal pleura of the lungs and anterior to the vertebrae, the posterior mediastinum contains the descending thoracic aorta, azygos and hemiazygos veins, thoracic duct, and esophagus.

HEART

The heart is a hollow muscular organ enclosed in a fibroserous sac within the middle mediastinum. Shaped somewhat like a cone, the heart lies obliquely in the chest with two thirds of its mass to the left of the median plane and one third located to the right. About the size of a person's clenched fist, the heart weighs approximately 250 to 300 gm. Superficial relationships include an apex, base, three surfaces, and four borders.

Pericardium

A fibroserous sac, the **pericardium,** surrounds the heart and proximal portions of the great vessels that enter and leave the heart. There are essentially two types of pericardium—fibrous

and serous. The external, strong **fibrous pericardium** is composed of tough fibrous connective tissue. Superiorly, at its apex, the fibrous pericardium blends with the tunica externa, the fibrous connective tissue outer layer of the great vessels. At its base the fibrous layer fuses with the central tendon of the diaphragm so that respiratory movements influence the movement of the pericardial sac. In the anterior midline the fibrous pericardium is attached to the posterior surface of the sternum by a strong **sternopericardial ligament.**

The double-layered **serous pericardium** is composed of a thin, transparent serous membrane. The outer, or parietal, layer of serous pericardium, sometimes called **parietal pericardium,** forms a smooth, moist lining for the fibrous pericardium. The fibrous and parietal serous pericardia are closely adherent and difficult to separate, and together they make up the pericardial sac. The inner, or visceral, layer of serous pericardium covers the cardiac muscle of the heart wall. Because it forms the outer layer of the heart wall, the visceral serous pericardium is often called **epicardium.**

The two layers of serous pericardium, parietal and visceral, form a continuous closed sac around the heart in the same way as the pleura surrounds the lungs. Between the parietal and visceral pericardia is a potential space, the **pericardial cavity,** which contains a small amount of serous fluid distributed as a capillary film on the opposing surfaces. The lubricating action of this fluid keeps the surfaces moist and reduces friction so that they glide easily over each other during heart movements.

Heart Wall

The heart wall consists of three layers. The outermost layer is the **epicardium,** which is the visceral layer of serous pericardium. Heart muscle, called cardiac muscle, makes up the middle layer, the **myocardium.** This layer makes up the bulk of the heart wall and is the layer that contracts to perform the pumping action of the heart. The thickness of the myocardium in the heart wall varies. The harder a particular chamber has to work to pump blood, the thicker the wall. The atria have relatively thin walls because they are primarily "receiving" chambers rather than "pumping" chambers. Ventricles have thick walls because they forcefully eject blood from the heart. The left ventricle has the thickest wall because it pumps blood into systemic circulation throughout the whole body. The **endocardium** is the innermost layer. This is a thin, smooth layer of simple squamous epithelium called the *endothelium.* The endothelial lining of the heart also covers the heart valves and is continuous with the endothelial lining of the blood vessels.

Superficial Features of the Heart

Superficial features of the heart include an apex, base, three surfaces, and four borders. The **apex,** formed entirely by the left ventricle, points downward and to the left. Located in the fifth intercostal space, at the level of the eighth thoracic vertebra, it is the most inferior region of the heart, and it is to the left of midline. These positions vary and are dependent on the phase of respiration.

The **base** of the heart is the broad superior portion of the heart that is opposite the apex. This means that the base projects superiorly, posteriorly, and to the right. It extends between the fifth and eighth thoracic vertebrae. The two atria are the primary components of the base, and the posteriorly positioned left atrium is the predominate portion of the base. The ascending aorta, pulmonary trunk, and superior vena cava emerge from the base. The base is sometimes referred to as the **posterior surface.**

In addition to the posterior surface, or base, there are two other surfaces of the heart. The anterior **sternocostal surface** is created primarily by the right atrium and right ventricle, although the left auricular appendage and left ventricle contribute a small portion. The two ventricles resting on the diaphragm comprise the **diaphragmatic surface.**

The right atrium, in line with the superior and inferior venae cavae, forms the **right border.** The **left border** is more convex and is outlined by the left ventricle. The right ventricle, with a small contribution from the left ventricle near the apex, forms the horizontal **inferior border.** The **superior border,** where the great vessels enter and leave the heart, is formed by both atria.

Chambers and Valves

The heart is divided into four chambers: the right and left atria, and the right and left ventricles. On the surface a groove that encircles the heart separates the atria from the ventricles. This is the coronary sulcus, or atrioventricular sulcus. Similarly, an interventricular sulcus marks the division between the right and left ventricles.

Valves. A system of valves is required to keep blood flowing through the heart in the appropriate direction. There are two basic types of valves in the heart. Both types consist of cusps or flaps of fibrous tissue covered with endothelium. **Semilunar valves** are found at the exit ports of the ventricles. **Atrioventricular valves** function as inflow valves where the blood flows from the atria into the ventricles.

Semilunar valves consist of three cusps that balloon out from the vessel wall to prevent backflow of blood from the aorta and pulmonary trunk into the ventricles. When the ventricles contract, the increased pressure forces the valve cusps flat against the vessel wall, opening the valve to allow ejection of blood. After contraction, as ventricular pressure decreases, the cusps are caught in a passive backflow and balloon out from the walls to close the orifice. This prevents blood from flowing backward into the ventricles.

Atrioventricular valves are so named because they are located between the atria and ventricles. The atria have thin walls, do not contract strongly, and generate relatively little pressure. Consequently, the atrioventricular valves must open easily to allow blood to flow from the atria into the ventricles. These valves have thin cusps that move readily in the current of flowing blood. Stringlike structures called **chordae tendineae** attach the cusps to projections of myocardium called **papillary muscles.** When pressure in the ventricles increases because of contraction, these valves are forced back over the opening to prevent blood from going back into the atria. The papillary muscles contract with the ventricles, which creates a tension on the valve cusps and prevents them from protruding back into the atria. The valves of the heart are illustrated in Fig. 4-8.

Right Atrium. The most right-sided portion of the heart is the **right atrium.** This thin-walled chamber receives venous blood from the coronary and the systemic circulations. Openings into this chamber include the **superior** and **inferior venae cavae,** which return venous blood from systemic circulation, and the opening of the **coronary sinus,** which returns blood from the circulation that supplies blood to the heart wall.

The smooth-walled posterior region of the right atrium, where the venae cavae enter, is called the **sinus venarum.** Anteriorly, the atrial wall is roughened by muscular ridges called **pectinate muscle.** A small muscular pouch, the **auricle,** projects toward the left from the right atrium and covers the root of the aorta. The posterior wall of the right atrium is formed by the **interatrial septum,** the partition between the right and left atria. In fetal circulation there is an opening in the interatrial septum. This opening, called the **foramen ovale,** allows blood to pass directly from the right atrium into the left atrium and bypasses pulmonary circulation. After birth, higher pressure on the left side of the heart pushes a flap of tissue across the opening to close it. After a time the foramen is sealed off, but a depression, the **fossa ovalis,** remains. The left or medial wall of the right atrium contains the right atrioventricular valve. This valve has three cusps and is called the **tricuspid** valve. The tricuspid valve has a vertical orientation and is posterior to or slightly to the right of the sternum at the level of the fourth intercostal space between the fourth and fifth ribs.

Right Ventricle. The triangular-shaped **right ventricle** forms a major portion of the sternocostal, or anterior, surface of the heart. This chamber receives blood from the right atrium through the tricuspid valve and ejects the blood into the **pulmonary trunk** for oxygenation in the lungs. A **pulmonary semilunar valve** is located at the outflow from the right ventricle into the pulmonary trunk. An average surface projection places this valve at the third costal cartilage on the left side of the sternum. The upper anterior portion of the right ventricle, around the origin of the pulmonary trunk, is the smooth-walled **conus arteriosus.** The remainder of the right ventricular wall is roughened by muscular ridges called **trabeculae carneae** and projections called **papillary muscles.** Stringlike **chordae tendineae** extend from the three papillary muscles to the cusps of the right atrioventricular, or tricuspid, valve to prevent inversion of the valve when ventricular pressure increases.

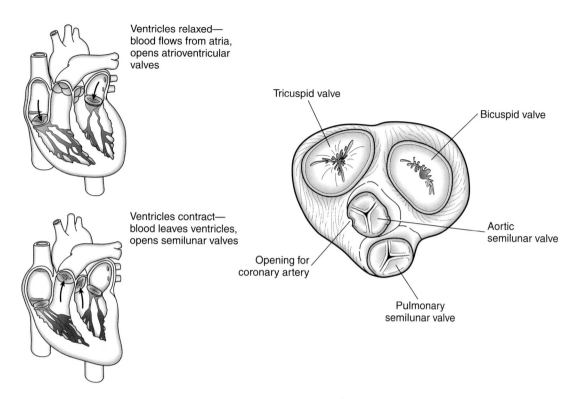

FIG. 4-8 Valves of the heart.

Left Atrium. The **left atrium** is the most posterior structure of the heart. It forms most of the base of the heart and consists of the atrium proper and its auricular appendage. The wall of the left atrium is slightly thicker than the right atrium, and its interior is smooth except for a few pectinate muscles in the auricle. Four **pulmonary veins,** two on each side, return oxygenated blood to the heart from the lungs and enter the left atrium at its superolateral aspect. The anterior wall of the left atrium is formed by the left atrioventricular valve. This valve has two cusps and is called the **bicuspid, or mitral,** valve. The mitral valve is the one most often affected by disease, especially rheumatic fever. The surface projection of the bicuspid, or mitral, is at the level of the fourth costal cartilage on the left side of the sternum.

Left Ventricle. From the left atrium, blood enters the **left ventricle** through the bicuspid, or mitral, valve. The left ventricle has much thicker walls than the right since it has to work harder to pump blood throughout the whole body via systemic circulation. Most of the internal surface of the left ventricle is covered with the muscular ridges of trabeculae carneae similar to those in the right ventricle. The wall is smooth in the **vestibule,** or aortic outflow region. The two papillary muscles, attached to the bicuspid valve by chordae tendineae, are usually larger than those in the right ventricle. From the left ventricle, blood enters the aorta to supply the body through systemic circulation. Between the left ventricle and the aorta there is an **aortic semilunar valve.** This valve is located at the level of the third intercostal

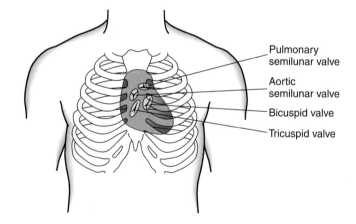

FIG. 4-9 Surface projections of the heart valves.

space, between the third and fourth ribs, on the left side of the sternum. Fig. 4-9 illustrates the surface projections of the heart valves.

The **interventricular septum** forms a partition between the right and left ventricles. The septum has an oblique orientation. Its position can be visualized on the surface of the heart by the anterior and posterior interventricular sulci, or grooves. Most of the septum is thick and muscular. There is a small, oval portion that is thin and membranous. This is located just inferior to the right cusp of the aortic semilunar valve. The membranous portion of the interventricular

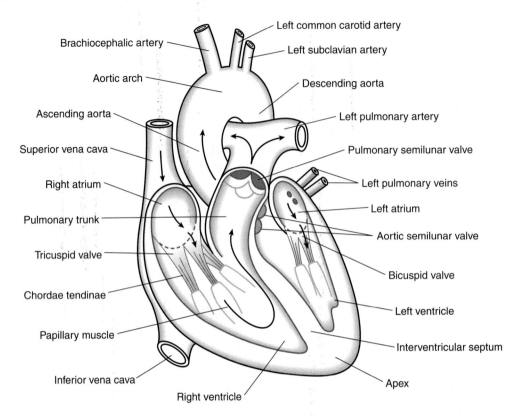

Brachiocephalic artery

Aortic arch

Ascending aorta

Superior vena cava

Right atrium

Pulmonary trunk

Tricuspid valve

Chordae tendinae

Papillary muscle

Inferior vena cava

Right ventricle

Left common carotid artery

Left subclavian artery

Descending aorta

Left pulmonary artery

Pulmonary semilunar valve

Left pulmonary veins

Left atrium

Aortic semilunar valve

Bicuspid valve

Left ventricle

Interventricular septum

Apex

FIG. 4-10 Features of the heart.

septum is the part most frequently involved in ventricular septal defect. This defect, either singly or in combination with other defects, is present in about half of the congenital cardiac abnormalities.

Valve location, as well as heart size and delineation, varies greatly depending on age, sex, body build, phase of respiration, and other factors. The locations and surface relationships stated here are for that "average" person who probably does not exist. The valve locations are anatomical projections and do not necessarily indicate the best position for listening to the heart sounds. Fig. 4-10 illustrates some of the features of the heart and the flow of blood through the heart.

Blood Supply to the Heart

The heart wall is muscle and requires a continuous supply of oxygenated blood to function effectively. Blood supply to the muscular wall of the heart is by way of the **coronary arteries** and their branches. The right and left coronary arteries originate from the aortic sinus at the root of the aorta, immediately superior to the aortic semilunar valve. Fig. 4-11 illustrates the coronary arteries.

Right Coronary Artery.   The **right coronary artery** passes slightly forward and to the right to emerge between the root of the pulmonary trunk and the right auricle. It then descends in the atrioventricular sulcus (coronary sulcus) to the inferior border. During its course the right coronary artery

gives off branches to the wall of the right atrium. Near the inferior border the right coronary artery gives off a **marginal branch** that proceeds toward the apex. The marginal branch supplies the right ventricle. After giving off the marginal branch, the right coronary artery continues in the coronary sulcus to the posterior surface, where it gives off a **posterior interventricular branch** that descends toward the apex in the posterior interventricular sulcus. This vessel gives off branches to supply the posterior wall of both ventricles and a portion of the interventricular septum.

Left Coronary Artery.   The **left coronary artery** is very short, usually only 2 to 3 cm in length. It emerges between the left auricular appendage and the pulmonary trunk and then divides. The **anterior interventricular (descending) branch** descends toward the apex in the anterior interventricular sulcus then turns toward the posterior surface to anastomose with the posterior interventricular branch of the right coronary artery. This branch supplies portions of both ventricles and the interventricular septum. The **circumflex branch** of the left coronary artery follows the left atrioventricular (coronary) sulcus around the left margin of the heart to the posterior surface, where it anastomoses with the right coronary artery. During its course, the circumflex branch gives off vessels to the left atrium and also supplies a portion of the left ventricle. The right coronary artery and its branches supply the right atrium, portions of both ventricles, and the posterior portion of the interventricular septum. The anterior interventricular branch of the left coro-

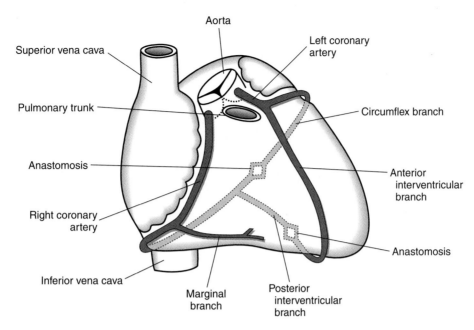

FIG. 4-11 Coronary arteries.

nary artery supplies both ventricles and a portion of the interventricular septum, whereas the circumflex branch supplies the left atrium and a portion of the left ventricle. It should be understood that variations in the branching patterns of the coronary arteries are very common.

Venous Drainage. The primary venous drainage of the heart wall is through veins that empty into the **coronary sinus,** which drains into the right atrium. The coronary sinus is a thin-walled venous dilation in the coronary sulcus on the posterior surface of the heart. The main tributary of the coronary sinus is the **great cardiac vein,** which begins at the apex and ascends in the anterior interventricular sulcus. When it reaches the atrioventricular sulcus (coronary sulcus), it passes to the left to enter the left end of the coronary sinus. Another vessel, the **middle cardiac vein,** is on the posterior surface and enters the coronary sinus on the right. It drains the posterior wall of both ventricles. Other small vessels may empty directly into chambers of the heart.

Conduction System of the Heart

The conduction system of the heart consists of specialized cardiac muscle fibers that initiate and coordinate the contractions of the chambers. Impulses for contraction are initiated in the **sinoatrial node** (SA node), which is located in the wall of the right atrium near the superior vena cava. Because it initiates the impulses, the SA node is called the pacemaker. From the SA node the impulses spread through the cardiac muscle cells of the atria, causing them to contract. The **atrioventricular node** (AV node), which is located in the interatrial septum, receives the impulses from the atrial cells and transmits them to the **atrioventricular bundle.** The AV bundle is short and branches into the **right** and **left**

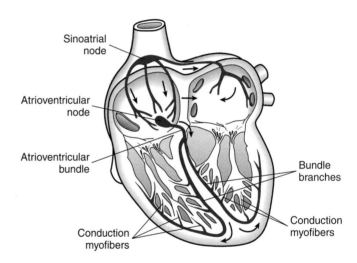

FIG. 4-12 Conduction system of the heart.

bundle branches, which extend along both sides of interventricular septum. From the bundle branches, the impulses are transmitted, by way of **conduction myofibers, Purkinje fibers,** to the papillary muscles and to the cardiac muscle cells of the ventricles. Even though the heart has its own rhythm established by the SA node, this rhythm can be altered by stimulation from the autonomic nervous system. Sympathetic stimulation speeds up the action of the SA node, and parasympathetic (vagal) stimulation decreases the heart rate. Fig. 4-12 illustrates the conduction system of the heart.

Great Vessels of the Heart

Aorta. For descriptive purposes, the aorta is divided into the ascending aorta in the middle mediastinum, aortic arch in the superior mediastinum, and descending aorta in the posterior mediastinum. The **ascending aorta** originates at the outflow orifice from the left ventricle. An **aortic semilunar valve** at the aortic orifice prevents backflow of blood from the aorta into the left ventricle. The right and left coronary arteries originate from the ascending aorta immediately superior to the aortic orifice in the region of the semilunar valve. The ascending aorta passes superiorly to the level of the sternal angle, at the level of the disk between the fourth and fifth thoracic vertebrae, where it continues as the arch of the aorta. In the superior mediastinum the **aortic arch** ascends to the middle of the manubrium then arches posteriorly and to the left so that it passes to the left of the trachea and esophagus. At the level of the intervertebral disc between the fourth and fifth thoracic vertebrae, the arch continues in the posterior mediastinum as the **descending thoracic aorta.** The brachiocephalic (innominate), the left common carotid, and the left subclavian arteries arise from the arch. The angiogram in Fig. 4-13 shows these vessels. The **brachiocephalic artery** (trunk) is the largest and most anterior of the three vessels that arise from the aortic arch. At its origin it is anterior to the trachea, but as it ascends, the vessel becomes more lateral. Posterior to the right sternoclavicular joint and lateral to the trachea, the brachiocephalic artery divides into the right subclavian and the right common carotid arteries. The **left common carotid artery** is the middle branch of the aortic

arch. It is to the left and slightly posterior to the brachiocephalic artery. In the superior mediastinum the left common carotid artery is at first anterior to the trachea, then it becomes more lateral. As it passes posterior to the left sternoclavicular joint to ascend in the neck region, it follows a course similar to the right common carotid artery. The **left subclavian artery** is the third and most posterior branch from the aortic arch. As the vessel passes through the superior mediastinum, it lies very near the pleura and left lung. In fetal circulation, a vessel called the **ductus arteriosus** extends from the left pulmonary artery to enter the inferior aspect of the aortic arch. This allows fetal blood to pass directly from the pulmonary artery into the aorta and bypass the lungs, which are not yet functioning. The fetal ductus arteriosus usually closes by the end of the third month after birth to become the **ligamentum arteriosum.**

There are numerous variations in the arch of the aorta and the origins of its branches. Some of these are asymptomatic, but others are not compatible with life and must be surgically corrected.

Pulmonary Trunk.   Arising from the right ventricle, the **pulmonary trunk** ascends on the left side of the ascending aorta to the level of the aortic arch. At its origin from the right ventricle, the pulmonary trunk is anterior to the ascending aorta, but as it ascends, the trunk becomes more posterior. When it reaches the aortic arch, at the level of

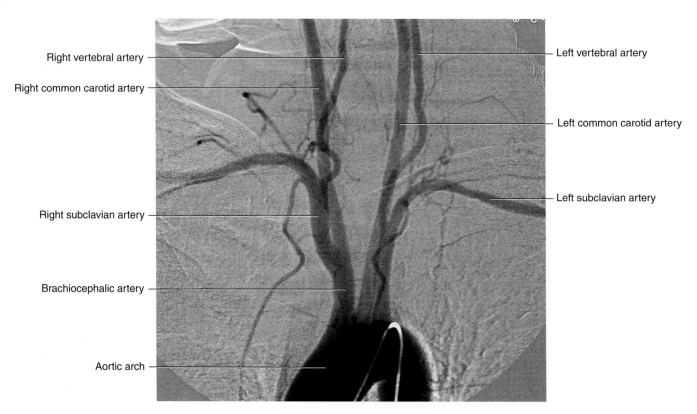

FIG. 4-13 Angiogram of the branches from the aortic arch.

the sternal angle, the pulmonary trunk divides into the right and left pulmonary arteries. The **right pulmonary artery** is longer and larger in diameter than the left. As it proceeds to the lungs, the right pulmonary artery passes posterior to the superior vena cava and the ascending aorta but anterior to the right bronchus. The **left pulmonary artery** courses horizontally to the left, anterior to the left bronchus and the descending aorta. At the hilus of the lung the pulmonary arteries divide according to the divisions of the bronchial tree.

Venae Cavae.   The **superior vena cava** (SVC) is formed in the superior mediastinum by the union of the **right** and **left brachiocephalic veins.** The left brachiocephalic vein crosses horizontally anterior to the aorta and pulmonary trunk to join with the vein on the right. The superior vena cava descends on the right side of the superior mediastinum to enter the right atrium vertically from above. The lower half of the vessel is enclosed within the pericardium in the middle mediastinum. It is located to the right of the aorta and anterior to the trachea and esophagus. The superior vena cava returns blood to the heart from structures above the diaphragm except the lungs.

The **inferior vena cava** ascends through the abdominal cavity to the right of the midline. It penetrates the diaphragm at vertebral level T8 and enters the middle mediastinum of the thoracic cavity. Here it enters the lowest part of the right atrium, almost in a vertical line with the superior vena cava. The inferior vena cava returns blood from the region below the diaphragm.

OTHER THORACIC STRUCTURES

Thymus

The **thymus** gland is located immediately behind the manubrium of the sternum in the superior mediastinum. In infancy and early childhood the gland is a prominent mass of lymphoid tissue that may extend downward into the anterior mediastinum. After puberty it gradually decreases in size and is replaced by fatty tissue until it may be hardly recognizable in the adult. The thymus has a major role in the development and maintenance of the immune system.

Trachea

Beginning as a continuation of the larynx in the neck, the **trachea** descends in front of the **esophagus** to enter the superior mediastinum a little to the right of midline. At the level of the sternal angle the trachea bifurcates into the **right** and **left primary bronchi.** Each bronchus is posterior to its corresponding pulmonary artery. The region of bifurcation is known as the **carina.** A series of C-shaped cartilages keeps the trachea open for the passage of air. The posterior soft tissue of the trachea allows for expansion of the esophagus during swallowing.

Esophagus

The **esophagus** extends from the pharynx at the level of the cricoid cartilage (C6) in the neck to the **stomach** in the upper left quadrant of the abdomen. As it descends through the neck and superior mediastinum, the esophagus is in a near midline position between the trachea anteriorly and the vertebral bodies posteriorly. The **left bronchus** passes in front of, or anterior to, the esophagus. In the posterior mediastinum the esophagus descends anterior and to the right of the descending aorta. In this region its anterior relationships are to the pericardium and the **left atrium.** In the lower regions of the posterior mediastinum, the esophagus curves to the left to penetrate the diaphragm at the T10 vertebral level. As it curves, the esophagus passes anterior to the aorta.

There are four clinically significant constrictions in the esophagus: (1) at its beginning, (2) at the level of the aortic arch, (3) at the level of the carina where the left bronchus crosses it, and (4) where it passes through the diaphragm. Objects tend to lodge in these constricted areas.

Thoracic Duct

The **thoracic duct** is the primary duct of the lymphatic system. It collects lymph from the whole body except the upper right quadrant. The thoracic duct begins in the abdomen as the **cisterna chyli.** From there, it ascends on the right side of the aorta, just anterior to the vertebral column. At level T12 it passes through the diaphragm in the same opening as the descending aorta and enters the posterior mediastinum of the thorax. The relative position of the thoracic duct in the posterior mediastinum of the lower thoracic region is illustrated in Fig. 4-14. At the level of the fifth thoracic vertebra, it deviates to the left, posterior to the esophagus, and enters the superior mediastinum, where it ascends into the neck on the left side. The thoracic duct empties into the venous system at the junction of the left internal jugular and left subclavian veins.

Azygos Vein

The **azygos vein** begins in the abdomen and enters the posterior mediastinum of the thorax along with the thoracic duct. In the thorax the azygos vein ascends just anterior to the vertebral column. It is posterior to the esophagus and to the right of the aorta and thoracic duct. The relative position of the azygos vein is illustrated in Fig. 4-14. At the level of T4, it arches over the root of the right lung to enter the **superior vena cava** in the superior mediastinum. A smaller **hemiazygos vein** ascends on the left side to the level of T9, then crosses the midline behind the aorta and esophagus to empty into the azygos vein. These veins drain the thoracic wall and posterior abdominal wall.

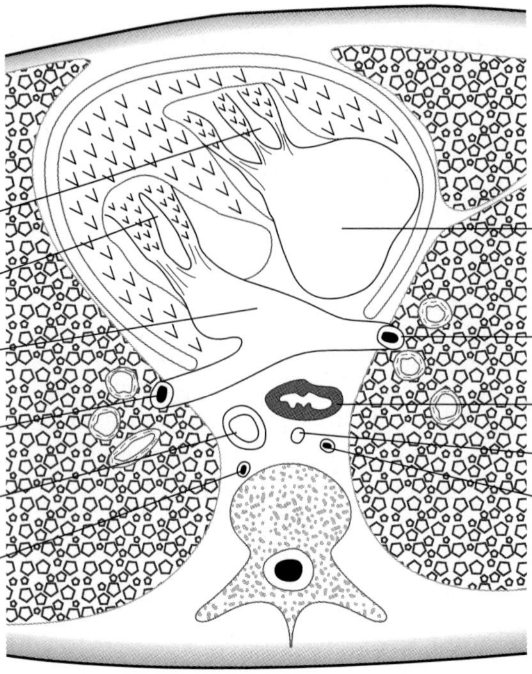

FIG. 4-14 Relationships of structures in the posterior mediastinum.

Sectional Anatomy of the Thorax

TRANSVERSE SECTIONS

Section Through the Thoracic Inlet

Sections through the superior thoracic aperture or thoracic inlet, illustrated in Fig. 4-15, show the structures passing through the root of the neck into the thorax and the shoulder region with the pectoral girdle and upper extremity. Since the superior thoracic aperture slopes inferiorly from posterior to anterior, a transverse section through the first thoracic vertebra typically does not intersect the manubrium of the sternum.

Anteriorly in sections through the thoracic inlet, the **sternocleidomastoid** muscles are thin straps anterior to the lobes of the **thyroid gland.** The horseshoe-shaped **tracheal cartilage** is between the thyroid lobes and the **esophagus.** The **internal jugular veins** are lateral to the **common carotid arteries.** Also of interest at this level are the **clavicle, scalene muscles, brachial plexus,** and **first rib.**

The components of the humeroscapular joint will be discussed in more detail in a later chapter, but because of their relationship to the wall of the thorax, they will also be mentioned here.

At the level of the thoracic inlet the most superficial muscle of the back is the **trapezius** as it goes from the vertebral column to the scapula. Lying directly beneath the trapezius are the **rhomboideus muscles.** Throughout the length of the vertebral column the **erector spinae** muscles will be seen in the groove between the spinous and trans-

verse processes. The large **deltoid** muscle forms a semicircle around the humerus from the clavicle to the spine of the scapula. Depending on the angle of the slice you will see either two or three muscles directly related to the scapula. At some angles, when only the spine of the scapula is seen, there is a more superficial **infraspinatus** muscle and a deeper **supraspinatus** muscle. When the cut is below the scapular spine, through the blade or body of the scapula, the more superficial muscle is still the infraspinatus but the muscle deep to the body is the **subscapularis.** Occasionally the angle of the slice is such that both the spine and the body of the scapula are seen. In this case, all three muscles are present. The infraspinatus appears superficial to the spine, the supraspinatus appears to be between the spine and the body, and the subscapularis is deep to the body of the scapula. These muscles are illustrated in Fig. 4-15.

Section Through the Apex of the Lung

Particular attention should be given to vascular relationships in this and the following few sections. As the aorta goes from the ascending to descending portions, it arches in an anterior-posterior direction, as well as in a right-to-left direction. This means that the vessels closely associated with the aortic arch will assume corresponding arch-shaped positions. At the level of the apex of the lung, illustrated in Fig. 4-16, the **right common carotid artery** and the **right subclavian artery** are seen as two separate vessels close together on the right side of the trachea. The close proximity of the two vessels indicates that they are near the bifurcation of the brachiocephalic vein, and, in sections inferior to this, illus-

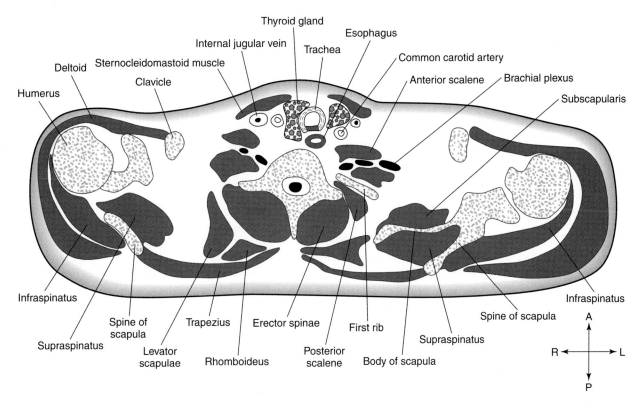

FIG. 4-15 Section through the thoracic inlet.

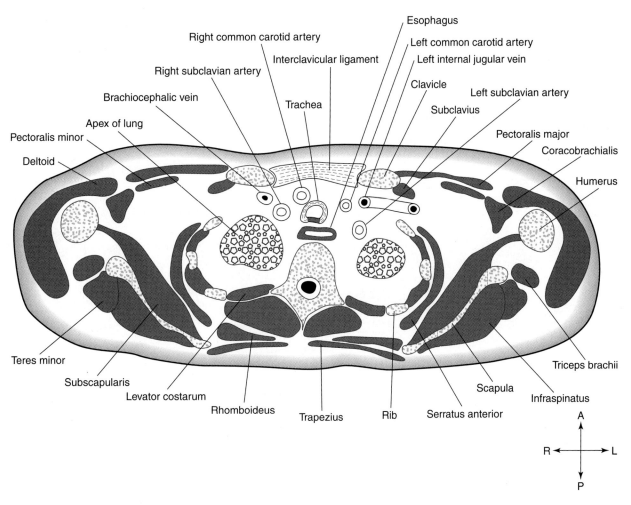

FIG. 4-16 Transverse section through the apex of the lung.

trated in Fig. 4-17, there is the single **brachiocephalic (innominate) artery.** The brachiocephalic artery is the first and most anterior branch from the arch of the aorta. On the left the anterior vessel is the **left common carotid artery.** The **left subclavian artery** is also on the left but is more posterior. This is the third and most posterior branch from the aortic arch. The **subclavian vein** is seen joining with the **internal jugular vein** to form the **left brachiocephalic (innominate) vein** on the left. On the right the brachiocephalic vein has already formed. The computed tomographic image in Fig. 4-18 shows the relationships of the common carotid and subclavian arteries.

The anterior thoracic wall at the level of the lung apex is formed by the **pectoralis major and minor** muscles and the two clavicles joined by an **interclavicular ligament.** A **subclavius muscle** is associated with each clavicle.

In addition to the intercostal muscles, two other muscles associated with the rib cage are illustrated in Figs. 4-16 and 4-17. The **serratus anterior** muscles that form the medial walls of the axillae appear much like parentheses enclosing the ribs and intercostal muscles. The **levator costarum** muscle connects a rib to its appropriate transverse vertebral

process. Muscles associated with the scapula and upper extremity include the **teres major** and the **teres minor.** The teres minor is closely associated with the **infraspinatus** muscle, and it is sometimes difficult to distinguish between them except by location. The teres minor is at the lateral end of the infraspinatus muscle. Teres major is lateral to the teres minor. Both of these muscles are illustrated in Fig. 4-17.

Section Through the Aortic Arch

A section through the arch of the aorta probably will intersect the manubrium of the sternum. When looking at an inferior view through the arch of the aorta, as illustrated in Fig. 4-19, there should be three holes in the arch representing the three branches, the anterior **brachiocephalic artery,** the posterior **left subclavian artery,** and in the middle the **left common carotid artery.** The **left brachiocephalic vein** crosses anterior to the aortic arch to join the **right brachiocephalic vein.** The right and left brachiocephalic veins join to form the **superior vena cava.** The computed tomographic image in Fig. 4-20 shows the right and left brachiocephalic veins and the three vessels from the aortic arch.

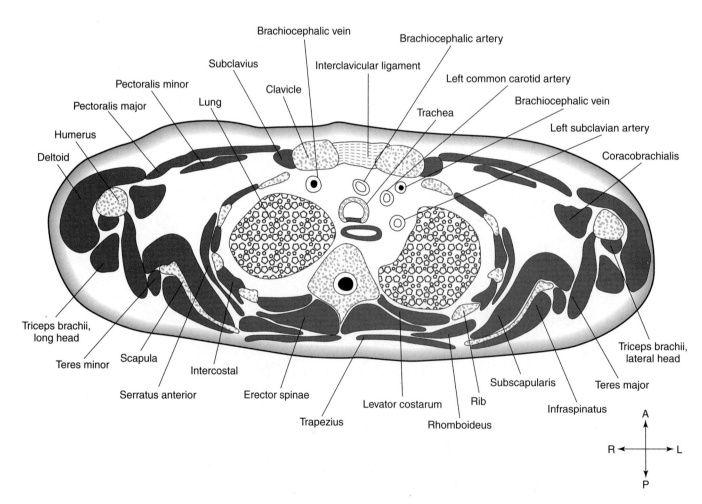

FIG. 4-17 Transverse section that shows the brachiocephalic artery.

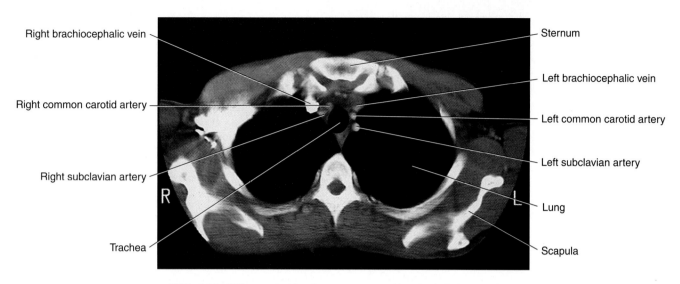

FIG. 4-18 CT image showing the common carotid and subclavian arteries.

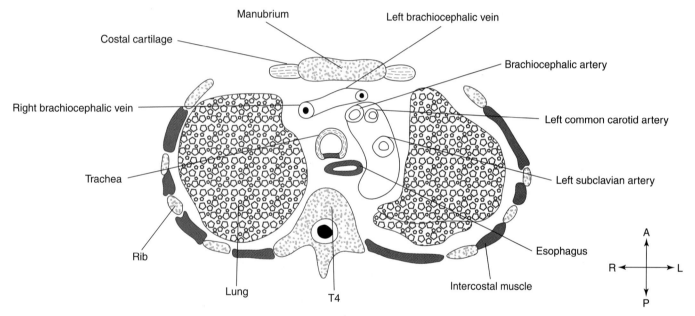

FIG. 4-19 Transverse section through the aortic arch.

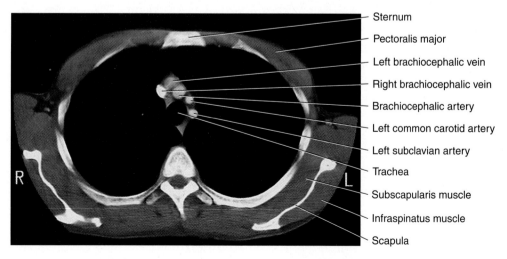

FIG. 4-20 CT image showing the three vessels from the aortic arch.

Section Through the Sternal Angle

The **sternal angle** (angle of Louis), at the T4-T5 vertebral level, is an easily palpable landmark. Transverse sections at this level show an anteriorly located **ascending aorta** and posteriorly situated **descending aorta** on the left side of the mediastinum. This is illustrated in Fig. 4-21. The right-sided **superior vena cava** is opposite the ascending aorta. Posterior to the ascending aorta and superior vena cava the **trachea** begins to bifurcate into the **main stem (primary) bronchi.** The **esophagus**. is between the tracheal bifurcation and the descending aorta. The **azygos vein** is seen for the first time at this level as it makes a loop over the root of the right lung to enter the superior vena cava. The computed tomographic image in Fig. 4-22 shows the vessels and the bifurcation of the trachea that are described above.

Section Through the Pulmonary Trunk

The **pulmonary trunk** appears on the left side within the pericardium at approximately level T5. In sequence from right to left, the great vessels are the **superior vena cava, ascending aorta,** and **pulmonary trunk,** as shown in Fig. 4-23. At this level the pulmonary trunk may be slightly posterior to the ascending aorta, but at more inferior levels it becomes anterior. Even though the pulmonary trunk is the outflow from the right ventricle, it is the most left-sided of the three great vessels. The **right pulmonary artery,** as it branches from the pulmonary trunk, must pass horizontally, posterior to the ascending aorta and superior vena cava, to enter the right lung (see Fig. 4-23). Since the pulmonary trunk is on the left, the right pulmonary artery is longer and more horizontal than the left. The right and left pulmonary arteries are anterior to the right and left main stem bronchi, respectively. In the posterior mediastinum the large vessel on the left is the **descending aorta.** The **esophagus** is anterior and slightly to the right of the descending aorta, and the **azygos vein** is to the right of the esophagus. The **thoracic duct** is usually between the azygos vein and the descending aorta but may be difficult to locate. The computed tomographic image in Fig. 4-24 shows the right pulmonary artery as it passes horizontally, posterior to the superior vena cava and the ascending aorta.

Section Through the Base of the Heart

Sections through the base of the heart show the three great vessels at or near their attachment to the heart. As you follow the three great vessels from higher levels down to their origin from the chambers of the heart, you will notice that they keep the same right-to-left sequence (superior vena cava, ascending aorta, pulmonary trunk), but the anterior-posterior relationship of the ascending aorta and pulmonary trunk appears to change. At higher levels the ascending aorta is anterior to the pulmonary trunk (see Fig. 4-23). At lower levels the ascending aorta is posterior to the pulmonary trunk (Fig. 4-25). The pulmonary trunk courses in a posterior direction as it ascends from the right ventricle. The outflow orifice is guarded by the **pulmonary semilunar valve.** The superior vena cava remains on the right side as it enters the right atrium, the most right-sided chamber of the heart. The **left atrium** is the most posterior chamber of the heart, and the vessels entering the left atrium are the **pulmonary veins** carrying freshly oxygenated blood from the lungs. The **esophagus, azygos vein,** and **descending aorta** are in the posterior mediastinum. The computed tomographic image in Fig. 4-26 shows the relationships of the superior vena cava, ascending aorta, pulmonary trunk, and left atrium.

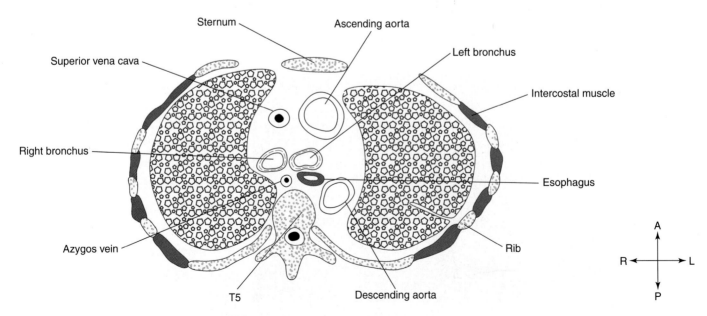

FIG. 4-21 Transverse section through the sternal angle.

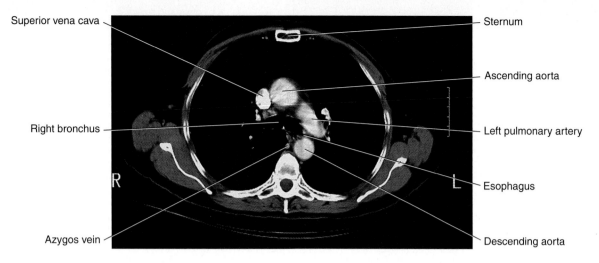

FIG. 4-22 CT image through the sternal angle.

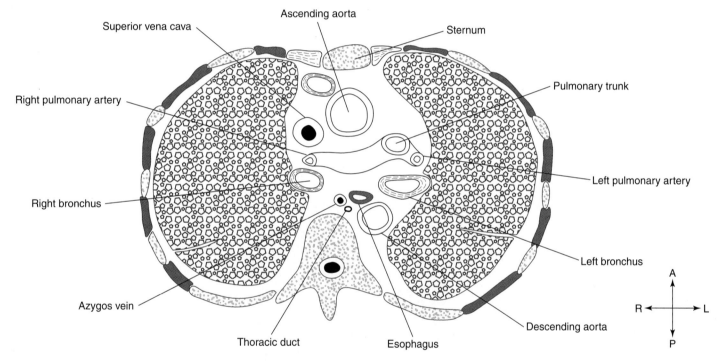

FIG. 4-23 Transverse section through the pulmonary trunk.

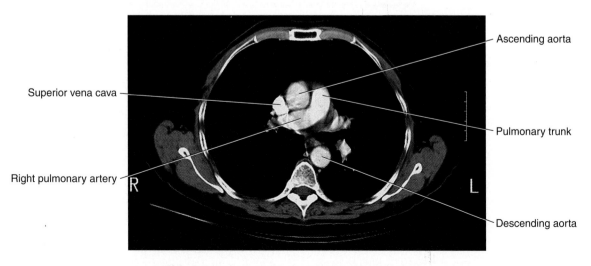

FIG. 4-24 CT image showing the right pulmonary trunk.

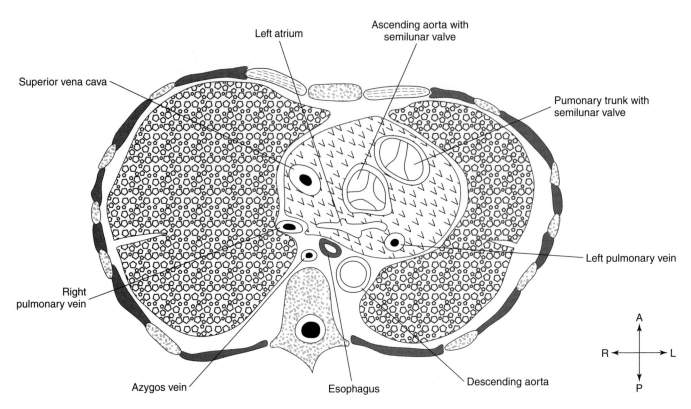

FIG. 4-25 Transverse section through the base of the heart.

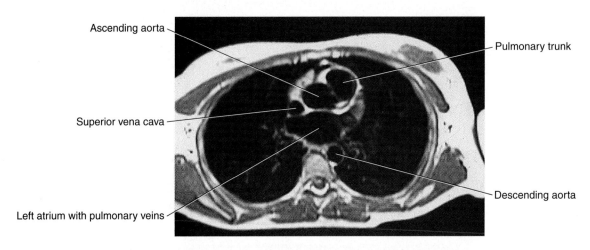

FIG. 4-26 CT image through the base of the heart.

Section Through the Chambers of the Heart

Transverse sections through the chambers of the heart show the **left atrium** to be the most posterior chamber. Posteriorly the left atrium is related to the **esophagus.** Anteriorly the left atrium is related to the centrally located aortic outflow region of the left ventricle. The **right atrium** is the most right-sided chamber. The cavity of the right atrium is anterior and perpendicular to that of the left atrium so the **interatrial septum** is in a coronal plane. The most anterior chamber is the **right ventricle,** which is immediately to the left of the right atrium. Blood flow from the right atrium through the **tricuspid valve** into the **right ventricle** is pri-

marily passive and is directed to the left and slightly anteriorly. The **bicuspid valve** between the left atrium and **left ventricle** is directed inferiorly, anteriorly, and to the left. The thick **interventricular septum** is predominately in a coronal plane. The **right coronary artery** is seen in the fat-filled sulcus between the right atrium and right ventricle. The **coronary sinus** is a venous dilation that receives blood from the coronary circulation and empties into the right atrium. It is located in the left atrioventricular sulcus along the posterior surface of the heart. These features of the heart are illustrated in Fig. 4-27 and by the computed tomographic scan and sonogram in Fig. 4-28.

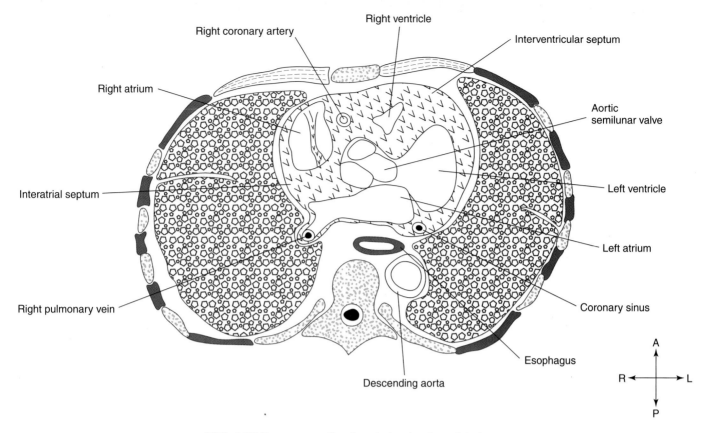

FIG. 4-27 Transverse section through the chambers of the heart.

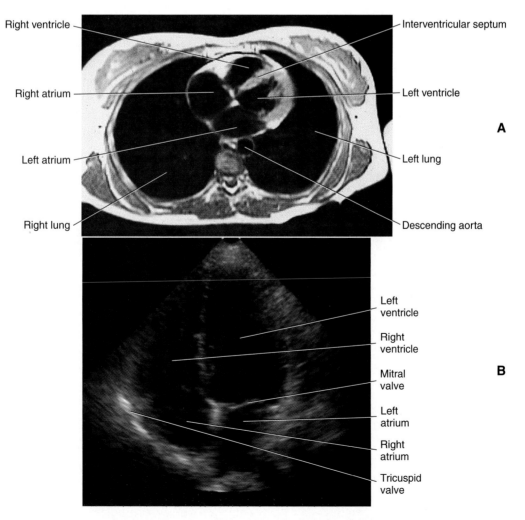

FIG. 4-28 **A,** CT image through the chambers of the heart. **B,** Sonogram of the heart.

SAGITTAL SECTIONS

Section Through the Right Lung

Sagittal sections to the right of the midline that intersect the **right lung** show the upper lobe separated from the middle lobe by a **horizontal (minor) fissure.** The middle lobe is separated from the lower lobe by an **oblique (major) fissure.** Sections in this region usually show the relationship of the **scapula** to the **infraspinatus, supraspinatus,** and **subscapularis muscles.** The infraspinatus muscle fills the fossa below the scapular spine, and the supraspinatus fills the space above the scapular spine. The subscapularis muscle is deep to the plate or body of the scapula. Anteriorly the **pectoralis major** and **minor muscles** form the thoracic wall. **Axillary vessels,** which are a continuation of the subclavian vessels, are deep to the pectoralis muscles. These features are shown in Fig. 4-29.

Section Through the Right Atrium

Since the right atrium is the most right-sided chamber of the heart, it is the first chamber seen when making serial sagittal sections from right to left. The sagittal section illustrated in Fig. 4-30 is approximately 2 cm to the right of the midline. It shows the **inferior vena cava** and **superior vena cava** draining into the cavity of the **right atrium.** A continuation of the right atrium into the pectinate region of the **right auricle** is evident. The **left atrium** is seen as a posterior chamber with a **pulmonary vein** draining into it. Just superior to the left atrium, the **right pulmonary artery** and **right main bronchus** are sectioned as they course to the right, posterior to the superior vena cava. The artery is anterior to the bronchus. This section also shows the **azygos** vein as it enters the superior vena cava. The myocardium in the anterior region of the heart is the **right ventricle.** The **right coronary artery** is in the sulcus between the right atrium and right ventricle.

Midsagittal Section

A midsagittal section through the thorax, illustrated in Fig. 4-31, usually cuts through the **aorta** as it ascends from the left ventricle. Remember that the aorta is to the right of the pulmonary trunk as they ascend from the heart. A portion of the **tricuspid valve,** between the right atrium and right ventricle, should be seen since it is near the midline or slightly to the right. It is the most inferior of the four valves of the heart and is generally at the level of the intercostal space between the fourth and fifth ribs. The sound of the tricuspid valve is heard over the right half of the inferior

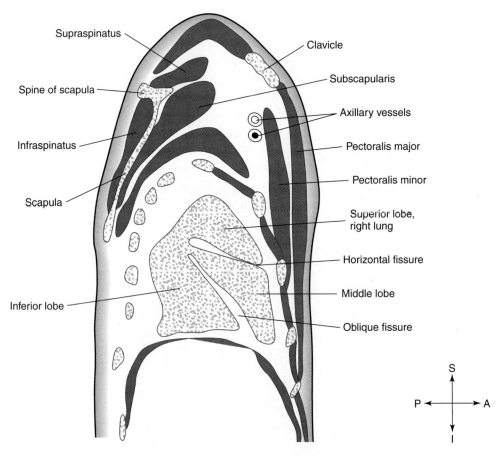

FIG. 4-29 Sagittal section through the right lung.

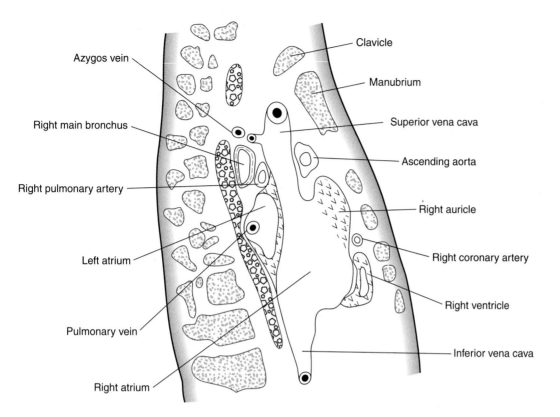

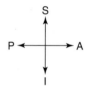

FIG. 4-30 Sagittal section through the right atrium.

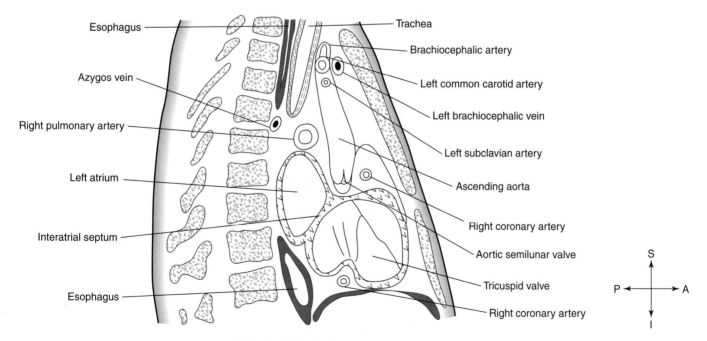

FIG. 4-31 Midsagittal section through the thorax.

portion of the body of the sternum. Near the bottom of the ascending aorta, at the level of the third intercostal space, the **aortic semilunar valve** guards the orifice between the left ventricle and aorta. The aortic valve sound is heard on the right edge of the sternum in the second intercostal space. More superiorly, where the aorta arches, are the openings for the **left subclavian, left common carotid,** and **brachiocephalic arteries.** The **left brachiocephalic vein** is cut as it courses horizontally in front of the aorta to meet its counterpart on the right side. The **right pulmonary artery** is located posterior to the aorta. Recall that the right pulmonary artery passes posterior to the aorta and superior vena cava as it goes toward the right lung.

Section Through the Pulmonary Trunk

Just to the left of midline the **pulmonary trunk** exits the **right ventricle** and curves posteriorly over the **left atrium.** This is illustrated in Fig. 4-32. Remember that the pulmonary trunk is to the left of the aorta as the vessels emerge from the heart. Since the aortic arch curves to the left, you may see a portion of the arch continuous with the **descending aorta.** The **left brachiocephalic vein** passes horizontally anterior to the pulmonary trunk and aortic arch so the vein is cut in cross section. The **left bronchus** is also cut in cross section as it courses on its path to the left lung. It is anterior

to the descending aorta and posterior to the pulmonary trunk. After the short **left coronary artery** branches from the aorta, it follows a horizontal path posterior to the pulmonary trunk. The **coronary sinus** is in the fat-filled sulcus inferior to the posteriorly located left atrium. Both the left coronary artery and coronary sinus are seen in cross section in sagittal sections to the left of median (see Fig. 4-32).

Section Through the Bicuspid Valve

Sagittal sections showing the bicuspid valve are 4 to 5 cm left of midline. These sections, illustrated in Fig. 4-33, show the **right ventricle** in an anterior position and separated from the **left ventricle** by an **interventricular septum.** Two cusps (anterior and posterior) of the **bicuspid (mitral) valve** are between the left atrium and left ventricle. Sections in this region usually show the two branches of the left coronary artery, the **anterior interventricular** (anterior descending) branch in the fat of the interventricular sulcus and the **circumflex** branch in the anterior part of the atrioventricular sulcus. The **coronary sinus** is still evident on the posterior aspect of the heart. Since this section is to the left of the pulmonary trunk, the **left pulmonary artery** is seen anterior to the descending aorta and superior to the left bronchus. The elongated but narrow left lung is divided into two lobes by the oblique fissure.

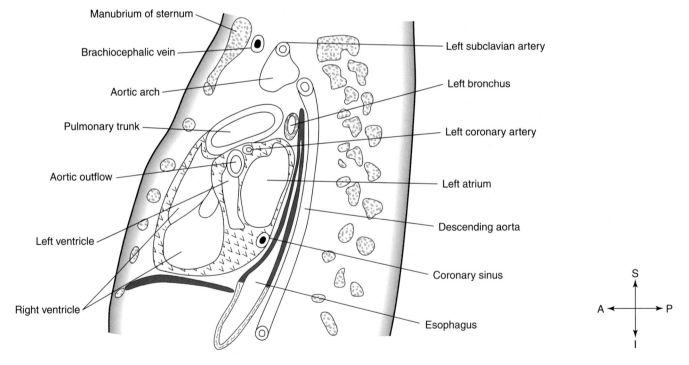

FIG. 4-32 Sagittal section through the pulmonary trunk.

CORONAL SECTIONS

The anterior-posterior relationships of the mediastinal structures evidenced in the transverse and sagittal sections should be kept in mind when studying a coronal series. Structures that have a definite anterior-posterior curvature, such as the azygos vein as it curves over the root of the lung and the aortic arch, will be cut perpendicular to their axis, as illustrated in Fig. 4-34. The posterior chamber of the heart, the left atrium, will be seen in posterior coronal sections, but the right ventricle will not be seen because it is an anterior chamber. The muscles that may be present will be discussed in a later chapter.

Section Through the Left Atrium

The **left atrium** is the most posterior chamber of the heart. It receives newly oxygenated blood from the lungs via the pulmonary veins. If the section is just right, these veins may be seen entering the left atrium, as illustrated in Fig. 4-34. Superior to the left atrium, the **trachea** descends slightly to the right of midline. In some sections through the left atrium the bifurcation of the trachea into **right** and **left main stem bronchi** may be evident. In more posterior sections the esophagus will be seen instead of the trachea. To the left of the trachea the posterior part of the **aortic arch** is evident as it is cut across its axis. The most posterior of the three aortic arch tributaries, the **left subclavian artery,** may be seen as it branches from the arch. This vessel is in close relationship to the left lung. The **left vertebral artery** branches from the left subclavian artery and ascends in the neck. The **left pulmonary artery** is inferior to the aortic arch and to the left of the trachea. In some views the right pulmonary artery may also be seen. The descending aorta is evident as it enters the abdomen through the diaphragm. The azygos vein parallels the aorta in this region. Superiorly the azygos vein arches over the root of the right lung to empty into the superior vena cava.

Section Through the Right Atrium and the Left Ventricle

Fig. 4-35 illustrates a plane through the right atrium and left ventricle. It shows the **superior vena cava** in a straight line with the **right atrium** on the right side of the heart. The superior vena cava is formed when the **right** and **left brachiocephalic veins** join. The azygos vein empties into the superior vena cava. The apex of the heart, formed by the **left ventricle,** displaces the left lung so it is narrower than the right lung. The right-to-left arrangement of the superior vena cava, ascending aorta, and pulmonary trunk is evident.

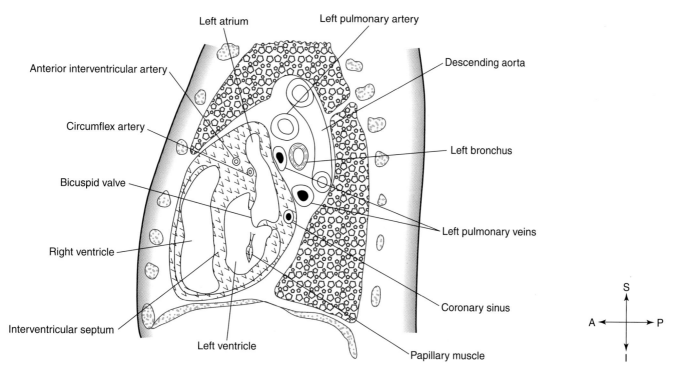

FIG. 4-33 Sagittal section through the bicuspid valve.

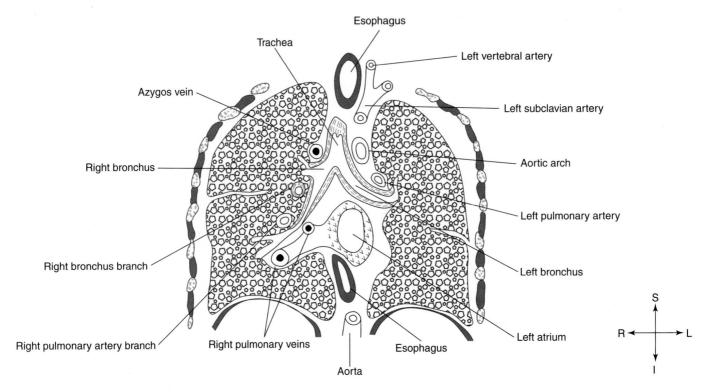

FIG. 4-34 Coronal section through the left atrium.

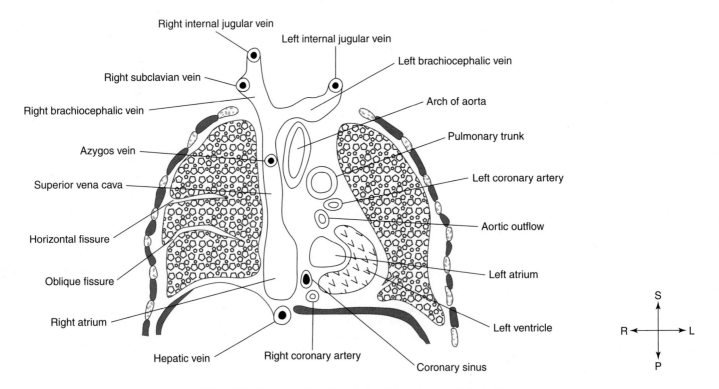

FIG. 4-35 Coronal section through the right atrium and left ventricle.

Pathology

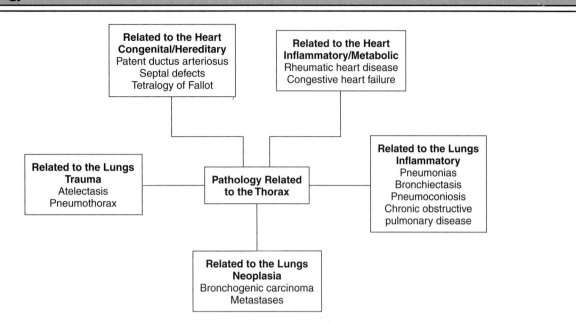

Patent Ductus Arteriosus

A patent ductus arteriosus results if the lumen of the ductus arteriosus persists after birth. The ductus arteriosus, a channel between the aorta and pulmonary trunk, is open during the prenatal period to allow most of the blood to bypass the lungs. Normally this channel closes shortly after birth. When it remains open, much of the cardiac output is diverted from the aorta to the pulmonary circulation, causing the left ventricle to work harder to maintain systemic circulation. This may result in cardiomegaly and increased vascular congestion. Symptoms may be slight and unnoticed in the infant, but as the child grows older and becomes more active, there may be evidence of dyspnea.

Septal Defects

A defect in either the interatrial or interventricular septum allows blood to pass between the chambers, usually from left to right because of the higher pressures on the left side. The more common type of septal defect is an opening in the interventricular septum, often described as a hole in the heart. The opening may be small and of little significance. Larger openings permit blood to flow from the left ventricle into the right ventricle, placing an increased load on the right ventricle with subsequent enlargement. Bacterial endocarditis also may develop around the edges of the opening. In these cases, surgical repair may be indicated.

Tetralogy of Fallot

Tetralogy of Fallot is a congenital defect of the heart that combines four structural anomalies: (1) pulmonary stenosis resulting in an obstruction to pulmonary flow; (2) ventricular septal defects, or abnormal opening between the right and left ventricles; (3) dextroposition of the aorta in which the aortic opening overrides the ventricular septum and receives blood from both the right and left ventricles; and (4) hypertrophy of the right ventricle. Infants with this condition are sometimes referred to as blue babies because of the presence of cyanosis. The cyanosis occurs because poorly oxygenated blood

from the right ventricle enters the overriding aorta and mixes with the oxygenated blood from the left ventricle. Treatment involves surgical correction whenever possible.

Rheumatic Heart Disease

Rheumatic heart disease is the most important and constant cardiac complication of rheumatic fever. It begins as endocarditis, an inflammation of the inner lining of the heart, including the membrane covering the valves. As the inflammation heals, scar tissue forms on the valves, usually the mitral (bicuspid) and aortic valves, causing damage in the form of stenosis, insufficiency, and/or incompetency. Stenosis results when the scarred valve cusps adhere to one another. If blood leaks through the valve, it is classified as insufficiency. If the valve does not close properly, allowing blood to reflux during contraction, it is classified as incompetency. These conditions usually are manifest only in the adult because it takes several years for the scarring to develop enough to alter valve function. If the condition becomes severe, the compromised valve may have to be surgically replaced with an artificial valve.

Congestive Heart Failure

Congestive heart failure is an inclusive term for conditions in which the heart is unable to pump blood at a sufficient rate and volume to maintain good blood supply to the tissues. It may be caused by any disease process that overburdens the heart, may involve either side of the heart, and may develop gradually or quickly. Left ventricular failure occurs when the left ventricle fails to pump an amount of blood equal to venous return on the right side. As a result, blood backs up in the pulmonary circulation with subsequent increased pulmonary venous pressure, and fluid leaks from the capillaries into the interstitial tissue of the lungs (pulmonary edema). In addition, there is decreased output to the systemic circulation, which decreases kidney perfusion, resulting in increased sodium and water retention and increased blood volume. Left side failure is often due to coronary artery disease, valvular disease, or hypertension. Right

Continued

Pathology—cont'd

ventricular failure occurs when the right ventricle is unable to pump an amount of blood equal to the venous return in the right atrium. As a result, there is increased venous pressure in systemic circulation as blood backs up in the superior vena cava, inferior vena cava, and systemic veins. The liver may enlarge and become tender because blood accumulates in its substance. Ascites and edema in the extremities may be evident. Common causes of right side failure include pulmonary valve stenosis and emphysema.

Atelectasis
Atelectasis is a collapsed or airless state of the lung. It is not a disease process, but is the result of an abnormal process and occurs when the lungs fail to expand properly or when there is excessive resorption of air from the alveoli. Fetal atelectasis is common in premature births when the lungs do not fully expand. In the adult, atelectasis is commonly the result of an obstruction by foreign objects or mucus, or compression of the airways by tumors, pleural effusion, or air. It may also occur as a complication following chest or abdominal surgery caused by a lack of deep breathing.

Pneumothorax
Pneumothorax is the accumulation of air in the pleural cavity. The air may come from inside the lungs, usually when a weakened area of the lung, such as an emphysematous bulla, ruptures. Air may also enter the pleural cavity from the outside as the result of a perforating wound or fractured rib. In any case, the presence of air compresses the lung and may lead to collapse (see atelectasis).

Pneumonias
Pneumonia refers to an inflammation of the lung tissue and may be caused by any irritant that results in inflammation. The most common causative agents are bacteria and viruses. Three main categories of pneumonia are recognized: lobar or bacterial pneumonia, lobular or bronchopneumonia, and interstitial or viral pneumonia. Lobar or bacterial pneumonia affects the alveoli or a segment of or an entire lobe of a lung and is usually caused by *Streptococcus pneumoniae* (pneumococcus) bacteria. The onset is rapid with cough, chest pain, blood-streaked sputum, rapid pulse and respiration, and high fever. Lobular pneumonia or bronchopneumonia, usually caused by *Streptococcus pneumoniae, Streptococcus hemolyticus,* or *Staphylococcus aureus,* begins in the bronchi and may progress into the bronchioles and alveoli. It appears in patchy areas rather than involving an entire segment or lobe. Bronchopneumonia is more common than lobar pneumonia, and the onset of symptoms is more gradual and less dramatic. Interstitial or viral pneumonia differs from the other two types because it is caused by a virus and no exudate is formed in the alveoli. It is the most common type and may occur in epidemic proportions; however, it is usually less severe than the others. Viral pneumonia also occurs as a complication of other viral diseases such as measles, influenza, and chickenpox.

Bronchiectasis
Bronchiectasis is a dilation of a weakened area in the wall of the smaller bronchi, similar to an aneurysm of an artery. The weakened area in the wall is caused by chronic inflammation.

As the bronchus dilates, it forms a sac in which infection can occur. In chronic conditions the wall of the bronchus may be destroyed and an abscess results.

Pneumoconiosis
Pneumoconiosis refers to a group of lung diseases caused by long-continued irritation by certain substances, usually industrial dusts, that results in chronic interstitial inflammation. Examples of pneumoconiosis include silicosis, caused by silica dust, anthracosis (black lung), caused by coal dust, and asbestosis, caused by asbestos dust.

Chronic Obstructive Pulmonary Disease (COPD)
Chronic obstructive pulmonary disease (COPD) is a general term for a group of conditions that result in a chronic obstruction of airflow in the bronchi. It is associated with long-term respiratory disorders such as asthma, chronic bronchitis, and emphysema. Bronchial asthma is marked by dyspnea, wheezing, and difficulty with expiration caused by spasmodic constriction of the bronchi. The attacks often are in response to allergens but may also occur as a result of emotional disturbances and bronchial infections. Chronic bronchitis produces inflammation in the bronchi with increased secretion of mucus, which interferes with airflow and causes persistent coughing and shortness of breath. It appears to be common in individuals who smoke cigarettes over a period of years. Pulmonary emphysema also is associated with long-term cigarette smoking and often exists concurrently with chronic bronchitis, although it is anatomically different. Emphysema is characterized by a destruction of the alveolar walls to create large saccules, some of which may resemble large balloons called bullae (see pneumothorax). As the alveolar walls deteriorate and coalesce, the lungs become less efficient and gaseous exchange between alveoli and pulmonary capillaries is compromised. The individual may develop an enlarged or barrel chest, and cardiac complications eventually occur.

Bronchogenic Carcinoma
Bronchogenic carcinoma is the most common fatal primary malignancy in the United States. Statistical evidence indicates that the degree of risk for developing bronchogenic carcinoma is directly proportional to the number of cigarettes smoked. The tumors arise in the major bronchi and metastasize by way of the lymph nodes and bloodstream. One of the devastating features of lung cancer is the formation of metastases to the lymph nodes, liver, brain, bone marrow, and adrenal gland. Often the first indication of lung cancer is a dysfunction caused by a secondary tumor outside the lungs. The symptoms of bronchogenic carcinoma are due to obstruction of the airways and metastases.

Metastases
It is important to remember that not all tumors in the lungs are primary tumors (bronchogenic carcinoma). Many primary malignancies in other organs develop metastases in the lungs. These secondary lung tumors often arise from the breast, kidneys, and colon. By the time these tumors are identified, it is often too late for therapeutic measures to be of benefit.

· REVIEW QUESTIONS ·

1. What bones form the thoracic cage?
2. Where is the sternal angle relative to the jugular notch?
3. What marks the anterior boundary of the inferior thoracic aperture?
4. What are the three muscles that form thoracic boundaries?
5. Numerous muscles are evident in transverse sections through the thorax. (a) name four muscles in the pectoral region; (b) name two superficial back muscles; (C) name four deep back muscles; and (f) name six muscles in the scapular region.
6. Name five nerves that emerge from the brachial plexus.
7. What is the effect of estrogen, progesterone, prolactin, and oxytocin on the female breast?
8. Where is the pleural cavity (pleural space) located?
9. Indicate whether each of the following is a feature of the right lung or a feature of the left lung:
   a. Cardiac notch
   b. Three lobes
   c. Horizontal fissure
   d. Larger volume
   e. Narrow and longer
10. Identify the specific portion of the mediastinum that contains each of the following:
    a. Brachiocephalic veins
    b. Superior vena cava
    c. Descending thoracic aorta
    d. Heart
    e. Esophagus
11. Identify the chamber of the heart described by each of the following:
    a. Posterior chamber
    b. Pectinate muscle
    c. Chamber on the right side
    d. Receives oxygenated blood through pulmonary veins
    e. Most anterior chamber
    f. Forms the apex of the heart
    g. Has the thickest wall
    h. Blood passes through the aortic semilunar valve when it leaves this chamber
    i. Blood passes through the tricuspid valve to enter this chamber
    j. Receives blood from the superior vena cava
12. Where do the right and left coronary arteries originate?
13. List in sequence, from fastest to slowest, the components of the conduction system of the heart.
14. What are the three branches of the aortic arch?
15. List in sequence, from right to left, the three large vessels at the base of the heart.
16. What is the function of the azygous vein?

· CHAPTER QUIZ ·

Name the Following:

1. The junction between the manubrium and body of the sternum
2. The anterior boundary of the inferior thoracic aperture
3. The layer of the heart wall that contains cardiac muscle
4. The two major branches of the left coronary artery
5. The most posterior chamber of the heart
6. The pacemaker of the heart
7. The nerve plexus that supplies innervation to the arm
8. The muscles between the ribs
9. The blood vessels that return oxygenated blood from the lungs to the left atrium
10. The most posterior branch of the aortic arch

True/False:

1. The left lung is longer and narrower than the right lung, and it is divided into three lobes.
2. The middle mediastinum is a subdivision of the inferior mediastinum, and it contains the heart.
3. The parietal layer of serous pericardium lines the fibrous pericardium of the pericardial sac.
4. The right ventricle makes up most of the right border of the heart.
5. The pulmonary semilunar valve is on the left side of the sternum at the level of the third costal cartilage.
6. The most posterior chamber of the heart is the left atrium, which receives oxygenated blood from the pulmonary arteries.
7. The vessel that passes horizontally, posterior to the aorta and the superior vena cava, is the right pulmonary artery.
8. The ascending aorta is to the right of the pulmonary trunk.
9. The left bronchus is posterior to the esophagus.
10. The azygos vein drains into the superior vena cava.

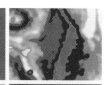
OBJECTIVES

Upon completion of this chapter, the student should be able to do the following:

- State the boundaries of the abdomen.
- Define the transpyloric, subcostal, transumbilical, interiliac median, and midclavicular planes and then use these planes to divide the abdomen into four quadrants and nine regions.
- Describe the features of lumbar vertebrae.
- Describe the structure of the diaphragm, name and give the vertebral levels of the three major openings in the diaphragm, and identify the structures that pass through each opening.
- Name the four muscles that form the anterolateral abdominal wall and the three muscles associated with the posterior abdominal wall.
- Discuss the topography of the posterior abdominal wall and the effect this has on organ position and fluid accumulation.
- State the level of origin of the visceral branches of the abdominal aorta and identify the regions each one supplies.
- Identify and trace the pathway of the tributaries of the inferior vena cava.
- Trace the pathway of blood through the hepatic portal system of veins.
- Discuss the peritoneum and its extensions, including mesentery, omenta, ligaments, and cul-de-sacs.
- Discuss the structure and relationships of the liver, including its lobar subdivisions and blood supply.
- Discuss the visceral relationships of the gallbladder.
- Describe the external features of the stomach, its peritoneal extensions, its relationships, and its blood supply.

- Name the regions of the small intestine and discuss the relationships of each region.
- Identify the regions of the large intestine and discuss the relationships of each region.
- Describe the location of the spleen and its relationship to other organs.
- Discuss the location and relationships of the head, neck, body, and tail of the pancreas.
- Describe the location and relationships of the kidneys, ureters, and suprarenal glands.
- Identify the abdominal viscera, muscles, and blood vessels on transverse, sagittal, and coronal sections.

General Anatomy of the Abdomen

SURFACE MARKINGS

The ventral body cavity is divided into two distinct subdivisions that are separated by the dome-shaped diaphragm. This is illustrated in Figure 5-1. The upper portion, superior to the diaphragm, is the thoracic cavity. The lower portion, inferior to the diaphragm, is the abdominopelvic cavity. For the sake of convenience, the large abdominopelvic cavity may be divided into an upper abdominal cavity and a lower pelvic cavity. This is an artificial division since there is no partition between the two cavities and some structures may move from one region to the other.

Boundaries

The **abdominal cavity,** the upper portion of the abdominopelvic cavity, is the largest cavity in the body. It extends from the **diaphragm** above to the **superior pelvic aperture** below. Because the dome of the diaphragm extends superiorly under the ribs to the level of the fifth intercostal space, the contents of the superior portion of the abdominal cavity are protected by the thoracic cage. Portions of the liver, stomach, and spleen are in this region. Inferiorly, the large wings, or **alae,** of the iliac bones offer some protection for the soft tissue. The superior peripheral boundaries are the **xiphoid process** of the sternum and the sloping **costal cartilages** of the false ribs. The inferior peripheral margins of the cavity are the **iliac crest, inguinal ligament,** and **symphysis pubis.** The iliac crest is the highest portion, or margin, of the ilium bone, and it terminates anteriorly in the anterior superior iliac spine. The inguinal ligament is the folded inferior margin of the broad, flat tendon, or **aponeurosis,** of the external oblique muscle. This ligament extends from the anterior superior iliac spine to the pubic tubercle, a small elevation about 2 cm lateral to the pubic symphysis. Just superior to the pubic tubercle, there is an opening in the aponeurosis to form the inguinal canal.

Umbilicus

The most obvious surface marking on the anterior abdominal wall is the **umbilicus,** or naval. The umbilicus is the scar that results from the closure of the umbilical cord shortly after birth. It represents the site of attachment of the umbilical cord in the fetus. The position of the umbilicus varies depending on such factors as muscle tone, obesity, body build, and age. In general, however, it is located at the level of the intervertebral disc between the third and fourth lumbar vertebrae.

Linea Alba

When the skin of the abdomen is removed, a light colored line that extends from the xiphoid process to the symphysis pubis is evident. This is the **linea alba,** and its position is indicated on the surface by a shallow groove in the midline. The linea alba is formed by the fusion of the sheets of tendon that extend from the anterolateral muscles of the abdominal wall.

Abdominal Planes

Superficial landmarks are used to identify the various abdominal planes that are used as indicators of vertebral levels and to describe the location of deeper structures. Vertical and horizontal planes divide the abdomen into regions that are used to describe the location of organs or, in the clinical setting, the location of pain, tenderness, swelling, or abnor-

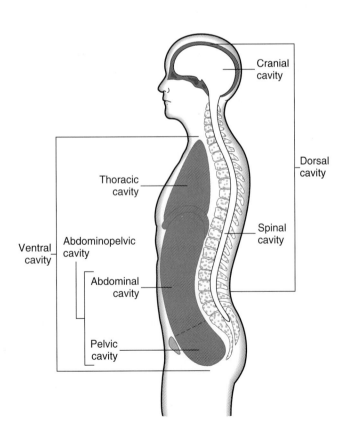

FIG. 5-1 Divisions of the ventral body cavity.

mal growths. Five horizontal and three vertical planes will be described. These planes are summarized in Table 5-1.

Vertical Planes. The **right midclavicular plane** extends vertically from the midpoint of the right clavicle to the midpoint of a line joining the right anterior superior iliac spine and symphysis pubis, or midinguinal point. The **left midclavicular plane** is in the same position as the right midclavicular plane except that it is on the left side. It extends from the midpoint of the left clavicle to the left midinguinal point. The **midsagittal plane,** or **median plane,** is a vertical plane through the umbilicus. It divides the body into right and left halves. These planes are illustrated in Fig. 5-2.

Horizontal Planes. The **transpyloric plane** is the most superior of the horizontal planes. It is located about halfway between the jugular notch and the symphysis pubis or, more simply, midway between the xiphoid and umbilicus. This plane typically intersects the **pyloric region of the stomach,** which accounts for the name. Passing laterally to the right on this plane gives the location of the **first part of**

the **duodenum** and the **top of the head of the pancreas.** Proceeding farther to the right, this plane intersects the **ninth costal cartilage,** which gives the location of the **fundus of the gallbladder** and then the upper portion of the hilus of the **right kidney.** Going to the left of the midline, the transpyloric plane gives the location of the **neck of the pancreas** and middle portion of the **hilar region of the left kidney.** Usually this plane marks the level of the **first lumbar vertebra.**

A line through the most inferior point of the rib cage gives the position of the **subcostal plane,** which marks the level of the **third lumbar vertebra.** The subcostal plane intersects the **third part of the duodenum** and **lower border of the pancreatic head.** There is no good method of locating the L2 vertebral level except that it is halfway between the transpyloric and subcostal planes.

The **transumbilical plane** passes horizontally through the umbilicus. In individuals with relatively normal abdominal contour, this marks the level of the intervertebral disc between the third and fourth lumbar vertebrae. The **interiliac plane** passes through the most superior point of the iliac crests. This plane marks the level of the **fourth**

TABLE 5-1 *Horizontal and Vertical Abdominal Planes*

Plane	Description	Vertebral Level
Transpyloric	Horizontal plane halfway between the xiphoid and the umbilicus	Indicates vertebral level L1
Subcostal	Horizontal plane through the most inferior point of the rib cage	Indicates vertebral level L3
Transumbilical	Horizontal plane through the umbilicus	Indicates the disc between L3 and L4
Interiliac	Horizontal plane between the highest points of the iliac crests	Indicates vertebral level L4
Transtubercular	Horizontal plane between the tubercles of the iliac crests	Indicates vertebral level L5
Midclavicular	Vertical plane from the midpoint of the clavicle to the midpoint of the inguinal ligament; right and left	
Median	Vertical plane through the umbilicus; divides body into right and left halves	

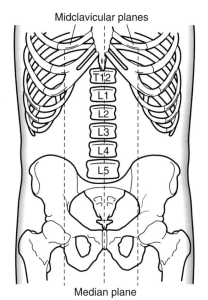

Midclavicular planes

Median plane

FIG. 5-2 Vertical planes of the abdominal cavity.

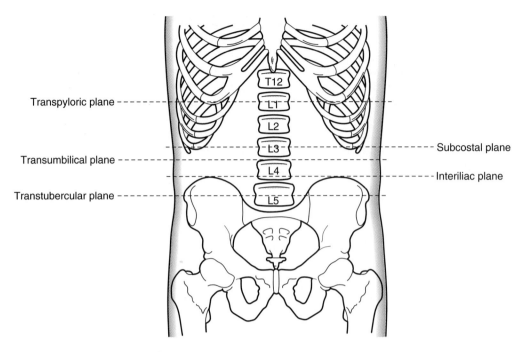

FIG. 5-3 Horizontal planes of the abdominal cavity.

lumbar vertebra. The **transtubercular plane** passes through the tubercules of the iliac crests. The tubercles are small projections on the crests about 5 cm posterior to the anterior superior iliac spine. This plane marks the level of the **fifth lumbar vertebra.** The horizontal planes are illustrated in Fig. 5-3.

Abdominal Quadrants and Regions

Abdominal Quadrants. The horizontal transumbilical plane and the vertical median plane divide the abdomen into four quadrants for descriptive purposes. For example, the pain of acute appendicitis usually localizes in the lower right quadrant. See Fig. 1-4 for an illustration of the four abdominopelvic quadrants.

Abdominal Regions. Nine abdominal regions are described using the horizontal subcostal and transtubercular planes and the vertical right and left midclavicular planes. On the right and left sides the regions are, from superior to inferior, **hypochondriac, lumbar** or **lateral,** and **iliac** or **inguinal.** The three regions in the midline are, from superior to inferior, the **epigastric, umbilical,** and **hypogastric.** See Fig. 1-5 for an illustration of the nine abdominopelvic regions.

OSSEOUS COMPONENTS

The only osseous components of the abdomen are the lumbar vertebrae in the posterior wall. Some abdominal organs extend upward under the thoracic cage but the components of the thoracic cage are not considered part of the abdomen.

Five large lumbar vertebrae with their intervertebral discs form the skeletal support for the posterior abdominal wall.

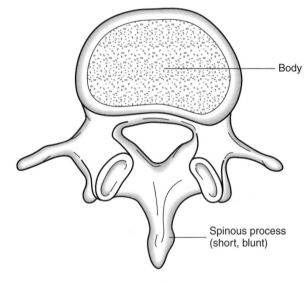

FIG. 5-4 Lumbar vertebra.

Lumbar vertebrae, illustrated in Fig. 5-4, have large bodies with short, thick, blunt spinous processes. The transverse processes are also thicker than in other vertebrae. The shape of the vertebrae and discs gives a normal lumbar curvature that is convex anteriorly. This curvature develops during the second year as a child begins to walk and puts increased weight on the lumbar region. An exaggeration or increase in the convex curvature is called **lordosis.**

The spinal cord within the vertebral foramen ends at the level of the third lumbar vertebra at birth. Due to the different growth rates of the cord and vertebral column, the spinal cord ends at the level of the **second lumbar vertebra** in the adult. Even though the spinal cord ends at L2, the meninges, subarachnoid space, and cerebrospinal fluid continue to the second sacral vertebra. This is of clinical importance when doing a spinal tap to remove cerebrospinal fluid for laboratory examination. The needle is inserted between the third and fourth lumbar vertebrae, or sometimes between the fourth and fifth lumbar vertebrae, to remove the fluid from the subarachnoid space. This minimizes the possibility of damage to the spinal cord. Remember that the location of L4 is determined by the interiliac plane, through the superior points of the iliac crests.

Muscular Components

The muscular components of the abdomen include the diaphram, the muscles of the anterolateral wall, and the muscles of the posterior wall. The musculotendinous diaphram forms a movable partition between the thoracic and abdominal cavities. The anterolateral abodominal wall is formed by four muscles and their aponeuroses. The posterior abdominal wall is formed primarily by two pairs of muscles and their attachments to the vertebrae, ribs, and ilium.

Diaphragm

The musculotendinous diaphragm extends superiorly under the rib cage to the level of the fifth intercostal space when the individual is supine. Because of the large right lobe of the liver, the diaphragm usually rises to a slightly higher level on the right side than on the left. The central portion of the diaphragm consists of tendinous fibers that form a strong **central tendon.** All the muscular fibers of the diaphragm converge and insert on the central tendon. The muscular portion of the diaphragm is divided into three regions according to the origin of its fibers. A short and narrow **sternal portion** arises from the back of the xiphoid process. The extensive **costal portion** originates from the inner surface of the lower six costal cartilages. These costal muscular fibers form the two domes or **hemidiaphragms.** The **vertebral or lumbar portion** arises from the upper lumbar vertebrae as a pair of **muscular crura.** Each crus is a thick, fleshy muscular bundle that tapers inferiorly and becomes tendinous. Fibers from each crus spread out and ascend to attach to the central tendon. The right crus encircles the esophagus.

Since structures passing from the thoracic cavity into the abdominal cavity must penetrate the diaphragm, its continuity is interrupted by three large and several small apertures. Each opening is called a hiatus. At the level of the eighth thoracic vertebra, the wide **caval hiatus** for the inferior vena cava is located within the central tendon about 3 cm to the right of the median plane. Not only is the caval hiatus the most superior of the three openings, it is also the most anterior. In addition to the inferior vena cava, this opening transmits the right phrenic nerve and lymph ves-

sels. Occasionally, the right hepatic vein passes through this opening before it enters the inferior vena cava.

The oval **esophageal hiatus,** at the level of the tenth thoracic vertebra, is an opening in the muscular diaphragm posterior to the central tendon. It is 2 or 3 cm to the left of the midline and is surrounded by the right crus of the diaphragm. In addition to the esophagus, the esophageal hiatus transmits the the vagus nerve and esophageal branches of the left gastric blood vessels.

The long, oblique **aortic hiatus** is located between the right and left crura of the diaphragm and begins at the level of the twelfth thoracic vertebra. The aortic hiatus is the most posterior of the three large openings in the diaphragm. Technically the aorta does not penetrate the diaphragm. Instead it passes between the crura slightly to the left of midline. In addition to the aorta, this opening transmits the azygos vein and thoracic duct.

Muscles of the Anterolateral Abdominal Wall

The anterior and lateral abdominal wall consists of four muscles and their aponeuroses with a covering of fascia and skin. The muscles, illustrated in Fig. 5-5 and by the computed tomography image in Fig. 5-6, are the rectus abdominis, the external oblique, the internal oblique, and the transverse abdominis. The skin and muscles of the anterior and lateral abdominal wall are innervated by intercostal nerves.

Anteriorly, on each side of the linea alba, the long, vertical **rectus abdominis** muscles extend the length of the abdominal wall from the symphysis pubis to the xiphoid process. The rectus abdominis is enclosed in a rectus sheath formed by the aponeuroses of the three lateral muscles.

The outermost layer of the lateral muscles is formed by the **external oblique.** Fibers of this muscle originate from the ribs and extend downward and medially. Most of the fibers terminate in a broad aponeurosis that inserts on the linea alba, iliac crest, and pubic tubercle. The inferior margin of this aponeurosis forms the inguinal ligament.

In contrast to the external oblique, the fibers of the **internal oblique** extend upward and medially, perpendicular to the external oblique, from the iliac crest to the inferior borders of the ribs. Medially the aponeurosis of the internal oblique splits into two layers to enclose the rectus abdominis.

The **transverse abdominis** is the innermost of the three flat muscles. These fibers pass in a transverse or horizontal direction. This arrangement of the three flat muscles provides maximum support for the abdominal viscera and diminishes the risk of tearing the muscles.

Muscles of the Posterior Abdominal Wall

Two pairs of muscles and their attachments to the vertebrae, ribs, and ilium form the musculature of the posterior abdominal wall. The long, thick **psoas major muscle** is lateral

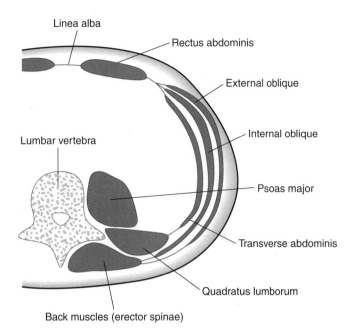

FIG. 5-5 Muscles of the abdominal wall.

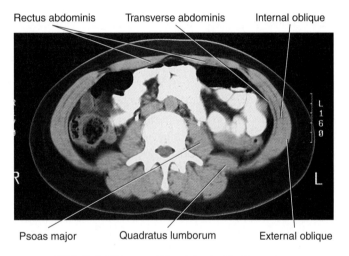

FIG. 5-6 CT image of the abdominal wall muscles.

to the lumbar region of the vertebral column. Its fibers originate on the transverse processes, borders, and intervertebral discs of the lumbar vertebrae, pass along the brim of the pelvis, and enter the thigh to insert on the lesser trochanter of the femur. In transverse sections the psoas muscles appear as large muscular masses adjacent to the lumbar vertebral bodies. The psoas muscles are innervated by branches of the lumbar nerves.

The second muscle associated with the posterior abdominal wall is the **quadratus lumborum.** This thick muscular sheet originates on the iliac crest and transverse processes of the lower lumbar vertebrae and ascends to insert on the transverse processes of the upper lumbar vertebrae and twelfth rib. It is innervated by branches of the lumbar nerves. In transverse sections this muscle appears lateral and posterior to the psoas muscle. The arrangement of the pos-

terior wall muscles is illustrated in Fig. 5-5 and in the computed tomographic image in Fig. 5-6.

The **iliacus muscle** is a large, triangular sheet of muscle in the iliac fossa on the medial side of the alae, or wings, of the ilium. It originates in the iliac fossa and inserts with the psoas major on the lesser trochanter. This muscle is a part of the posterior abdominopelvic wall but does not appear in sections of the abdomen. It is located in the false pelvis and is evident in pelvic sections. The iliacus and psoas muscles are closely associated, and together they often are referred to as the **iliopsoas.** The iliopsoas is the most powerful flexor of the thigh.

An examination of the posterior abdominal wall reveals a single longitudinal ridge and two oblique ridges. The **longitudinal ridge line,** sometimes called the longitudinal divide, is especially evident in transverse sections (see Figs. 5-5 and 5-6). It is formed by the **lumbar vertebrae,** the **normal lumbar lordosis,** the **psoas major muscles,** the **inferior vena cava,** and the **aorta.** On either side of the elevated longitudinal ridge there is a paravertebral groove, or gutter. In superior regions of the abdomen, this groove is occupied by the liver on the right side and the spleen on the left side. The kidneys, ureters, and portions of the colon also are located in the paravertebral grooves. Whenever an organ crosses the midline, it is moved anteriorly because of the elevation of this longitudinal ridge. For example, the right lobe of the liver is rather posterior in position, whereas the left lobe is more anterior because it is moved forward by the longitudinal ridge. The pancreas offers another example of this anterior displacement. The tail of the pancreas is in a relatively posterior position, near the spleen. As the gland courses to the right, it is pushed forward by the longitudinal ridge so that the head and neck are more anteriorly situated.

Inferiorly, the longitudinal ridge divides to form two **oblique ridges** that mark the location of the pelvic inlet. These oblique ridges are formed by the **bony pelvic inlet,** the **psoas major muscles,** and the **iliac blood vessels.**

In addition to influencing organ position, the longitudinal and oblique ridges, to some extent, determine regions of fluid accumulation. Fluids will tend to flow off the sides of the longitudinal ridges to accumulate in the paravertebral "valleys" or grooves. The paravertebral grooves slope posteriorly from the oblique ridges so that fluids tend to flow down the abdominal portions of the oblique ridges and accumulate in the superior regions of the paravertebral grooves when the patient is supine.

VASCULAR COMPONENTS

Vasculature of the Abdominal Wall

The principal arterial supply of the anterolateral abdominal wall comes from branches of the internal thoracic arteries and the parietal branches of the abdominal aorta. In addition to these, branches of the intercostal and subcostal arteries contribute to the arterial supply at higher levels. All of these vessels branch and anastomose freely. Venous

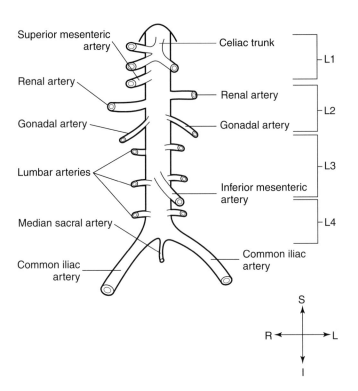

FIG. 5-7 Abdominal aorta and its branches.

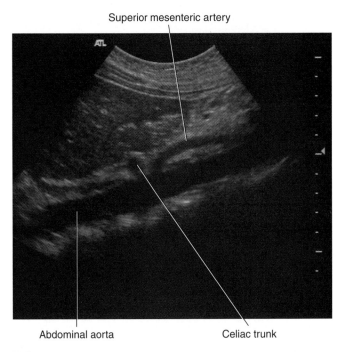

FIG. 5-8 Sonogram of the celiac trunk and superior mesenteric artery.

drainage is accomplished primarily through branches of the superficial epigastric and lateral thoracic veins. The posterior abdominal wall is supplied and drained by lumbar arteries and veins. These are direct tributaries of the aorta and inferior vena cava, respectively. Azygos veins also contribute to the venous drainage of the abdominal wall.

Abdominal Aorta and Its Branches

The abdominal aorta begins about 2.5 cm above the transpyloric lines at the aortic hiatus in the diaphragm. At this level it is usually slightly left of midline, but as the aorta descends, it assumes a more midline position. At the L4 vertebral level, marked by the interiliac line, the aorta bifurcates into the right and left common iliac arteries. The branches of the abdominal aorta may be divided into four groups: unpaired visceral, paired visceral, unpaired parietal, and paired parietal. The visceral branches supply the viscera or organs of the abdominal cavity, whereas the parietal branches supply the abdominal wall. The branches of the abdominal aorta are illustrated in Fig. 5-7.

Unpaired Visceral Branches. The unpaired visceral branches of the abdominal aorta are the celiac, the superior mesenteric artery (SMA), and the inferior mesenteric artery. The **celiac trunk** (artery) is the first major branch of the abdominal aorta. It arises from the ventral surface of the aorta just above the transpyloric line, near the upper margin of the first lumbar vertebra. The celiac trunk is only 1 to 2 cm in length before it divides into the **left gastric, hepatic,** and **splenic arteries.** The **left gastric artery,** the

smallest branch of the celiac, passes to the left to supply the cardiac region of the stomach and then descends along the lesser curvature. Its branches anastomose with those of the right gastric artery, a branch of the hepatic artery. Intermediate in size, the **common hepatic artery** is directed to the right and enters the porta of the liver, where it divides into right and left branches. During its course, the common hepatic artery gives off the **right gastric, gastroduodenal,** and **cystic arteries.** The third and largest branch of the celiac is the **splenic artery.** This long, tortuous vessel passes horizontally to the left, behind the stomach and along the upper border of the pancreas, to enter the hilus of the spleen. As it passes along the upper border of the pancreas, the splenic artery gives off numerous **pancreatic branches.**

The second unpaired visceral branch of the aorta is the **superior mesenteric artery** (SMA). This vessel arises just below the transpyloric line at the level of the lower border of the first lumbar vertebra. The superior mesenteric artery branches and anastomoses freely to supply all of the small intestine except for the duodenum. In addition, it supplies the cecum, ascending colon, and most of the transverse colon. At its origin the superior mesenteric artery is separated from the aorta by the left renal vein. The splenic vein and body of the pancreas are anterior to the superior mesenteric artery. The sonogram in Fig. 5-8 shows the celiac trunk and superior mesenteric artery as they branch from the aorta.

The third unpaired visceral vessel arising from the aorta is the **inferior mesenteric artery.** This branch originates from the ventral surface of the abdominal aorta at the L3 vertebral level marked by the subcostal plane. Near its origin the inferior mesenteric artery descends anterior to the aorta, then it curves to the left to supply the distal portion of the transverse colon and all of the descending colon, sigmoid colon, and rectum.

Paired Visceral Branches.   The paired visceral branches of the aorta are the suprarenal, renal, and gonadal arteries. The small suprarenal arteries arise from the aorta, one vessel on each side, at the level of the superior mesenteric artery. The suprarenal arteries course laterally and slightly superiorly to supply the suprarenal (adrenal) gland.

A large renal artery arises from each side of the aorta at the upper L2 vertebral level, just inferior to the superior mesenteric artery. Each vessel passes laterally at right angles to the aorta and enters the hilus of the kidney on that side. Since the aorta is slightly left of midline, the right renal artery is longer than the left. As it proceeds to the right kidney, the right renal artery passes posterior to the inferior vena cava, the right renal vein, the head of pancreas, and the second, or descending, part of the duodenum. The right renal artery is usually at a slightly lower level than the left renal artery because the right kidney is generally displaced downward by the liver and is at a lower level than the left kidney. As it passes to the kidney, the left renal artery lies posterior to the body of the pancreas, the left renal vein, and the splenic vein. One or two accessory renal arteries may be present. These usually arise directly from the aorta.

The paired visceral gonadal vessels, testicular arteries in the male and ovarian arteries in the female, branch from the aorta just inferior to the renal vessels. This places their origin in the lower margin of the second lumbar vertebra. Each testicular artery descends along the psoas muscle and passes over the ureters and the lower part of the external iliac artery to reach the deep inguinal ring, where it enters the spermatic cord. Along with the other contents of the spermatic cord, the testicular artery enters the scrotum to supply the testes. In the female the ovarian arteries descend along the psoas muscle to the pelvic brim. Here they cross over the external iliac vessels to enter the pelvic cavity, where they continue in the suspensory ligament to supply the ovary.

Unpaired Parietal Branch.   The unpaired parietal branch of the abdominal aorta is the **middle sacral artery.** This vessel arises from the posterior surface of the aorta, just proximal to the aortic bifurcation. As it descends along the anterior surface of the L4 and L5 vertebrae, the middle sacral artery gives off a pair of lumbar arteries, which supply a portion of the posterior abdominal wall.

Paired Parietal Branches.   Four pairs of **lumbar arteries** constitute the paired branches of the aorta. These vessels arise from the posterolateral surface of the aorta along the upper four lumbar vertebrae. Lumbar arteries supply the posterolateral abdominal wall.

Bifurcation of the Aorta.   At the L4 vertebral level the aorta divides into the **right** and **left common iliac arteries,** which diverge along the bodies of the fourth and fifth lumbar vertebrae. At the level of the disc between the fifth lumbar vertebra and sacrum, each common iliac artery divides into internal and external branches. The **internal iliac artery** supplies the wall and viscera of the pelvis, perineum, and gluteal region. The **external iliac artery** supplies the lower limb.

Inferior Vena Cava and Veins of the Abdomen

Anterior to the fifth lumbar vertebra the right and left common iliac veins join to form the inferior vena cava (IVC), which is the largest vein in the body. The inferior vena cava receives tributaries as it ascends through the abdomen along the vertebral column. After passing along the posterior surface of the liver, the inferior vena cava passes through the caval hiatus of the diaphragm at the T8 vertebral level. In the mediastinum it penetrates the pericardium to drain into the lower part of the right atrium. There are no valves in the inferior vena cava, but there is a rudimentary semilunar valve at its atrial orifice.

In general the inferior vena cava is slightly to the right of the aorta. Near its origin at the L5 vertebral level, the inferior vena cava is posterior to the aorta, but as it ascends, it becomes more anterior so that in superior regions of the abdomen, it is anterior to the aorta. As the inferior vena cava ascends the abdomen, it is anterior to the right psoas muscle, the right renal artery, the right suprarenal gland, and the right crus of the diaphragm. The inferior vena cava is retroperitoneal and is posterior to the superior mesenteric vessels, the head of the pancreas, and the horizontal third part of the duodenum. Tributaries of the inferior vena cava include the common iliac, lumbar, right gonadal, renal, right suprarenal, inferior phrenic, and hepatic veins.

Common Iliac Veins.   Anterior to the sacroiliac joint, the external and internal iliac veins join to form a common iliac vein. The right and left common iliac veins drain the same regions that are supplied by the arteries of the same name. The common iliac veins pass obliquely upward from the sacroiliac joint to the fifth lumbar vertebra, where they join to form the inferior vena cava.

Lumbar Veins.   The lumbar veins consist of four or five pairs of vessels that collect blood from the muscles and skin of the abdominal wall. The arrangement of these veins varies. Some drain directly into the inferior vena cava, whereas others may enter the azygos system.

Gonadal Veins.   The testicular veins in the male begin on the dorsal side of the testes and ascend in the spermatic cord to enter the abdomen. In the abdominal cavity the veins ascend retroperitoneally along the psoas muscle and anterior to the ureter. On the right side the testicular vein

Superior mesenteric vein   Superior mesenteric artery

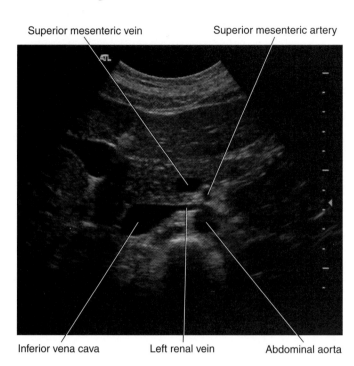

Inferior vena cava   Left renal vein   Abdominal aorta

FIG. 5-9 Sonogram showing relationship of the left renal vein to the superior mesenteric artery and the aorta.

Middle hepatic vein   Left hepatic vein

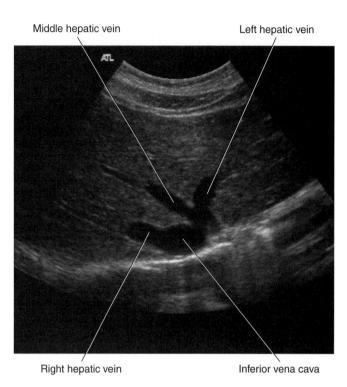

Right hepatic vein   Inferior vena cava

FIG. 5-10 Sonogram showing the right, left, and middle hepatic veins near their entry into the inferior vena cava.

opens directly into the inferior vena cava. On the left side it opens into the left renal vein. The ovarian veins in the female follow the same pattern as the testicular veins in the male, except they begin at the ovaries.

Renal Veins.   The renal veins drain the kidneys and empty into the inferior vena cava at the L2 vertebral level. They are usually anterior to the renal arteries because the inferior vena cava is anterior to the aorta at this level. Since the inferior vena cava is to the right side of midline, the left renal vein is considerably longer than the right. The left renal vein passes posterior to the splenic vein and body of the pancreas. It crosses in front of (anterior to) the aorta, just below the origin of the superior mesenteric artery so that the left renal vein is posterior to the superior mesenteric artery but anterior to the aorta. The sonogram in Fig. 5-9 shows the relationship of the left renal vein to the superior mesenteric artery and the aorta. The left renal vein receives the left gonadal (testicular or ovarian) vein from below and the left suprarenal vein from above before it enters the inferior vena cava. The right renal vein is slightly more inferior than the left because the right kidney is lower than the left kidney in position. The right renal vein passes posterior to the second or descending part of the duodenum.

Suprarenal Veins.   The right suprarenal vein is a short vessel emerging from the right suprarenal gland and emptying directly into the posterior aspect of the inferior vena cava. The left suprarenal vein is usually longer and drains

into the left renal vein. There is considerable variation in the arrangement of the suprarenal veins.

Inferior Phrenic Veins.   These veins drain blood from the inferior or abdominal surface of the diaphragm. The left inferior phrenic usually joins the left suprarenal vein, but the right inferior phrenic generally drains directly into the inferior vena cava.

Hepatic Veins.   The **hepatic veins** drain blood from the liver and return it to the inferior vena cava. The **central veins** of the liver lobules collect blood from the **intralobular venous sinusoids.** The central veins merge to form the hepatic veins, which exit from the posterior surface of the liver and empty immediately into the inferior vena cava. Sometimes the right hepatic vein passes through the caval hiatus before entering the inferior vena cava. The sonogram in Fig. 5-10 shows the right, left and middle hepatic veins as they drain into the inferior vena cava.

Hepatic Portal System.   Blood from the digestive system is carried to the liver by a hepatic portal system of veins before it enters the inferior vena cava. Blood from the inferior mesenteric vein, superior mesenteric vein, and splenic vein enters the hepatic portal vein as illustrated in Fig. 5-11. In the liver the hepatic portal vein branches until it ends in small capillary-like spaces, called sinusoids, within the liver lobule. From the sinusoids, the blood enters the central veins, which merge to form the hepatic veins as described above.

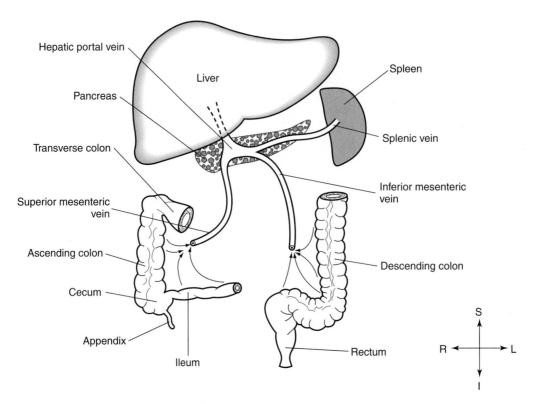

FIG. 5-11 Hepatic portal system.

The **inferior mesenteric vein** drains blood from the descending colon, sigmoid colon, and rectum. The vessel begins at the rectum and ascends to the left of the inferior mesenteric artery. As it courses upward, it is retroperitoneal and anterior to the left psoas muscle. The inferior mesenteric vein usually empties into the splenic vein, posterior to the body of the pancreas.

The **superior mesenteric vein** collects blood from the small intestine, cecum, ascending colon, and transverse colon. It begins in the right iliac fossa and ascends on the right side of the superior mesenteric artery. Both the superior mesenteric artery and superior mesenteric vein, along with their numerous branches, are enclosed within the layers of the mesentery. The superior mesenteric vein terminates behind the neck of the pancreas, where it joins the splenic vein to form the hepatic portal vein.

Four or five small vessels emerge from the hilus of the spleen and join to form a single **splenic vein.** As it courses to the right, inferior to the splenic artery and posterior to the body of the pancreas, the splenic vein receives numerous tributaries from the pancreas. The splenic vein terminates behind the neck of the pancreas, where it joins the superior mesenteric vein to form the hepatic portal vein.

There are some important vascular relationships to remember in this region. As the splenic vein courses to the right from the spleen to the hepatic portal vein, it passes anterior to the superior mesenteric artery near that vessel's origin from the aorta. It was mentioned earlier that at this level the superior mesenteric artery is separated from the aorta by the left renal vein. Sections at this level will show, in order from anterior to posterior, the **splenic vein, superior mesenteric artery, left renal vein,** and **aorta.**

The **hepatic portal vein** is formed behind the neck of the pancreas at the L2 vertebral level by the union of the **superior mesenteric vein** and the **splenic vein.** From this point the hepatic portal vein ascends obliquely to the right, posterior to the duodenum and anterior to the inferior vena cava. It is usually 7 to 8 cm long and is enclosed in the free border of the lesser omentum along with the **hepatic artery** and **bile duct.** At the porta of the liver the hepatic portal vein divides into right and left branches and enters the substance of the liver. Since the left lobe of the liver is more anterior than the right, the left branch of the portal is more anterior in position than the right. In the lesser omentum the portal vein is posterior to the hepatic artery and bile duct and the bile duct is to the right of the artery. The portal vein typically is surrounded by connective tissue, which makes it quite echogenic and easy to identify.

PERITONEUM

The wall of the abdominal cavity is lined with a thin, translucent serous membrane called the parietal peritoneum. This forms a peritoneal sac and a peritoneal cavity, both enclosed within the abdominal cavity, which is delineated by the muscular abdominal walls.

Peritoneal Sac

During development, some organs of the abdominal cavity protrude from the abdominal wall into the peritoneal cavity and carry a covering of peritoneum with them. The layer around the organs is called the visceral peritoneum and is continuous with the parietal peritoneum lining the walls. The space between the two layers of peritoneum is the peritoneal cavity. As the organs continue to develop, the peritoneal cavity is obliterated, leaving only a potential space between the visceral and parietal layers of peritoneum. The two layers of peritoneum are separated by only a capillary film of serous fluid for lubrication. This permits the organs to move against each other without friction. Normally the peritoneal cavity has a very small volume and contains only a few drops of serous fluid. Abnormal accumulations of serous fluid, called ascites, may exaggerate the volume to form a real space of several liters in volume. In males the peritoneal cavity is a closed cavity, but in females it communicates with the exterior through the uterine tubes, uterus, and vagina.

Terminology Relating to the Peritoneum

The extent and character of the peritoneum are complex, and specific terms are used to describe different parts. **Mesentery** is the double layer of peritoneum that encloses the intestine and attaches it to the abdominal wall. Blood and lymphatic vessels, nerves, lymph nodes, and fat cells are found between the two layers of a mesentery. An **omentum** is a mesentery, or double layer of peritoneum, that is attached to the stomach. The lesser omentum joins the lesser curvature of the stomach and proximal duodenum to the liver. The space behind the lesser omentum and stomach is the **omental bursa,** or **lesser sac.** The remainder of the peritoneal cavity is the **greater sac.** The omental bursa is closed at the end near the spleen but open at the right edge. The opening into the omental bursa is the **epiploic foramen,** which allows communication between the lesser and greater sacs of the peritoneal cavity. The **hepatic artery,** the **portal vein,** and the **bile duct** are enclosed within the layers of peritoneum at the free margin of the lesser omentum. The greater omentum hangs from the greater curvature of the stomach like an apron over the intestines.

Anything that is not a mesentery or omentum usually is referred to as a **peritoneal ligament.** These are double layers of peritoneum that connect one organ to another or to the anterior abdominal wall. An example of this is the **falciform ligament,** which extends from the liver to the anterior abdominal wall. Fig. 5-12 illustrates the continuity of the peritoneum and its extensions, the mesenteries and omenta.

As might be expected, numerous exceptions exist to these generalizations. This is particularly true with the peritoneal attachments associated with the stomach. Although called *ligaments,* many of these actually are a part of the omenta.

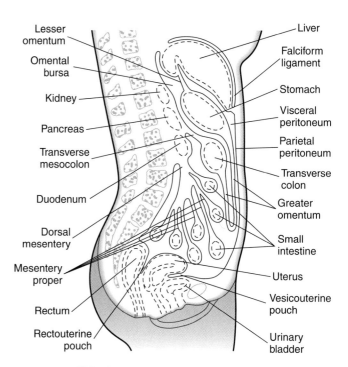

FIG. 5-12 Peritoneum and its extensions.

Cul-de-sacs

In certain places peritoneal folds form blind pouches, or cul-de-sacs. The largest of these is the omental bursa or lesser sac, which already has been described. In the pelvic region of the female peritoneal cavity a cul-de-sac exists between the rectum and uterus. This is the **rectouterine pouch,** or pouch of Douglas. A **vesicouterine pouch** is formed by the reflection of peritoneum from the uterus to the superior surface of the bladder. In males a **rectovesical pouch** lies between the rectum and posterior surface of the bladder.

Retroperitoneal Structures

Some organs of the abdominal cavity are not included within the peritoneal sac but are found behind the peritoneum as illustrated in Fig. 5-12. Their location is described as *retroperitoneal*. Only the anterior surfaces of these organs will be covered with peritoneum. The kidneys, pancreas, duodenum, ascending and descending colon, abdominal aorta, and inferior vena cava are retroperitoneal.

VISCERA OF THE ABDOMEN

Liver

The liver is the largest organ in the abdominal cavity. The large right lobe occupies the right hypochondriac region and fills the right paravertebral groove. From the right hypochondriac region, the liver extends across the epigastric region into the left hypochondriac region. As the liver mass extends across the midline it is moved forward by the longitudinal ridge line, so the smaller left lobe is more anteriorly positioned.

Surfaces and Aspects.   The anterior, superior, and posterior aspects of the liver are related to the diaphragm and follow its configuration. The convex superior aspect usually bulges upward more on the right side than on the left. The inferior or visceral surface is flatter than the superior aspect but has depressions where it is in contact with the abdominal viscera. The inferior surface is not in a horizontal plane but instead is situated at a 45-degree angle to both the longitudinal and horizontal planes so that the more inferior portions are more anteriorly positioned and the superior portions are more posteriorly located. The visceral surface of the right lobe is related to the right kidney, right colic flexure, gallbladder, and duodenum. The left lobe has a large depression for the stomach and a smaller one for the colon.

Peritoneal Relationships.   Most of the liver is enclosed in visceral peritoneum. An exception to this is a triangular space on the posterior surface, called the **bare area,** that is devoid of peritoneum and is in direct contact with the diaphragm. A deep groove exists in the bare area for the inferior vena cava. As the peritoneum around the bare area is reflected onto the diaphragm it forms the **cardinal ligaments,** which represent the margins of the bare area.

A small space exists between the visceral peritoneum of the liver and the parietal peritoneum on the diaphragm, both anteriorly and posteriorly. Anteriorly, this is part of the **greater sac** and is called the **subphrenic recess.** Posteriorly, to the left of midline, the space is part of the **omental bursa,** or lesser sac (see Fig. 5-12).

On the right side the peritoneum is reflected from the liver over the surface of the right kidney forming a **hepatorenal recess.** This recess is clinically significant because it represents the most posterior portion of the peritoneal cavity. Fluids and pus tend to accumulate in the hepatorenal recess when the patient is supine.

The lesser omentum from the lesser curvature of the stomach and first part of the duodenum is continuous with the visceral peritoneum of the liver. The left portion, between the stomach and the liver, is called the **gastrohepatic** (hepatogastric) ligament. The right portion, between the duodenum and liver is called the **duodenohepatic** (hepatoduodenal) ligament. To state this another way, the gastrohepatic and hepatoduodenal ligaments make up the lesser omentum. The portal vein, hepatic artery, and bile duct are enclosed within the right margin of the lesser omentum.

The **falciform ligament** is a thin anteroposterior fold of peritoneum attached to the convex surface of the liver, to the diaphragm, and to the anterior abdominal wall down to the level of the umbilicus. The falciform ligament marks the division between the right and left lobes on the anterior surface.

Configuration of the Visceral Surface.   An examination of the inferior, visceral surface of the liver reveals, with

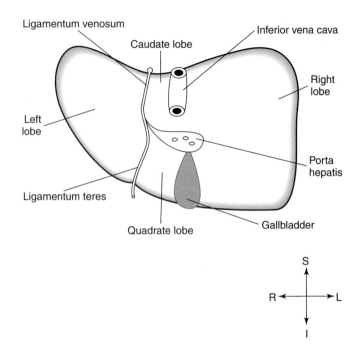

FIG. 5-13 Configuration of the visceral surface of the liver.

a little imagination, an H-shaped configuration separating the organ into four distinct regions. In addition to the right and left lobes, there is a caudate lobe and a quadrate lobe. The left arm of the H is formed by the **ligamentum teres** inferiorly and the **ligamentum venosum** superiorly. The ligamentum teres represents the obliterated umbilical vein, which carried blood from the placenta to the liver in fetal circulation. The ligamentum venosum is the remnant of the ductus venosus, which carried blood directly from the umbilical vein to the inferior vena cava to bypass the liver in fetal circulation. The left lobe is to the left of the line marked by the ligamentum teres and ligamentum venosum. The right arm of the H is formed inferiorly by the gall bladder and superiorly by the inferior vena cava. The right lobe is to the right of the line marked by these two structures. The **caudate** and **quadrate lobes** are between the two vertical lines. The cross bar of the H is formed by the porta hepatis, which includes the portal vein, hepatic artery, and hepatic duct. The caudate lobe is superior and posterior to the crossbar (porta hepatis) and the quadrate lobe is inferior and anterior to it (Fig. 5-13). The ligamentum venosum separates the left lobe from the caudate lobe, which is separated from the right lobe by the inferior vena cava. Inferiorly, the ligamentum teres separates the left lobe from the quadrate lobe and the gallbladder separates the quadrate lobe from the right lobe. In the central region, the caudate lobe is separated from the quadrate lobe by the porta hepatis.

A superficial anatomical examination indicates that the caudate and quadrate lobes are a part of the right lobe. The falciform ligament, anteriorly, and the ligamenta teres and venosum, posteriorly, mark the surface division between the right and left lobes. An investigation of the internal morphology and vasculature reveals that functionally the caudate and quadrate lobes are more closely related to the left lobe than to the right.

Blood Supply. Blood is brought to the liver by the **hepatic artery** and **hepatic portal vein.** Approximately 70% of the blood supply to the liver is nutrient-rich venous blood from the digestive system brought to the liver by the hepatic portal vein. The remaining 30% is oxygenated blood supplied by the hepatic artery. The blood passes through the **sinusoids of the liver** to enter the **central vein** of a liver lobule. The central veins converge to form **hepatic veins,** which transport the blood to the inferior vena cava.

Gallbladder

The gallbladder is a sac like reservoir for bile. It lies along the right edge of the quadrate lobe of the liver, as illustrated in Fig. 5-13. For descriptive purposes, it may be divided into fundus, body, and neck. The fundus is the inferior extremity of the sac that usually protrudes from the inferior margin of the liver. It is in contact with the anterior abdominal wall, duodenum, and transverse colon. The body extends upward from the fundus and is in direct contact with the visceral surface of the liver. It is also related to the duodenum and transverse colon. The neck is a narrow and constricted portion directed toward the porta of the liver. It is continuous with the cystic duct, which joins the hepatic duct to form the common bile duct. A hormonal feedback system controls the flow of bile from the common bile duct into the duodenum.

Esophagus

Most of the esophagus lies is the thoracic cavity with only the terminal portion located in the abdomen. While in the thoracic cavity, the esophagus lies anterior to the vertebral column and to the right of the descending aorta. At the T7 vertebral level, it deviates to the left, passing anterior to the aorta, on its way to the stomach. After penetrating the diaphragm at the T10 vertebral level, the abdominal portion of the esophagus forms a groove in the left portion of the liver and enters the stomach at the **cardiac orifice.** The right margin of the esophagus is continuous with the lesser curvature of the stomach. A **cardiac notch** separates the left margin of the esophagus from the fundus of the stomach. The **lower esophageal sphincter** at the cardiac orifice slows the passage of food from the esophagus into the stomach and also prevents reflux of gastric contents into the esophagus.

Stomach

The stomach pulverizes food and mixes it with gastric juice. It is located in the upper left quadrant of the abdomen. Under normal conditions the stomach cannot be palpated because the walls are rather flat and flabby. However, because the walls are distensible, the size and shape of the stomach varies with circumstances.

Curvatures. The stomach has two curvatures. The concave **lesser curvature** is directed to the right and superiorly. It is continuous with the right margin of the esophagus. The **greater curvature** is convex and forms the left and inferior margins of the stomach.

Regions. For descriptive purposes, the stomach is divided into four regions. The limited **cardiac portion** lies adjacent to the cardiac orifice, where the esophagus enters. The **fundus** is the rounded portion above the gastroesophageal junction. The major portion is the **body** of the stomach, which is between the fundus and pyloric regions. The distal portion which empties into the small intestine is the **pyloric region.** The junction of the body and pyloric region is marked by the **angular notch** or **incisura angularis,** a notch on the lesser curvature. The pyloric region is divided into a wider portion, the **pyloric antrum,** and a narrow **pyloric canal.** The sphincter region at the orifice between the stomach and duodenum is the **pylorus.**

Peritoneal Relationships. The stomach is completely covered by peritoneum and is attached to other organs by peritoneal folds and ligaments. The **gastrohepatic** portion of the lesser omentum radiates from the lesser curvature to attach to the liver. From the inferior and left greater curvature, the **greater omentum** falls like an apron over the intestines. A portion of the greater omentum is attached to the transverse colon and is called the **gastrocolic** ligament. The anterior surface of the stomach is related to the diaphragm, left lobe of the liver, and anterior abdominal wall. The posterior surface is related to many abdominal viscera including the spleen, left kidney and suprarenal gland, pancreas, and transverse colon.

Blood Supply. All three branches of the celiac trunk contribute to the vasculature of the stomach. The **left gastric artery** is the smallest branch of the celiac. It courses to the left along the lesser curvature, giving off branches along the way, to supply that region. The **right gastric** and **right gastroepiploic arteries** are branches of the common hepatic artery. The splenic artery contributes the **left gastroepiploic artery** and numerous short **gastric arteries.** The veins of the stomach follow the same pattern as the arteries, both in name and distribution. The venous blood from the stomach, like blood from other parts of the digestive tract, is taken to the liver by way of the hepatic portal vein, but the way gastric veins enter the portal system varies considerably. From the liver, the blood enters the hepatic veins, which carry it to the inferior vena cava.

Small Intestine

Most of the digestion of food and absorption of nutrients takes place in the small intestine. This long, convoluted tube is usually 6 or 7 m long and is divided into the **duodenum, jejunum,** and **ileum.** The jejunum and ileum are enclosed in peritoneum and are suspended from the posterior

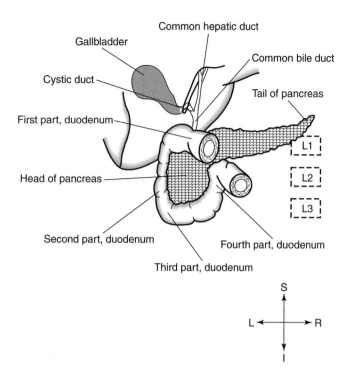

Gallbladder
Common hepatic duct
Cystic duct
Common bile duct
First part, duodenum
Tail of pancreas
Head of pancreas
Second part, duodenum
Fourth part, duodenum
Third part, duodenum
L1
L2
L3

S
L ← → R
I

FIG. 5-14 Divisions of the duodenum.

wall by a fan-shaped **dorsal mesentery.** The duodenum is retroperitoneal except for a small portion near the pylorus of the stomach.

Duodenum.   The first part of the small intestine, beginning at the pyloric valve, is the **duodenum.** About 25 cm long, this portion presents a C-shaped pattern as it curves around the head of the pancreas to become continuous with the jejunum. The duodenum is the most fixed part of the small intestine. For descriptive purposes the duodenum may be divided into four parts as illustrated in Fig. 5-14.

The **first,** or **superior, part** is horizontal, beginning at the pylorus and extending to the gallbladder. Anteriorly, the first part is related to the quadrate lobe of the liver and the gallbladder. The inferior vena cava, portal vein, bile duct, and gastroduodenal artery course along the posterior surface. The inferior border of the first (horizontal) part of the duodenum courses along the upper margin of the pancreatic head.

Posterior to the gallbladder, the duodenum turns sharply downward to become the **second,** or **descending, part.** It is against the posterior abdominal wall in the paravertebral groove, along the right side of the first three lumbar vertebrae. As it descends, it is to the right and parallel to the inferior vena cava. As the second part descends, it passes anterior to the hilus of the right kidney and posterior to the transverse colon. The second part, then, is related anteriorly to the right lobe of the liver and transverse colon, posteriorly to the right kidney, renal vessels, ureter, and psoas muscle, and medially to the bile duct and pancreas. The pancreatic and bile ducts enter the second part.

After descending to the lower margin of L3 or upper margin of L4, the duodenum again makes a sharp turn, this time to the left, to become the **third** or **inferior horizontal part.** As this part extends across the midline, from right to left, it is moved forward by the longitudinal ridge. As it courses horizontally, the third part passes anterior to the inferior vana cava, aorta, right ureter, right gonadal vessels, and psoas muscles, but posterior to the superior meseneric vessels. Superiorly, this part is related to the pancreas and inferiorly to the coils of jejunum.

The **ascending fourth part** ascends anterior and slightly to the left of the aorta. In addition to the aorta, the fourth part is related on its posterior aspect to the left psoas muscle, left renal, and left gonadal vessels. To its left are the left kidney and ureter and to its right is the pancreas. Superiorly, the fourth part is related to the body of the pancreas. The fourth or ascending part ascends only to the second lumbar vertebra then ends abruptly in the duodenojejunal flexure. This flexure is directed anteriorly and is attached to the posterior abdominal wall by a fibromuscular band called the *suspensory muscle* of the duodenum or the *ligament of Treitz.*

Jejunum.   The second division of the small intestine is the **jejunum.** This is a tightly coiled tube that begins at the duodenojejunal flexure and continues until it imperceptibly changes into the ileum. Most of the jejunum is located in the umbilical region of the abdomen.

Ileum.   No obvious structural changes occur at the junction between the jejunum and **ileum;** however, the tissues that form the wall do change. The mucosa of the ileum lacks circular folds. Accumulations of lymphoid tissue called *Peyer's patches* are also evident in the wall of the ileum. Most of the ileum lies in the hypogastric region with distal parts usually in the pelvis. The ileum terminates in the right iliac region by opening into the cecum through the ileocecal valve.

Both the ileum and jejunum are enclosed in peritoneum and are suspended from the posterior abdominal wall by fan-shaped folds of mesentery. The duodenojejunal flexure and the iliocecal valve are fixed points, but between these two points the jejunum and ileum are highly mobile and fill any available space in the abdominopelvic cavity. Because of their mobility, the jejunum and ileum are the regions frequently involved in hernias.

Large Intestine

The large intestine extends from the ileocecal valve to the anus, a length of approximately 1.5 m. It consists of the cecum, colon, rectum, and anal canal. These regions are illustrated in Fig. 5-15. The large intestine forms an arch for the loops of small intestine.

Cecum.   Located in the right iliac region of the abdominopelvic cavity, the **cecum** is a blind saclike pouch that extends 5 to 7 cm below the ileocecal valve. The ver-

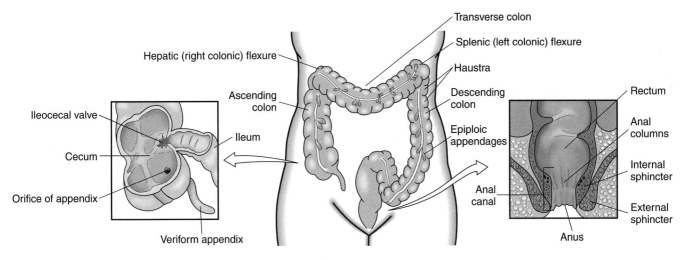

FIG. 5-15 Regions of the large intestine.

miform appendix is a blind tubular projection from the cecum. Although the position of the appendix varies considerably, it is commonly inferior and posterior to the cecum. The cecum is retroperitoneal and has no mesentery.

Ascending Colon.   From the cecum, the large intestine passes superiorly on the right side of the abdominal cavity to the liver. When it reaches the visceral surface of the liver, the **ascending colon** bends sharply to the left in the **right colic** or **hepatic flexure.** The ascending colon lies on the posterior abdominal wall, where it is separated from the muscles by the right kidney. It is retroperitoneal and has no mesentery.

Transverse Colon.   The **transverse colon** extends across the abdomen from the right colic (hepatic) flexure to the **left colic (splenic) flexure.** It is the longest part of the large intestine. Suspended by a mesentery, the **transverse mesocolon,** the transverse colon is the most movable part of the large intestine. Between the two flexures, the position of the transverse colon is variable but typically forms a loop that is directed inferiorly. This loop may be on the transpyloric plane or extend down to the pelvic brim. As the transverse colon extends across the abdominal cavity, it becomes more superior and more posterior so that the **splenic flexure** is the most superior part of the large intestine and is also relatively posterior in position. At the left colic or splenic flexure, the large intestine turns sharply downward as the descending colon.

Descending Colon.   The **descending colon** extends form the left colic flexure to the iliac crest. As it descends it passes along the lateral border of the left kidney. The descending colon is of smaller diameter than either the ascending or transverse colon. It is retroperitoneal and has no mesentery. At the iliac crest, the descending colon becomes continuous with the sigmoid colon.

Sigmoid Colon.   The **sigmoid colon** begins at the pelvic brim, crosses the sacrum, then curves to the midline at the third sacral segment. It is enclosed in peritoneum and has a long mesentery, the **sigmoid mesocolon.** Because of its mesentery, the sigmoid colon is movable. It is usually located in the pelvis but may extend upward into the abdomen.

Rectum.   The **rectum** extends from the third sacral segment to the pelvic diaphragm just below the tip of the coccyx, a length of about 12 cm. Here the rectum turns dorsally to become the anal canal. The rectum is partially covered with peritoneum but has no mesentery, therefore it is considered to be retroperitoneal.

Anal Canal.   The **anal canal** is 2.5 to 4.0 cm in length and represents the final portion of the intestinal tract. As the canal penetrates the pelvic diaphragm to terminate at the anus in the perineum, it is supported by the **levator ani muscles.**

Spleen

The spleen is a highly vascular organ composed of lymphoid tissue in the left hypochondriac region of the abdomen. It is located posterior to the stomach and is protected by the ninth, tenth, and eleventh ribs. In addition to the stomach, the visceral surface of the spleen is related to the left kidney and transverse colon. The hilus of the spleen is closely related to the tail of the pancreas. The spleen is enclosed in peritoneum except at the hilus and is held in place by two peritoneal ligaments. The gastrosplenic ligament attaches to the hilus to the greater curvature of the stomach and the lienorenal ligament attaches to the hilus to the left kidney. The spleen varies considerably in size and shape depending on the distention of the stomach and colon. Vascular needs of the spleen are supplied by the splenic artery and vein, which penetrate the organ at the hilus.

Pancreas

The pancreas is an elongated, soft, pliable gland that has both exocrine and endocrine functions. Because it is covered with peritoneum only on its anterior surface, it is considered to be retroperitoneal. The pancreas extends across the posterior surface of the abdomen from the duodenum to the spleen. For descriptive purposes it is divided into the head, neck, body, and tail.

The **head** is the broad, flattened, right extremity of the pancreas that lies within the curve of the duodenum (see Fig. 5-14). A small **uncinate process** projects inferiorly and medially posterior to the duodenum so that it rests on the inferior vena cava and left renal vein. The superior mesenteric vessels are anterior to the uncinate process. The **neck** is a constricted portion to the left of the head. The splenic and superior mesenteric veins join to form the hepatic portal vein posterior to the neck of the pancreas. The neck merges imperceptibly with the **body.** As the body of the pancreas extends to the left and superiorly across the aorta, its posterior surface is related to the superior mesenteric artery, splenic artery and vein, left suprarenal (adrenal) gland, and left kidney with its vessels. It is separated from the stomach by the omental bursa. The **tail** of the pancreas is the left extremity in close proximity to the hilus of the spleen. The tail is the most superior and posterior portion of the pancreas.

The main **pancreatic duct,** or **duct of Wirsung,** begins in the tail of the pancreas and runs through the substance of the gland, then empties into the descending second part of the duodenum. Blood supply is by way of the splenic artery, which is a branch of the celiac trunk. The splenic vein carries blood from the spleen to the hepatic portal circulation before it returns to the inferior vena cava.

Kidneys

Location and Position.   The **kidneys** are paired, reddish-brown, bean-shaped organs just below the diaphragm in the superior part of the paravertebral grooves. They are behind the peritoneum (retroperitoneal) along the posterior body wall, against the psoas muscle, and adjacent to the vertebral column. The superior part of each kidney is protected by the ribs. Each adult kidney is approximately 12 cm long and 6 cm wide and extends from the level of the twelfth thoracic vertebra to the third lumbar vertebra. This level changes during respiratory movements and with changes in posture. Because it is pushed down by the liver, the right kidney is generally slightly lower than the left. A cushion of **perirenal fat** surrounds each kidney, and the ribs, muscles, and intestines serve as protective barriers. Occasionally a kidney slips from its normal position and is no longer held securely in place by adjacent organs or its covering of fat. This condition is known as *floating kidney*, or ptosis, and may cause a kinking or twisting of the ureter with a subsequent obstruction of urine flow. In addition, the kidneys become more susceptible to physical trauma when they drop below the rib cage.

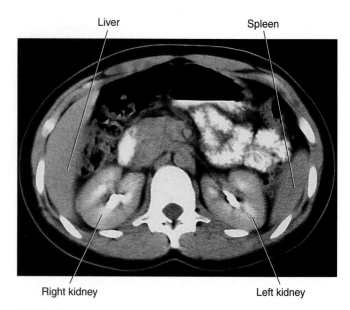

FIG. 5-16 CT image showing some of the relationships of the kidney to surrounding structures.

Hilus.   The region where the blood vessels enter and leave and where the ureter exists to descend to the bladder is called the **hilus of the kidney.** The hilus is generally at the level of the transpyloric plane with the plane intersecting the mid-hilar region of the left kidney and upper hilar region of the right kidney.

Relationships.   On its posterior or dorsal surface, the kidney is related to the diaphragm superiorly and to the quadratus lumborum and psoas muscles inferiorly. The computed tomographic image in Fig. 5-16 shows some of the relationships of the kidneys to surrounding structures. The anterior and medial surface of the superior pole of each kidney is covered by a **suprarenal (adrenal) gland.**

The anterior or ventral relationships are different for the right and left kidneys. On the right, the kidney forms a renal impression on the visceral surface of the liver. The second or descending part of the duodenum descends across the hilar region, and the right colic (hepatic) flexure of the colon covers the inferior pole of the kidney. The anterior or ventral surface of the left kidney is related to the left suprarenal gland, stomach, pancreas, spleen, left colic (splenic) flexure, and coils of the small intestine.

Ureters.   The **ureters** are muscular ducts that transport urine from the kidneys to the urinary bladder. Originating at the renal pelvis, the ureters descend retroperitoneally along the psoas muscle. The right ureter is in close relationship with the inferior vena cava as it descends. The abdominal portion of the ureter crosses the pelvic brim and the external artery just distal to the bifurcation of the common iliac artery, then continues as the pelvic ureter to enter the posterior surface of the urinary bladder. The ureter is vulnerable during pelvic and abdominal surgery, because it sometimes resembles a blood vessel and because it is in close proximity to the pelvic organs.

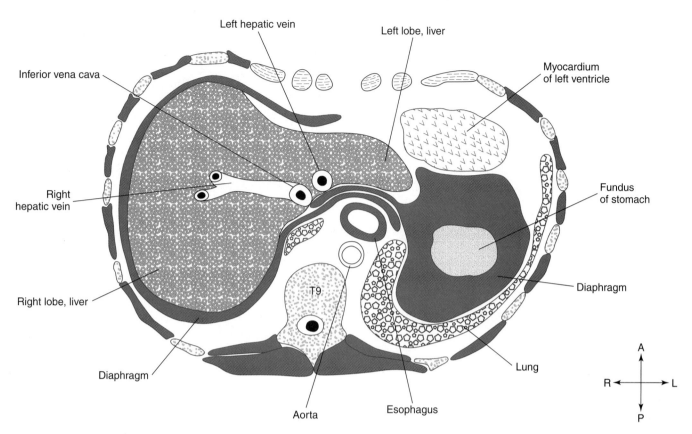

FIG. 5-17 Transverse section through the upper abdomen, level T9.

Suprarenal Gland

A **suprarenal (adrenal) gland** lies on each side of the vertebral column in close relation to the superior pole of the corresponding kidney. The suprarenal gland is separated from the kidney by fatty connective tissue. The right gland is somewhat pyramidal in shape, whereas the left is more semilunar. On the right, the suprarenal gland is limited by the liver laterally, the inferior vena cava anteriorly, and the diaphragm medially. The left suprarenal gland is related to the left crus of the diaphragm medially and the left kidney posteriorly and laterally. Anteriorly it is related to the stomach and pancreas. Each gland has an abundant blood supply from the suprarenal arteries, which branch directly from the aorta. Branches of the renal and inferior phrenic arteries also supply the suprarenal glands.

Sectional Anatomy of the Abdomen

TRANSVERSE SECTIONS

Sections Through Upper Abdomen, T9

Transverse sections through the superior regions of the abdomen will also intersect portions of the heart in the pericardial sac and lungs in the pleural cavity as illustrated in Fig. 5-17. The hiatus in the diaphragm for the inferior vena cava is at vertebral level T8, so in this region of the abdominal cavity, the inferior vena cava may be embedded in the substance of the liver. The right and left hepatic veins are short vessels that drain into the inferior vena cava near the caval hiatus in the diaphragm. Fig. 5-17 illustrates the right hepatic vein as it drains into the inferior vena cava. The left hepatic vein is slightly anterior to the right hepatic vein and inferior vena cava, because the left lobe of the liver is more anteriorly positioned.

Sections Through Level T10

The three most noticeable structures in transverse sections at level T10 are the liver, stomach, and spleen. The relationships of these organs are illustrated in Fig. 5-18 and in the computed tomographic image shown in Fig. 5-19.

The right lobe of the liver fills the right paravertebral groove. The left lobe is moved anteriorly as it crosses the longitudinal ridge to the left side. The falciform ligament attaches the anterior surface of the liver to the anterior abdominal wall and separates the right and left lobes superficially. Posteriorly the bare area of the liver is closely related to the diaphragm. The inferior vena cava is on the posterior surface, just the right of midline, near the vertebral body. The fissure for the ligamentum venosum separates the caudate lobe from the left lobe. Within the parenchyma of the liver, branches of the portal vein are surrounded by connective tissue.

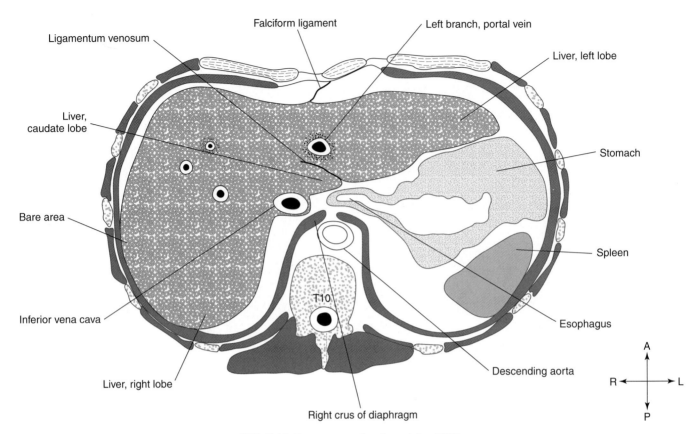

FIG. 5-18 Transverse section through level T10.

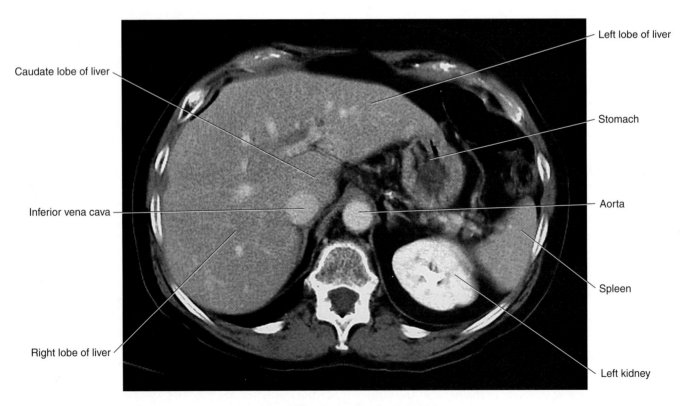

FIG. 5-19 CT image through level T10.

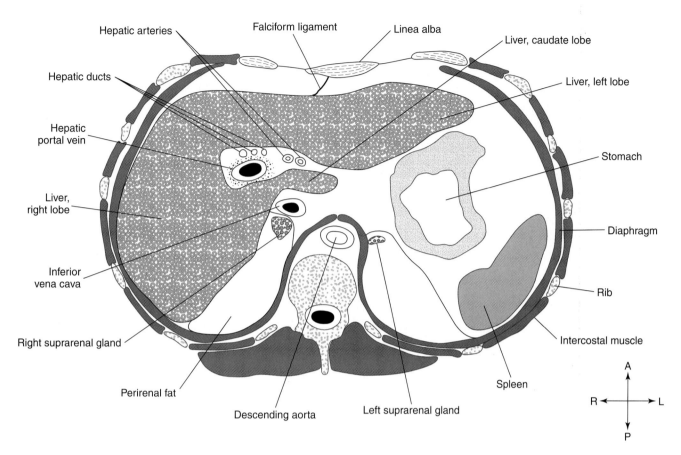

FIG. 5-20 Transverse section through the porta hepatis.

Fig. 5-18 also shows the esophagus as it enters the cardiac region of the stomach. Anteriorly the stomach is related to the left lobe of the liver and posteriorly to the spleen. The lateral surface is next to the diaphragm. The spleen is against the posterior abdominal wall, in the left paravertebral groove, posterior to the stomach.

Sections Through the Porta Hepatis

The relationship of structures in transverse sections through the porta of the liver is significant. The most obvious structure at the porta hepatis is the hepatic portal vein. The portal vein is formed behind the neck of the pancreas then courses obliquely toward the liver. It is enclosed in the free margin of the lesser omentum. At the porta hepatis, the portal vein is posterior to the hepatic arteries and hepatic ducts. The common hepatic artery, a branch of the celiac trunk, also ascends toward the liver in the right free margin of the lesser omentum. Near the porta, the common hepatic artery branches to form the right and left hepatic arteries, which are anterior to the portal vein and to the left of the hepatic ducts. Within the liver parenchyma, bile canaliculi merge to form progressively larger hepatic ducts until a right and left hepatic duct emerge from the porta. The hepatic ducts are anterior to the portal vein and to the right of the hepatic

arteries. Posterior to the portal vein a narrow piece of liver, the caudate process, connects the caudate lobe with the right lobe. These relationships are illustrated in Fig. 5-20.

Transverse sections at the level of the porta hepatis may also show suprarenal (adrenal) gland. The right suprarenal gland is somewhat pyrimidal in shape. It is limited anteriorly by the inferior vena cava, posteriorly by the kidney, laterally by the liver, and medially by the right crus of the diaphragm. The gland on the left is thinner and more semilunar in shape as it drapes along the margin of the kidney. Anteriorly and laterally it is related to the stomach and pancreas. Medially it is related to the left crus of the diaphragm.

Sections Through the Gallbladder

Transverse sections inferior to the porta, through the gallbladder, show the anteriorly located quadrate lobe delineated by the gallbladder and ligamentum teres. Relationships at this level are illustrated in Fig. 5-21. Because the celiac trunk branches from the aorta just above the transpyloric line, which intersects the gallbladder, the trunk or some of its three branches will probably be evident at this level. The tail of the pancreas frequently reaches this level, because the tail is the most superior portion of the pancreas.

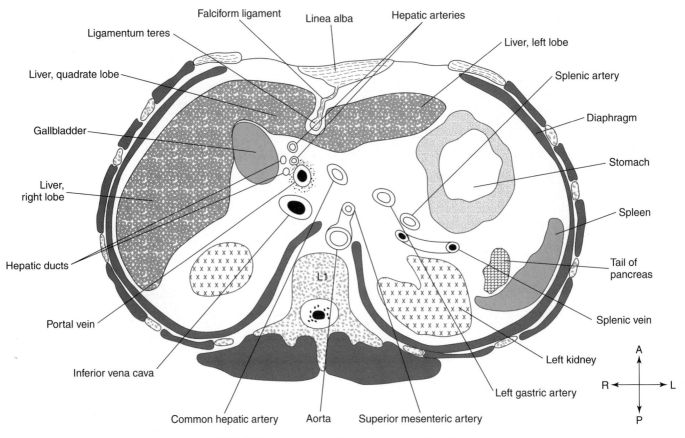

FIG. 5-21 Transverse section through the gallbladder.

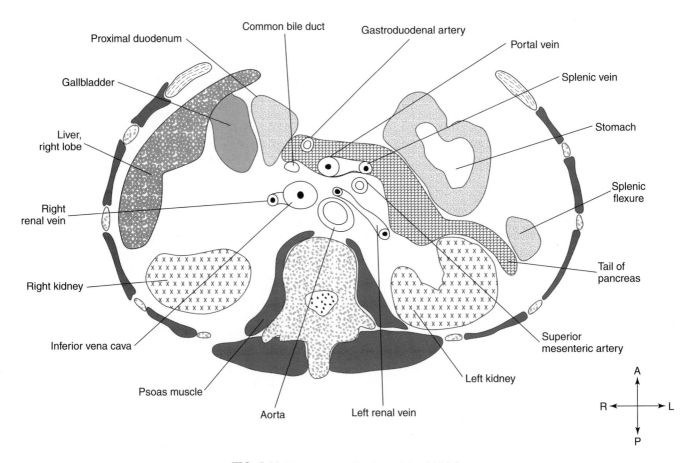

FIG. 5-22 Transverse section through level L1/L2.

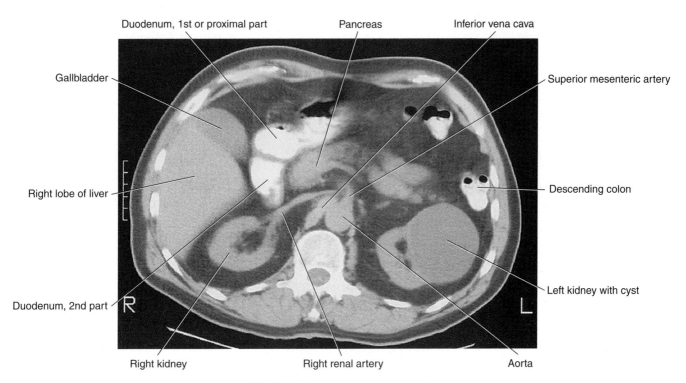

Duodenum, 1st or proximal part   Pancreas   Inferior vena cava

Gallbladder

Superior mesenteric artery

Right lobe of liver

Descending colon

Duodenum, 2nd part

R   L

Left kidney with cyst

Right kidney   Right renal artery   Aorta

FIG. 5-23 CT image through level L1/L2.

Sections Through L1/L2

Numerous interesting relationships exist at the level of the lower part of the first and upper part of the second lumbar vertebrae. The duodenum becomes evident next to the gallbladder. The head of the pancreas is closely butted against the duodenum. The common bile duct forms a groove along the posterior surface of the pancreatic head, whereas the gastroduodenal artery, a branch of the common hepatic artery, courses along the anterior surface. The portal vein is formed posterior to the neck of the pancreas when the splenic and superior mesenteric veins join. These relationships are illustrated in Fig. 5-22.

A classic vascular arrangement evident at the L1/L2 level is also shown in Fig. 5-22. The long left renal vein passes between the aorta and superior mesenteric artery as the vein goes from the left kidney to the inferior vena cava. The left renal vein is anterior to the aorta and posterior to the superior mesenteric artery. The computed tomographic image in Fig. 5-23 is at a similar level and shows some of these relationships.

Sections Through the Head of the Pancreas

Fig. 5-24 shows the head of the pancreas between the second and fourth parts of the duodenum. The third part will appear in sections inferior to this level. The uncinate process of the pancreas projects from the pancreatic head and extends posterior to the superior mesenteric vessels. The descending colon appears in the left paravertebral groove. The larger ascending colon, in the right paraverte-

bral groove, is more anterior than the descending colon. The kidneys are against the posterior abdominal wall and are related to the psoas and quadratus lumborum muscles. Notice also that the aorta and inferior vena cava add height to the longitudinal ridge line. The computed tomographic image in Fig. 5-25 also shows some of these relationships.

SAGITTAL SECTIONS

Sections Through the Ascending Colon

The most lateral sections on the right side of the abdomen show the right lobe of the liver conforming to the shape of the diaphragm and protected by the rib cage. Sections taken 2 cm or so more medially will intersect the kidney and ascending colon. Fig. 5-26 illustrates the organ relationships in this region. The predominant structure is the right lobe of the liver. The right kidney forms an indentation on the posterior visceral surface of the liver. The ascending colon extends from the cecum to the hepatic flexure. The quadratus lumborum and iliacus muscles form the posterior wall of the abdomen. Anteriorly the external oblique, internal oblique, and transverse abdominus muscles form the abdominal wall.

Sections Through the Gallbladder

Saggital sections approximately 6 or 7 cm to the right of midline typically intersect the gallbladder. A large portion of the right lobe of the liver with the right branch of the

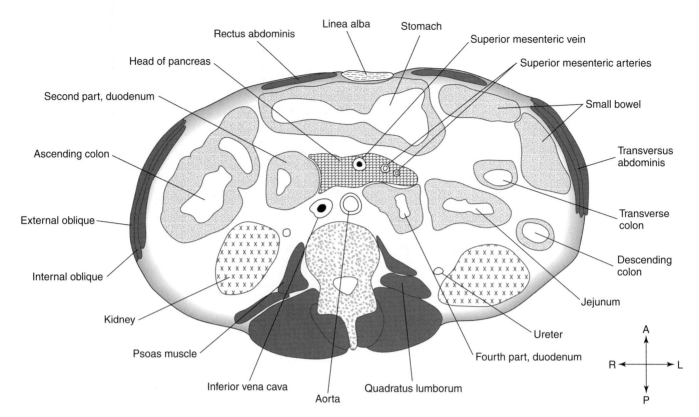

FIG. 5-24 Transverse section through the head of the pancreas.

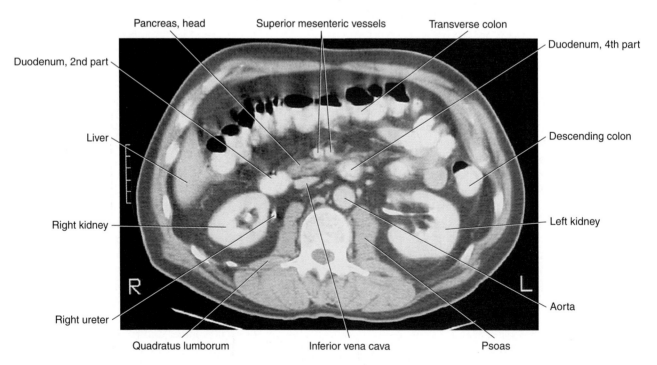

FIG 5-25 CT image through the head of the pancreas.

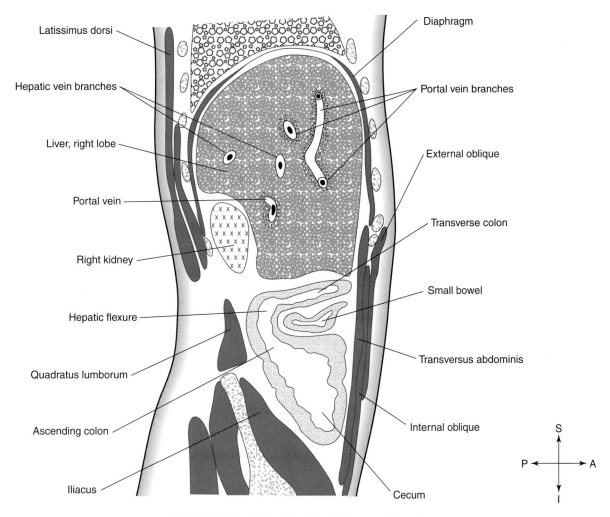

FIG. 5-26 Sagittal section through the ascending colon.

portal vein is visible. Fig. 5-27 illustrates the relationship of the duodenum to the gallbladder and kidney. The descending second part of the duodenum is related to the gallbladder anteriorly and rests on the kidney posteriorly. This illustrates the posterior position of the second part of the duodenum. The large psoas muscle, adjacent to the vertebral bodies, is evident in this region.

Sections Through the Head of the Pancreas

Because the head of the pancreas is surrounded by the four parts of the duodenum, it is logical that saggital sections through this region will be medial to the descending second portion of the duodenum but will intersect the horizontal first and third parts. This is illustrated in Fig. 5-28, which shows the first part of the duodenum superior to the pancreatic head and the third part inferior to it. Also in this region, the right adrenal gland is delineated by the right kidney and liver. The right renal artery and vein course to the right, posterior to the pancreatic head. Sections in this region show the anterior position of the transverse colon and

the segmented nature of the rectus abdominus muscle. The porta of the liver separates the caudate lobe posteriorly from the quadrate lobe anteriorly.

Sections Through the Inferior Vena Cava

The inferior vena cava ascends to penetrate the diaphragm and empty into the right atrium of the heart 1 or 2 cm to the right of midline. Fig. 5-29 illustrates the relationships of the inferior vena cava. It is related anteriorly to the caudate lobe of the liver, pancreas, and horizontal third part of the duodenum.

Midsagittal Section

A little to the left of the inferior vena cava, in more of a midline position, the aorta descends along the vertebral column. The classic relationship of the aorta, superior mesenteric artery, and left renal vein is usually evident in this region. Watch for the superior mesenteric artery as it branches from the aorta at approximately a 60-degree angle. The left

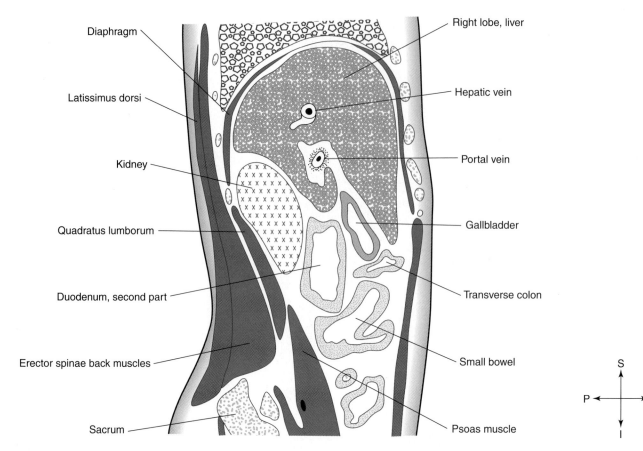

Diaphragm

Latissimus dorsi

Kidney

Quadratus lumborum

Duodenum, second part

Erector spinae back muscles

Sacrum

Right lobe, liver

Hepatic vein

Portal vein

Gallbladder

Transverse colon

Small bowel

Psoas muscle

S
P ← → A
I

FIG. 5-27 Sagittal section through the gallbladder.

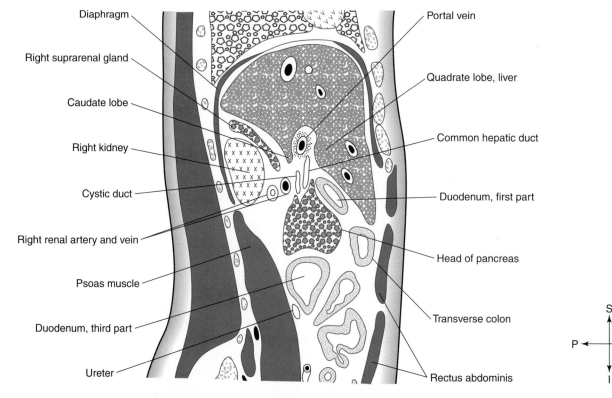

Diaphragm

Right suprarenal gland

Caudate lobe

Right kidney

Cystic duct

Right renal artery and vein

Psoas muscle

Duodenum, third part

Ureter

Portal vein

Quadrate lobe, liver

Common hepatic duct

Duodenum, first part

Head of pancreas

Transverse colon

Rectus abdominis

S
P ← → A
I

FIG. 5-28 Sagittal section head of the pancreas.

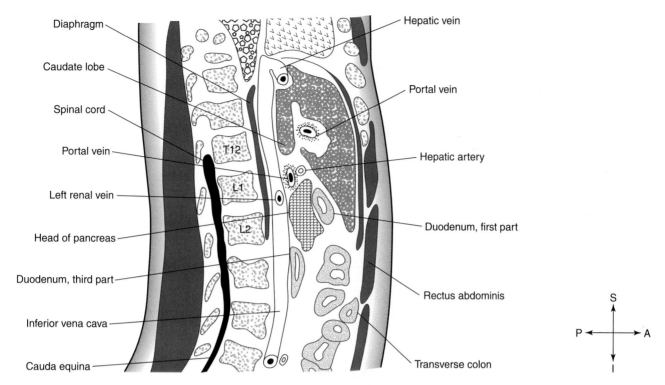

FIG. 5-29 Sagittal section through the IVC.

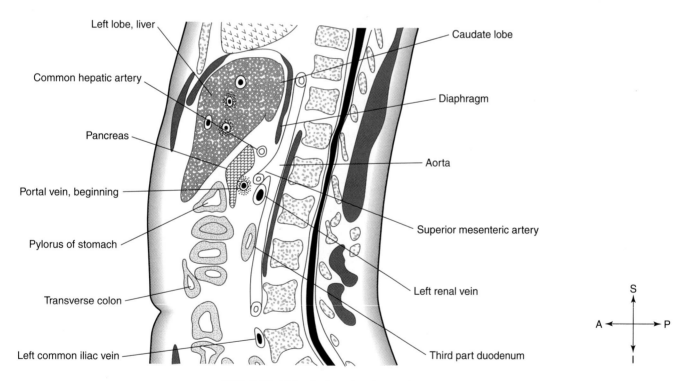

FIG. 5-30 Midsagittal section through the abdomen.

renal vein is neatly tucked in the angle between the two vessels as illustrated in Fig. 5-30. The horizontal third part of the duodenum, or possibly the ascending fourth portion, is just inferior to the left renal vein. Anteriorly the pylorus of the stomach is related to the inferior portion of the left lobe of the liver.

Left Parasagittal Sections

Proceeding to the left from the midline, the relationships of the liver, stomach, spleen, pancreas, and kidney become evident. Fig. 5-31 illustrates some of these relationships. Centrally located in the superior portion of the abdomen, the stomach is related anteriorly to the left lobe of the liver and

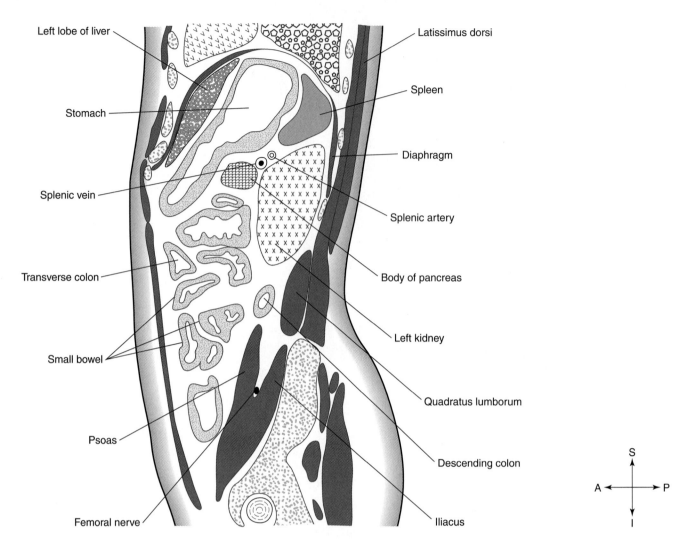

FIG. 5-31 Left parasagittal section through the abdomen.

posteriorly to the spleen. Just inferior to the spleen, the left kidney rests along the posterior abdominal wall. The body of the pancreas courses to the left posterior to the stomach and anterior to the kidney. The splenic artery and vein are located along the posterior superior margin of the pancreas.

CORONAL SECTIONS

Sections Through the Vertebral Canal

When considering coronal sections of the abdomen, remember the anterior-posterior relationships of the abdominal viscera. Because the spleen, kidneys, and right lobe of the liver are in the paravertebral grooves, against the posterior abdominal wall, they will be seen in the most posterior sections. This is illustrated in Fig. 5-32, which depicts a coronal section through the vertebral canal.

Sections Through Vertebral Bodies

Moving anteriorly from the vertebral canal to the vertebral bodies, structures related to the spleen become evident. These include the tail of the pancreas, stomach, and left

colic (splenic) flexure. The splenic vessels are typically related to the superior margin of the pancreas, so whenever any part of the pancreas is present, look for splenic vessels. Posterior sections such as the one depicted in Fig. 5-33 also illustrate the relationship of the kidneys to the psoas muscle. Because lordosis of the vertebral column is normal, coronal sections through lumbar vertebral bodies are more anterior than those through the thoracic vertebrae.

Sections Through the Anterior Abdomen

Anterior sections of the abdomen—for example, through the gallbladder—are likely to show both the right and left lobes of the liver and the structures related to them. The fundus of the gallbladder is the most anterior part. The body is slightly more posterior and is in contact with the visceral surface of the liver as shown in Fig. 5-34. The gallbladder is related to the right colic (hepatic) flexure and right side of the transverse colon. Medially, the body of the gallbladder is related to the pylorus of the stomach and duodenum. Because the pancreatic head is closely associated with the duodenum, it is usually seen in sections with the gallbladder. Coronal sections anterior to the gallbladder show only the liver.

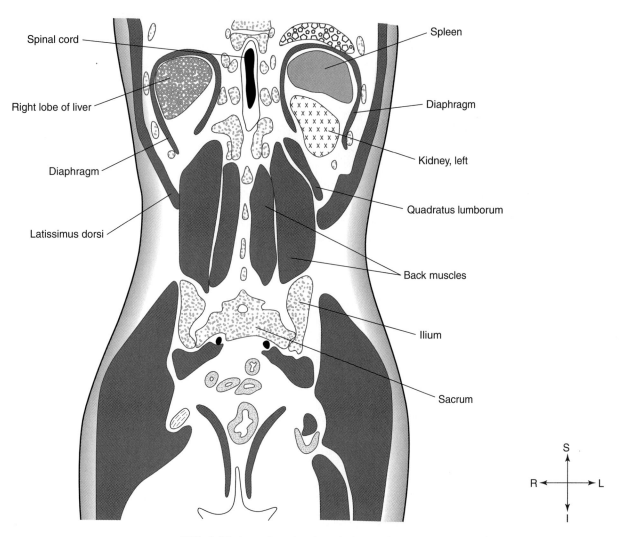

FIG. 5-32 Coronal section through the vertebral canal.

Spinal cord

Right lobe of liver

Diaphragm

Latissimus dorsi

Spleen

Diaphragm

Kidney, left

Quadratus lumborum

Back muscles

Ilium

Sacrum

S
R ← → L
I

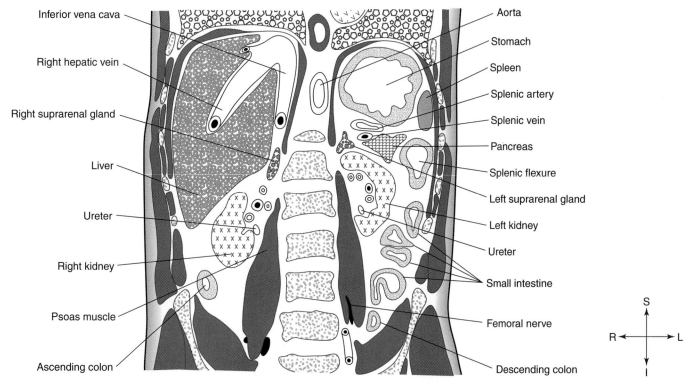

FIG. 5-33 Coronal section through the vertebral bodies.

Inferior vena cava

Right hepatic vein

Right suprarenal gland

Liver

Ureter

Right kidney

Psoas muscle

Ascending colon

Aorta

Stomach

Spleen

Splenic artery

Splenic vein

Pancreas

Splenic flexure

Left suprarenal gland

Left kidney

Ureter

Small intestine

Femoral nerve

Descending colon

S
R ← → L
I

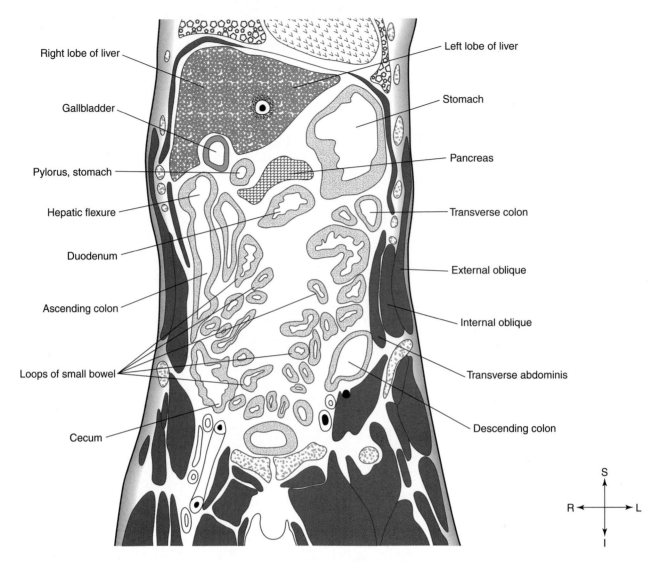

Right lobe of liver

Gallbladder

Pylorus, stomach

Hepatic flexure

Duodenum

Ascending colon

Loops of small bowel

Cecum

Left lobe of liver

Stomach

Pancreas

Transverse colon

External oblique

Internal oblique

Transverse abdominis

Descending colon

FIG. 5-34 Coronal section through the anterior abdomen.

Pathology

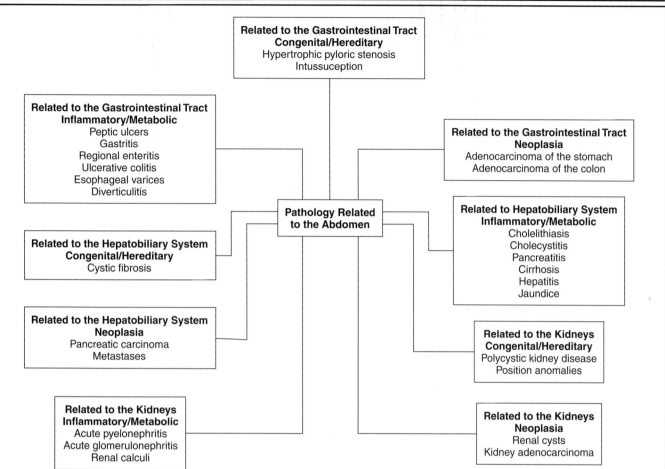

Hypertrophic Pyloric Stenosis

Hypertrophic pyloric stenosis is a congenital anomaly in which the pyloric canal is narrow because of a thickening of the pyloric sphincter. The initial sign is vomiting, at first mild then becoming more severe and projectile. The infant cries because of hunger, cramping, and constipation.

Intussusception

Intussusception is the prolapse of one part of the bowel into an adjacent distal region causing an obstruction. Most cases occur in children. If not treated, the bowel will become gangrenous because the blood supply is impeded.

Peptic Ulcers

A peptic ulcer is the erosion of the duodenal and/or gastric wall that is produced by gastric acid and proteolytic enzymes. The main symptom is pain that often radiates throughout the abdomen. If untreated, complications may occur, including peritonitis if the ulcer perforates into the abdomen, or life-threatening hemorrhage if blood vessels are involved in the perforation.

Gastritis

Gastritis is an inflammation of the stomach mucosa, which may be acute or chronic. Often related episodes of acute gastritis eventually lead to the chronic form. Etiologic agents include anything that irritates the stomach lining, such as alcohol, drugs, viruses, aspirin, and dietary irritants. If the condition becomes chronic, surgical intervention may be necessary.

Regional Enteritis

Regional enteritis, also known as Crohn's disease, is a chronic inflammation that may involve any part of the small intestine but usually affects the distal ileum and may extend into the proximal colon. The disease begins as an inflammation with regional scarring and thickening of the intestinal wall, which may lead to mechanical obstruction. Regional enteritis typically affects young adults and the initial symptoms may be similar to appendicitis. The etiology is unknown.

Ulcerative Colitis

Ulcerative colitis is an inflammatory disease that affects the mucosa of the colon, usually beginning in the rectal region and progressing into the sigmoid area. It is characterized by severe bloody diarrhea, which may lead to weight loss and electrolyte imbalances. The etiology is unknown, but some evidence suggests that it may have an autoimmune component.

Esophageal Varices

Esophageal varices are varicose veins of the esophagus. Conditions that create a resistance to blood flow through the liver result in a portal hypertension and inhibit normal venous

Continued

Pathology—cont'd

drainage through the portal system. The blood is directed through esophageal and gastric collateral veins and the increased blood flow through these vessels causes them to dilate.

Diverticulitis

A diverticulum is a protrusion of the mucosa and submucosa through the muscular layer at some point of weakness in the intestinal wall. The presence of diverticula is called *diverticulosis* and is usually asymptomatic. When inflammation occurs in the region of diverticula, the condition is called *diverticulitis*. Diverticula may occur in any portion of the intestine; however, they are more common in the sigmoid colon and may lead to bowel obstruction.

Adenocarcinoma of the Stomach

Adenocarcinoma is the most significant malignancy of the stomach. The symptoms are often vague but include bleeding, tiredness, loss of appetite, and weight loss. Blood tests may indicate anemia. Because the symptoms are vague, the individual may delay seeking medical intervention until the tumor is inoperable or has metastasized by way of lymphatic vessels or the bloodstream.

Adenocarcinoma of the Colon

Malignancies of the colon are typically adenocarcinomas, which are derived from the glandular epithelium in the lining of the wall. The majority of these tumors are in the rectum and sigmoid colon, which makes them fairly easy to detect with modern diagnostic techniques. Several predisposing factors have been proposed, including heredity, chronic ulcerative colitis, environment, and dietary habits.

Cystic Fibrosis

Cystic fibrosis is a hereditary disorder of the exocrine glands. The greatest threat is associated with the accumulation of excessively thick and adhesive mucus in the air passages, which obstructs bronchioles and restricts air movement, and from obstruction of the pancreatic ducts, which leads to inadequate enzymes for digestion and enzymatic necrosis of the pancreas with accompanying pancreatitis.

Cholelithiasis

Cholelithiasis is the presence or formation of gallstones, usually caused by the precipitation of substances out of the bile normally stored in the gallbladder. Generally, gallstones have a mixed composition, but most of them contain cholesterol, bilirubin, and calcium salts in varying proportions.

Cholecystitis

Cholecystitis is an acute inflammation of the gallbladder, often caused by obstruction of the cystic duct with gallstones. The condition is accompanied by a sudden onset of pain, fever, nausea, and vomiting. Repeated attacks of acute cholecystitis may damage the gallbladder and impair its function.

Pancreatitis

Pancreatitis is an inflammation of the pancreas resulting from autodigestion of pancreatic tissue by its own enzymes. The etiology is unknown, but it is associated with other conditions such as alcoholism, biliary tract obstruction, peptic ulcers, trauma, and certain drugs.

Cirrhosis

Cirrhosis is a liver condition characterized by the loss of normal liver tissue, which is replaced by fibrous bands of connective tissue. In its early stages it is asymptomatic, but as more and more liver tissue is replaced, functional impairments are evident, generally resulting in jaundice and portal hypertension. Cirrhosis of the liver is associated with chronic alcohol abuse, drugs, autoimmune disorders, metabolic and genetic disease, chronic viral infections, and chronic biliary tract obstructions.

Hepatitis

Hepatitis is a common condition characterized by inflammation of the liver tissue. It may be caused by alcoholism, toxic chemicals, parasites, and viruses. In a healthy individual, the liver will regenerate after hepatitis damage, but recurrent episodes may lead to permanent damage, including cirrhosis.

Jaundice

Jaundice is a yellowish discoloration of body tissues resulting from an accumulation of bile pigments (bilirubin), which are derived from the destruction of red blood cells and normally a component of bile. When bile is secreted into the small intestine, the pigments are eliminated in the feces. When a condition disturbs the normal flow of bile, the pigments accumulate in the blood and stain the tissues. The discoloration is most evident in the skin and eyes. Jaundice is not a disease entity but is evidence of a disease process.

Three general mechanisms can lead to jaundice. The first is obstructive jaundice, which is caused by an obstruction in the biliary system that impedes the flow of bile. The second mechanism is hemolytic jaundice, which is caused by excessive hemolysis of red blood cells, the source of the bile pigments. The third mechanism is hepatic jaundice, caused by liver disease, when the liver is unable to adequately process the bile pigments.

Pathology—cont'd

Pancreatic Carcinoma

Pancreatic carcinoma is a devastating malignancy of the pancreas, usually beginning in the head of the organ and progressing to the body and tail. It is rapidly progressive and often the symptoms are not apparent and diagnosed until the disease is in an advanced stage and has metastasized to other organs. Carcinoma in the head of the pancreas may impinge on the common bile duct and cause jaundice. Evidence indicates that smoking and high-fat diets increase the risk of pancreatic carcinoma.

Metastases

Primary tumors in abdominal organs, especially those that are drained by the hepatic portal system, frequently metastasize to the liver. Leukemias and lymphomas also affect the liver. Diffuse metastatic disease in the liver is not curable.

Polycystic Kidney Disease

Polycystic kidney disease is a hereditary disorder characterized by massive enlargement of the kidney and accompanied by the formation of cysts, which interferes with kidney function and ultimately results in renal failure. Renal dialysis and kidney transplant during end-stage renal failure may prolong life.

Development and Position Anomalies

Agenesis, the congenital absence of an organ, and hypoplasia, a congenital abnormally small organ, of the kidney are relatively uncommon. Occasionally the lower poles of the two kidneys are fused resulting in a congenital abnormality called *horseshoe kidney*. Renal function usually is not impaired in the horseshoe kidney. Position anomalies are more common than the development anomalies. In position anomalies, the kidneys are in an abnormal location or rotation. These anomalies usually do not impair renal function unless the ureter is twisted or blocked to impede the flow of urine.

Acute Pyelonephritis

Acute pyelonephritis (commonly called *kidney infection*) is a bacterial infection of the renal parenchyma and renal pelvis usually caused by *Escherichia coli*. This represents probably the most common kidney disease. Kidney infections are more common in women than in men because women have a shorter urethra, making it possible for bacteria from the outside to enter the bladder and progress up the ureters to the kidney. Any condition that causes stagnation of urine or obstructs urine flow predisposes to kidney infection. Antibiotic therapy is usually successful.

Acute Glomerulonephritis

Glomerulonephritis is an inflammation of the capillary loops in the glomeruli of the kidney. This differs from pyelonephritis, which is an inflammation of the interstitial tissue rather than the parenchyma (nephrons) of the kidney. It appears that most cases are the result of an immune response to an inflammatory agent. This may be an infection such as pyelonephritis, some other systemic disease, or toxic chemicals. The severity of the disorder depends on the number of glomeruli involved. Treatment is supportive to maintain electrolyte balance. In some cases, dialysis may be necessary.

Renal Calculi

Renal calculi, or kidney stones, precipitate from crystalline substances in the urine. Most often they form in the calyces or pelvis of the kidney but may occur in the urinary bladder. It is possible that those in the bladder actually developed in the kidney, passed down the ureter asymptomatically, and continued to grow in the bladder. Kidney stones are a common cause of urinary tract obstruction, particularly in adults. Predisposing factors include infections, inflammation, diet, metabolic disorders such as gout, and hyperactivity of the parathyroid gland.

Renal Cysts

Renal cysts are a common abnormality in the adult, particularly in those over the age of 50. Most cysts occur in the lower pole of the kidney and are asymptomatic.

Adenocarcinoma of the Kidney

Renal cell carcinoma (adenocarcinoma) is the most common malignant tumor of the kidney. It occurs twice as frequently in males as in females. Predisposing factors appear to be chronic inflammation, smoking, and exposure to hydrocarbons and other toxic chemicals. The tumors metastasize mainly through the bloodstream to the lungs, brain, bone, liver, and adrenal glands. The earliest symptom frequently is blood in the urine. If detected early enough, renal cell carcinomas are amenable to surgical treatment and may be cured.

Case Study A

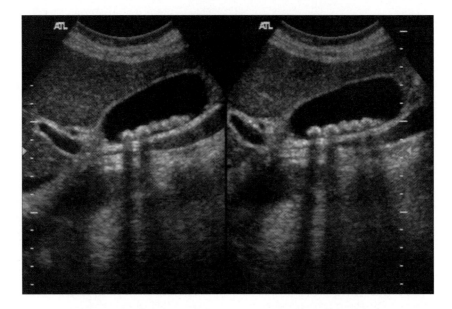

The patient presented to the emergency room with mid-epigastric and right shoulder pain, with nausea and indigestion. The symptoms had persisted for 2 days with an increase in severity. The patient had experienced this sort of "attack" several times within the past 6 years. The emergency physician sent the patient to the sonography department for a gallbladder ultrasound exam. The exam revealed the presence of multiple small stones seen within the gallbladder lumen, causing the classic "shadowing" artifact.

Case Study B

This is an upper gastrointestinal study that utilizes a combination of positive (liquid barium) and negative (air) contrast media. The three radiographs that are presented on the page opposite demonstrate the three-dimensional orientation of the stomach as one progresses distally from the fundus to the pylorus. Radiograph A is an anteroposterior (AP) projection (patient is supine) that demonstrates barium (light gray area) in the fundus and air (dark gray area) in the body and most of the pylorus. Note how the stomach is oriented in a superoinferior direction and from left to right. Radiograph B is a posteroanterior (PA) projection (patient is prone) that demonstrates barium in the body and pylorus and air in the fundus. Radiograph C is a lateral projection (patient is lying on the right side) that shows barium in the pylorus and a portion of the body and air in the fundus. Note that the stomach, in addition to being oriented in a superior to inferior direction, has a posteroanterior orientation. Part of the fundus is superimposed over the thoracic vertebrae. These three images demonstrate the position of the stomach within the abdominal cavity. When the patient lies supine (radiograph A), the liquid barium will flow to the lowest (most posterior) portion of the stomach, which is the fundus, and the air will rise to the highest (most anterior) portion, which is the body and pylorus. When the patient lies prone (radiograph B), the opposite occurs: the liquid barium again flows to the lowest portion, but this time, because of the prone position, this is the most anterior portion, which is the body and pylorus, and the air rises to the highest (or most posterior) region, which is the fundus. Radiographs A and B demonstrate the left to right trajectory of the stomach. When the patient lies on the right side (radiograph C), the liquid barium will flow to the region that is located more to the right, which is the pylorus and part of the body, and the air will rise to the fundus, which is located in the upper left quadrant of the abdominal cavity.

Continued

Case Study B—cont'd

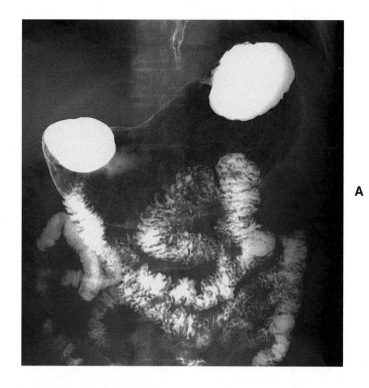

A

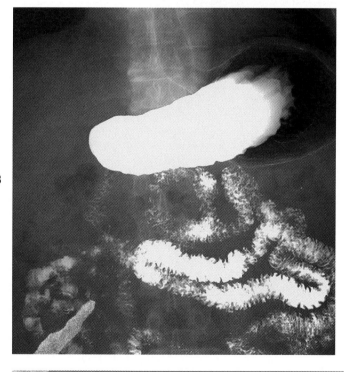

B

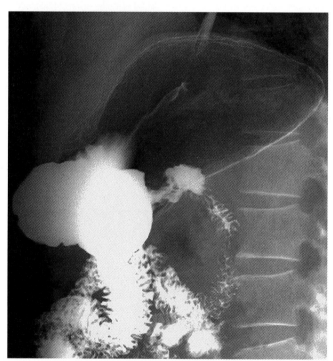

C

· REVIEW QUESTIONS ·

1. What is the superior boundary of the abdomen?
2. What vertebral level is indicated by each of the following planes?
   a. Transpyloric
   b. Subcostal
   c. Interiliac
   d. Transtubercular
3. What is the vertebral level for each of the following openings in the diaphragm?
   a. Aortic hiatus
   b. Caval hiatus
   c. Esophageal hiatus
4. What is the anterior abdominal wall muscle that is on either side of the linea alba?
5. What are the five features that contribute to the longitudinal ridge of the posterior abdominal wall?
6. What are the three unpaired visceral branches of the abdominal aorta and at what level does each one originate from the abdominal aorta?
7. Name six tributaries, in addition to the common iliac veins, that drain directly into the inferior vena cava.
8. What two vessels join to form the hepatic portal vein?
9. What term is used to denote an extension of peritoneum that is associated with the stomach?
10. In addition to portions of the small and large intestines, name two organs and two vessels that are retroperitoneal.
11. What separates the caudate lobe of the liver from the following?
    a. Right lobe
    b. Left lobe
    c. Quadrate lobe
12. What are the four regions of the stomach, and which region is most superior?
13. What portion of the small intestine is retroperitoneal?
14. What portion of the duodenum is most inferior?
15. What portions of the colon are rather mobile because they have a mesentery?
16. What portion of the pancreas is related to the spleen?
17. What branch of the common hepatic artery is located in the head of the pancreas?
18. The ureters are usually associated with what large muscle?
19. What is the anterior relationship of the right suprarenal gland?
20. What is the most superior and posterior portion of the spleen?

· CHAPTER QUIZ ·

Name the Following:

1. The superior abdominal region in the midline.
2. The innermost muscle of the anterolateral abdominal wall.
3. The structure or feature that separates the quadrate lobe of the liver from the right lobe.
4. The most superior portion of the colon.
5. The blood vessel that branches from the aorta just below the transpyloric line.
6. The three structures in a portal triad.
7. The portion of the stomach that superior to the entrance of the esophagus.
8. The portion of the duodenum that is at the L1 vertebral level.
9. The three branches of the celiac trunk.
10. The major blood vessel that is immediately anterior to the right suprarenal gland.

True/False

1. Portions of the liver, stomach, and spleen extend superiorly under the ribs and are protected by the thoracic cage.
2. The aortic hiatus is located at the level of the tenth thoracic vertebra.
3. The kidneys, the pancreas, and the stomach are retroperitoneal.
4. The celiac trunk arises from the aorta just above the transpyloric plane near the superior margin of the first lumbar vertebra.
5. The renal arteries are paired and arise from the aorta at the level of the third lumbar vertebra.
6. The hepatic veins, renal veins, and the left gonadal vein drain directly into the inferior vena cava.
7. Blood normally flows from the inferior mesenteric vein into the superior mesenteric vein.
8. The greater curvature of the stomach is directed inferiorly and to the right, and it has the greater omentum attached to it.
9. The third part of the duodenum is horizontal and is related to the inferior margin of the head of the pancreas.
10. The head of the pancreas is the most superior portion and is located on the right side of the midline, adjacent to the spleen.

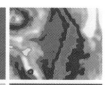

OBJECTIVES

Upon completion of this chapter, the student should be able to do the following:
- Define the term *pelvis.*
- Differentiate between the greater, or false, pelvis and the lesser, or true, pelvis.
- Describe the features of the sacrum and coccyx.
- Name the three bones that form the os coxa and describe the features of the os coxa.
- Compare the structure of the os coxa in the child and in the adult.
- Identify the two principal muscles that line the wall of the true pelvis.
- Describe the structures that support the pelvic viscera and prevent them from falling through the pelvic outlet.
- Describe the vascular supply to the pelvis.
- Name two nerves that emerge from the sacral plexus and state the importance of each.
- Describe the anterior relationships of the rectum both in the male and in the female.
- Compare the relationships of the urinary organs both in the male and in the female.
- Describe the normal location and attachments of the ovaries and factors that may alter the location.
- Identify the largest ligament that supports the uterus and name three smaller supporting ligaments.
- Describe the normal position and relationships of the uterus.
- Describe the relationships of the fornix of the vagina to the cervix.
- Describe the structure and location of the testes and the epididymis.
- Describe the structure of the scrotum and the spermatic cord.
- Identify three accessory glands of the male reproductive system and describe the location of each gland.
- Discuss the relationships of the seminal vesicles and prostate glands.
- Identify and compare the three muscles in the urogenital region of the perineum in the male and in the female.
- Describe and discuss the relationships of the female external genitalia.

- Compare the dorsal and ventral columns of erectile tissue in both the body and in the root of the penis.
- Compare vessel and muscle relationships in transverse sections through the sacroiliac joint and in transverse sections through the lower part of the sacrum.
- Distinguish between the rectovesicle pouch, the vesicouterine pouch, and the rectouterine pouch.
- Identify the muscles, viscera, blood vessels, and skeletal components of the female pelvis in transverse, sagittal, and coronal sections.
- Identify the muscles, viscera, and blood vessels, and skeletal components of the male pelvis in transverse, sagittal, and coronal sections.

General Anatomy of the Pelvis

The term *pelvis* is ambiguous and confusing because it has a variety of meanings in modern usage. First of all, pelvis is used to describe a loosely defined region of the body where the trunk meets the lower limbs. The term is also applied to the bony ring formed by the sacrum, the coccyx, and the two hip bones. This structure is sometimes referred to as the *bony pelvis*. The term also can describe the cavity that is enclosed by the bony pelvis. This is the pelvic cavity. Generally the context of the discussion clarifies the meaning.

PELVIC CAVITY

The bony pelvis encloses a funnel, or basin-shaped, cavity that is the inferior portion of the larger abdominopelvic cavity. The pelvic cavity is divided into a pelvis major, or false pelvis, and a pelvis minor, or true pelvis. The cavity of the pelvis major is the space between the iliac fossae and its inferior boundary is defined by the pelvic brim. It is considered to be a part of the abdominal cavity and it contains abdominal viscera, such as portions of the small intestine and the sigmoid colon. The iliac crest is such an obvious dividing point on transverse sections that the pelvis major is included in the discussion of pelvis rather than with the abdomen.

The minor pelvis is the space below the pelvic brim and is enclosed by the sacrum, the ischium, the pubis, and the pelvic portions of the ilium. It contains the urinary bladder, the rectum, the internal reproductive organs, and portions of the mobile intestinal tract that may be able to reach it.

OSSEOUS COMPONENTS

The bony framework of the pelvis is formed by the sacrum, the coccyx, and the paired os coxae, or hip bones.

Sacrum

The sacrum and the coccyx, which are illustrated in Fig. 6-1, make up the posterior midline portion of the bony pelvis. The sacrum transmits the weight of the body to the hip bones and then to the lower extremities. Normally, five sacral vertebrae fuse into one triangular mass, called the *sacrum*, that articulates with the fifth lumbar vertebrae superiorly, the coccyx inferiorly, and the os coxae laterally. Where the sacrum meets the fifth lumbar vertebrae, the sacrum is tilted posteriorly to form a **lumbosacral angle.** In some individuals the first sacral vertebra remains separate from the other four, or the fifth lumbar vertebrae may fuse with the sacrum. Both conditions put a strain on the near-

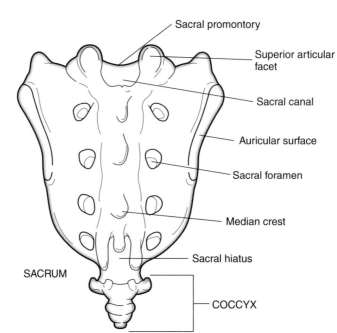

FIG. 6-1 The sacrum and coccyx.

Sacral promontory

Superior articular facet

Sacral canal

Auricular surface

Sacral foramen

Median crest

Sacral hiatus

SACRUM

COCCYX

est intervertebral articulation, which may result in joint degeneration and cause low back pain.

When the five sacral vertebrae fuse together they form a normal curvature so that the anterior or pelvic surface is concave. Anteriorly, the upper margin of the first sacral vertebrae forms the **sacral promontory,** which marks the posterior portion of the true pelvic inlet or pelvic brim. Both the anterior and posterior surfaces of the sacrum have two rows of four holes, or openings, called **sacral foramina.** Branches of the sacral nerves pass through the sacral foramina. On the posterior surface, between the sacral foramina, poorly defined and fused spinous processes form the **median crest.** The fifth sacral vertebrae has no spinous process or lamina. This deficiency in the neural arch leaves a midline opening called the **sacral hiatus.** Local anesthetics may be injected through the sacral hiatus. This procedure is called *extradural, epidural,* or *caudal anesthesia.*

On each side of the upper portion of the sacrum is a rather large **auricular surface** for articulation with the iliac bones to form the **sacroiliac (iliosacral) joint.** The connection between the bones is further enhanced by strong **interosseous ligaments** that act as cords to bind the bones together.

Coccyx

The most inferior portion of the vertebral column is the **coccyx,** or tailbone, which is joined to the sacrum by cartilage. It usually consists of four rudimentary vertebrae with no processes or foramina, although the number varies from three to five. During adulthood, the bones of the coccyx usually fuse to form a single structure. The coccyx offers no support for the vertebral column but does provide attachment for a portion of the gluteus maximus muscle and some of the muscles of the pelvic floor. Sometimes during child-

birth or a fall the sacrum and coccyx may separate, resulting in pain, especially when sitting.

Os Coxae

The **os coxae** (innominate bones) are commonly called the *hip bones.* Each os coxa consists of an **ilium, pubis,** and **ischium.** In the child these are three separate bones joined together by hyaline cartilage and each bone has its own ossification center within the cartilage. Ossification continues during childhood until the cartilage is replaced by bone. By puberty, only a small amount of cartilage remains as a Y-shaped region where the three bones meet in the acetabulum. When ossification is completed, the ilium, the ischium, and the pubis are fused together to form a single unit called the *os coxa,* which is illustrated in Fig. 6-2.

The **ilium** is the largest of the three bones of the os coxa. The superior part of the ilium presents a large, flaring, wing-like surface called the **ala.** The inner aspect of the ala is the **iliac fossa,** which is the origin of the iliacus muscle. The **iliac crest,** the most superior portion of the hip bone, is the superior margin of the ala. The crest terminates both anteriorly and posteriorly in short projections, the **superior** and **inferior iliac spines.** Posteriorly, the ilium articulates with the sacrum at the **sacroiliac joint.**

The bodies of the two **pubic bones** meet in the anterior midline at the **symphysis pubis.** A small projection that is just lateral to the body forms the **pubic tubercle** and from this point the **superior pubic ramus** extends laterally to meet the ilium. The pelvic surface of the superior margin of the superior pubic ramus is sharp and forms the **pectineal line,** which is continuous with the arcuate line of the ilium and the sacral promontory to mark the pelvic brim. The **inferior pubic ramus** extends inferiorly from the body to connect with the ischium. The inferior rami of the two pubic

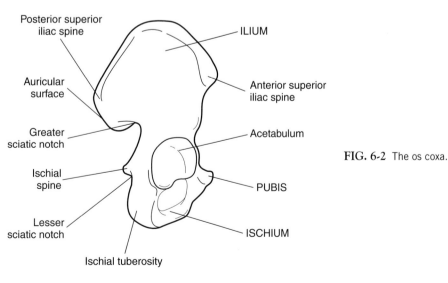

Posterior superior iliac spine

ILIUM

Auricular surface

Anterior superior iliac spine

Greater sciatic notch

Acetabulum

FIG. 6-2 The os coxa.

Ischial spine

PUBIS

Lesser sciatic notch

ISCHIUM

Ischial tuberosity

OS COXA (right, lateral view)

TABLE 6-1 *Important Markings on the Coxal Bones*

Marking	Description	Purpose
Acetabulum	Deep depression on lateral surface of coxal bone	Socket for articulation with head of femur (thigh bone)
Obturator foramen	Large opening between the pubis and ischium	Passageway for blood vessels, nerves, muscle tendons; largest foramen in the body
Ilium	Large flaring region that forms the major portion of the coxal bone	
Alae (wings)	Large flared portions of the ilium	Large area for numerous muscle attachments; forms false pelvis
Iliac crest	Thickened superior margin of the ilium	Muscle attachment; forms prominence of hips
Anterior superior iliac spine	Blunt projection at anterior end of the iliac crest	Attachment for muscles of trunk, hip, thigh; can be easily palpated
Posterior superior iliac spine	Blunt projection at posterior end of the iliac crest	Attachment for muscles of trunk, hip, thigh
Anterior inferior iliac spine	Projection on ilium inferior to the anterior superior iliac spine	Attachment for muscles of trunk, hip, thigh
Posterior inferior iliac spine	Projection on ilium inferior to the posterior superior iliac spine	Attachment for muscles of trunk, hip, thigh
Greater sciatic notch	Deep indentation inferior to the posterior inferior iliac spine	Passageway for sciatic nerve and some muscle tendons
Iliac fossa	Slight concavity on medial surface of alae	Attachment for iliacus muscle
Auricular surface	Large, rough region at posterior margin of iliac fossa	Articulates with sacrum to form the sacroiliac joint
Iliopectineal (arcuate) line	Sharp curved line at inferior margin of iliac fossa	Attachment for muscles; marks the pelvic brim
Ischium	Lower, posterior portion of the coxal bone	
Ischial spine	Projection near junction of ilium and ischium; projects into pelvic cavity	Attachment for a major ligament; distance between the two spines tells the size of the pelvic cavity
Ischial tuberosity	Large rough inferior portion of ischium	Muscle attachment; portion on which we sit; strongest part of the coxal bones
Lesser sciatic notch	Indentation below the ischial spine	Passageway for blood vessels and nerves
Pubis	Most anterior part of coxal bone	
Pubic symphysis	Anterior midline where two pubic bones meet	
Pubic rami	Armlike portions that project from the pubic symphysis	Form margins of the obturator foramen
Pubic arch	V-shaped arch inferior to the pubic symphysis formed by the inferior pubic rami	Broadens or narrows the dimensions of the true pelvis

bones meet at the symphysis pubis to form the **pubic arch,** or **subpubic angle.** This angle is usually less than 70 degrees in the male and greater than 80 degrees in the female.

The inferior portion of the os coxa is formed by the **ischium.** Anteriorly, the ramus of the ischium meets the inferior pubic ramus at an indistinct point; together they are often called the **ischiopubic ramus.** The posterior and inferior border of the ischium is formed by a bulky, rough area called the **ischial tuberosity.** A sharp, pointed **ischial spine** divides the space between the ischial tuberosity and ilium into the **lesser sciatic notch,** which is between the ischial tuberosity and the ischial spine, and the **greater sciatic** notch, which is between the ischial spine and the ilium. The notches are made into foramina by ligaments and they are closed by muscles.

The ilium, ischium, and pubis meet in the **acetabulum,** which is a deep fossa for articulation with the head of the femur. The three bones also surround an opening called the **obturator foramen,** which is directed inferiorly. This foramen is closed by the obturator membrane and muscles. The **pelvic outlet** (inferior pelvic aperture) must also be covered to give support and maintain the pelvic viscera in position. The features of the os coxa are summarized in Table 6-1. Refer to Figs. 6-2 and 6-3 to identify the features.

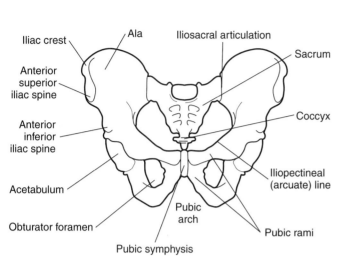

FIG. 6-3 Bones of the pelvis: sacrum, coccyx, and os coxae.

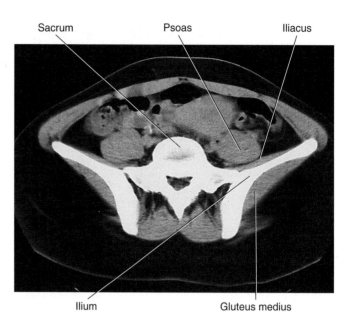

FIG. 6-4 CT image of the muscles in the wall of the false pelvis.

TABLE 6-2   *Pelvic Muscles*

Muscle	Origin	Insertion	Action	Innervation
Iliacus	Iliac fossa	Lesser trochanter of femur	Flexes thigh	Femoral nerve
Psoas	Lumbar vertebrae	Lesser trochanter of femur	Flexes thigh	Ventral rami of lumbar nerves
Obturator internus	Inner surface of pelvis	Greater trochanter of femur	Rotates thigh	Branches of L5 and S1
Piriformis	Anterior surface of sacrum	Greater trochanter of femur	Rotates and abducts thigh	Branches of S1 and S2
Levator ani	Inside pelvis from pubis to sacrum	Coccyx and levator ani on opposite side	Supports pelvic viscera	Pudendal nerve
Coccygeus	Spine of ischium	Sacrum and coccyx	Supports pelvic viscera	Branches of pudendal nerve

MUSCULAR COMPONENTS

Functionally, the muscles of the pelvic wall are associated with movements of the thigh. Other muscles, such as the gluteal muscles and the anterior thigh muscles, are external to the pelvis but are seen in pelvic sections. These muscles will be mentioned here and described in greater detail with the lower extremity. Table 6-2 summarizes the pelvic muscles.

Muscles in the Wall of the Greater (False) Pelvis

The muscles in the wall of the greater, or false, pelvis are actually abdominal muscles. The two principal muscles, **psoas** and **iliacus,** extend throughout the whole pelvic region and continue into the anterior thigh. The computed tomographic image in Fig. 6-4 illustrates these two muscles in a transverse plane.

The long, fleshy psoas muscle appears as a muscle mass lateral to the vertebral bodies as it continues from the abdomen into the pelvis. The muscle passes deep to the inguinal ligament as it continues from the pelvis into the thigh, where it inserts on the lesser trochanter of the femur. The psoas muscle acts with the iliacus muscle as a powerful flexor of the thigh. Lumbar nerves provide the innervation.

The iliacus is a fan-shaped muscle that originates along the crest and fossa of the ilium, and lines the iliac fossa. In the pelvis, it appears lateral to the psoas muscle. Fibers of the iliacus muscle insert on the femur with the psoas muscle. Because the iliacus and psoas muscles appear to merge into one muscle and they have a close functional relationship, the two muscles are often referred to as the single *iliopsoas muscle*. The iliacus is innervated by the femoral nerve, which is a branch of the lumbar plexus.

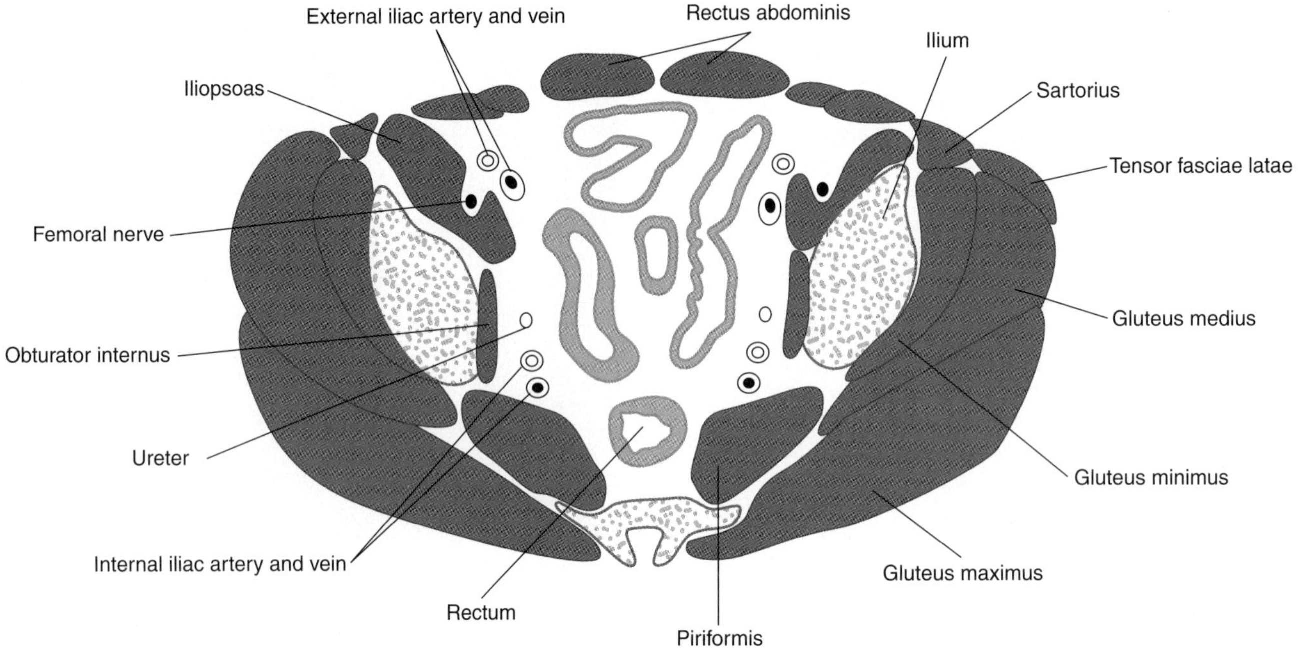

External iliac artery and vein

Rectus abdominis

Ilium

Iliopsoas

Sartorius

Tensor fasciae latae

Femoral nerve

Obturator internus

Gluteus medius

Ureter

Gluteus minimus

Internal iliac artery and vein

Gluteus maximus

Rectum

Piriformis

FIG. 6-5 Muscles associated with the true pelvis.

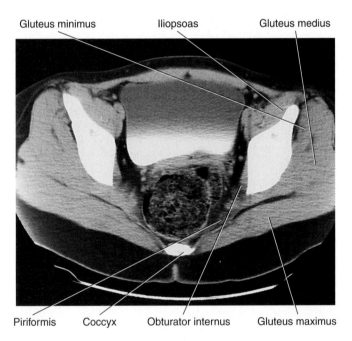

Gluteus minimus   Iliopsoas   Gluteus medius

Piriformis   Coccyx   Obturator internus   Gluteus maximus

FIG. 6-6 CT image of the muscles associated with the true pelvis.

Muscles in the Wall of the True Pelvis

Most of the inner surface of the bony true pelvis is lined with muscle. The **obturator internus** and **piriformis** muscles are the principal muscles that make up the wall of the true pelvis and form this lining. See the line drawing in Fig. 6-5 for an illustration of these two muscles. Fig. 6-6 is a computed tomographic image of these muscles.

The **obturator internus** muscle is a fan-shaped muscle that covers most of the lateral wall of the true pelvis. It originates on the inner surface of the pelvic bones and crosses over the **obturator foramen** to close off the opening, then leaves the pelvis through the **lesser sciatic notch.** As it passes through the lesser sciatic notch, it becomes tendinous and makes a sharp turn to insert on the medial surface of the greater trochanter. The obturator internus is innervated by branches from L5 and S1 that form the nerve to the obturator internus. This muscle rotates the thigh.

The **piriformis** muscle is located partially on the posterior wall of the true pelvis and partially external to the pelvis, posterior to the hip joint. It originates on the anterior surface of the sacrum and passes through the **greater sciatic notch** to insert on the greater trochanter of the femur. The piriformis is closely associated with the sacral nerve plexus and is innervated by sacral nerves. It rotates and abducts the thigh.

Muscles of the Pelvic Floor

The pelvic outlet (inferior pelvic aperture) must be covered to give support and to maintain the position of the pelvic viscera. The floor of the pelvis includes all structures contributing to this support, that is, the peritoneum, the pelvic diaphragm, and the urogenital diaphragm. The principal structure supporting the pelvic viscera is the **pelvic diaphragm,** which forms a muscular pelvic floor. It is a hammock-like structure consisting primarily of the **levator ani** and **coccygeus** muscles. Below (superficial to) the pelvic diaphragm, the urogenital diaphragm is formed by connec-

TABLE 6-3 *Extrapelvic Muscles*

Muscle	Description
Gluteus maximus	The largest and most superficial muscle of the gluteal region; forms most of the mass of the buttocks
Gluteus medius	A thick, broad muscle of the gluteal region; located deep to the gluteus maximus but originating more superiorly, which results in the covering of the inferior one third by the gluteus maximus
Gluteus minimus	The smallest and deepest muscle of the gluteal region; underlies both the gluteus maximus and the gluteus medius
Gemelli	Two small muscle masses inferior to the piriformis muscle and deep to the lower part of the gluteus maximus; associated with the obturator internus tendon
Quadratus femoris	A short, flat, rectangular muscle that is located inferior to the gemelli and the extrapelvic portions of the obturator internus muscles
Tensor fasciae latae	A superficial muscle of the superior lateral thigh; overlies the superior lateral portion of the gluteus medius
Sartorius	A long, straplike muscle that courses obliquely and inferiorly across the anterior thigh; most superficial muscle of the anterior thigh
Rectus femoris	A large ropelike muscle mass that extends the length of the anterior thigh; one of the quadriceps femoris muscle group
Vastus lateralis	A large muscle that forms the lateral portion of the thigh; partially covered by the iliotibial fascia; one of the quadriceps femoris muscle group
Vastus medialis	A large muscle that forms the medial portion of the thigh; one of the quadriceps femoris muscle group
Vastus intermedius	An elongated muscle next to the shaft of the femur; deep to the rectus femoris, between the other two vastus muscles; one of the quadriceps femoris group
Pectineus	A flat muscle, medial to the iliopsoas, in the floor of the femoral triangle; apparent anterior to the pubic bone in transverse sections
Adductor longus	A superficial, flat muscle that extends obliquely from the pubis to the femur; medial to the pectineus
Adductor brevis	A flat muscle deep to the adductor longus on the medial aspect of the thigh
Adductor magnus	The largest of the adductor muscles in the medial compartment of the thigh; deep to the adductor longus and adductor brevis
Obturator externus	A relatively small, fan-shaped muscle that covers the obturator foramen; closely associated with the adductor muscles
Gracilis	A thin, straplike, superficial band of muscle that extends down the medial aspect of the thigh from the pubis to the tibia
Biceps femoris	A large, elongated muscle on the posterior and lateral aspects of the thigh; the superior portion is deep to the gluteus maximus; one of the hamstring muscles
Semitendinosus	A superficial muscle medial to the biceps femoris; the superior portion is deep to the gluteus maximus; one of the hamstring muscles
Semimembranosus	A fleshy muscle, deep and medial to the semitendinosus; one of the hamstring muscles

tive tissue membranes located within the infrapubic angle between the ischiopubic rami.

Of the two muscles that form the pelvic diaphragm, the **levator ani** is the larger and more important. The integrity of the pelvic floor depends on the appropriate function of the levator ani muscles. In females, these muscles are particularly vulnerable during a strenuous delivery. When the muscles are damaged, support for the pelvic viscera is weakened. This may be followed by urinary incontinence and prolapse of the uterus. The levator ani muscles originate on the pelvic surface of the pubis and the spine of the ischium. The fibers converge to insert on the coccyx and some fibers insert on the muscle of the opposite side. The levator ani muscles are innervated by the pudendal nerve.

The **coccygeus** muscle is the smaller of the two muscles that form the pelvic diaphragm. From its origin on the spine of the ischium, the fibers fan out to form a triangular sheet that inserts on the sacrum and coccyx. Branches of the pudendal nerve innervate the coccygeus muscle.

Extrapelvic Muscles Seen in Pelvic Sections

Numerous muscles, such as the gluteal muscles and the thigh muscles, are external to the pelvis but are apparent in sections through the pelvis. These muscles are associated with the hip joint and movement of the lower extremity. Some of the more important and obvious extrapelvic muscles are named and described briefly in Table 6-3. They are discussed in more detail with the lower extremity. Some of these muscles are illustrated with the pelvic wall muscles in Figs. 6-5 and 6-6.

Vascular Components

At the level of the fourth lumbar vertebra, the abdominal aorta divides into the right and left **common iliac arteries.** These vessels descend to the pelvic brim, where they pass over the sacroiliac joint at the level of the disc between the fifth lumbar vertebra and the sacrum. At this point, the common iliac arteries divide into the **external** and **internal iliac arteries.** The external iliac artery follows the pelvic brim, then passes under the inguinal ligament to become the femoral artery, which continues through the thigh. The internal iliac artery, a short vessel that is only 4 cm long, branches profusely. Parietal branches supply blood to the pelvic wall and the visceral branches supply blood to the pelvic organs. Blood is drained from the pelvis primarily by the internal iliac veins and their tributaries.

Nerve Supply to the Pelvis

Portions of the fourth and fifth lumbar nerves unite to form a thick cord-like **lumbosacral trunk,** which descends obliquely over the sacroiliac joint to enter the pelvis. Within the pelvis, the lumbosacral trunk joins with the first four sacral nerves to form the **sacral plexus,** which lies on the piriformis muscle. Numerous nerves emerge from the sacral plexus to supply pelvic structures, the buttocks, and the lower limb. Two of these nerves, the sciatic nerve and the pudendal nerve, are included in this discussion. With a few exceptions, branches of the sacral plexus leave the pelvis through the greater sciatic notch (foramen).

Sciatic Nerve

The **sciatic** nerve, one of the branches of the sacral plexus, is the largest nerve in the body. The sciatic nerve passes through the greater sciatic notch (foramen) at the lower border of the piriformis muscle to enter the gluteal region, then it descends in the posterior compartment of the thigh. Its branches supply the flexor muscles of the thigh and all the muscles of the leg and foot. Because of its location, the sciatic nerve may be injured in dislocations and fractures of the hip. It is also vulnerable when giving intramuscular injections into the buttock.

Pudendal Nerve

The **pudendal** nerve, another branch of the sacral plexus, leaves the pelvis through the lesser sciatic notch (foramen) to supply the perineum, the external anal sphincter, and the sensory fibers of the external genitalia. This is the nerve anesthetized in a pudendal nerve block during childbirth and during surgical procedures on the female genitalia.

Obturator Nerve

The **obturator** nerve does not arise from the sacral plexus but from the lumbar plexus of nerves in the abdomen. It enters the pelvis and runs along the lateral pelvic wall then leaves through the obturator foramen. The obturator nerve supplies the obturator externus muscle and the adductor muscles of the thigh. It also sends branches to the hip and knee joints. Because of its proximity to pelvic lymph nodes, it is vulnerable to injury during surgery for malignant disease in the pelvis. It may also be affected by changes in the ovary, which is near the nerve. Because the nerve supplies both the hip and knee joints, pain from the hip may be referred to the knee, making it difficult to locate the cause.

Viscera of the Pelvis

Gastrointestinal Organs

Most of the length of the gastrointestinal tract is located in the abdomen. Loops of the mobile small intestine, especially the ileum, may extend into the pelvis. Portions of the colon are normally located within the false pelvis and if the mobile transverse colon is particularly pendulous, it may extend down into the true pelvis. Because of the mobility of the portions of the gastrointestinal tract that have a mesentery, the amount in the pelvis is variable.

The cecum and ascending colon are normally found within the greater or false pelvis on the right side. The descending colon on the left side becomes continuous with the sigmoid colon at the pelvic brim. In contrast to the descending colon, which is retroperitoneal, the sigmoid colon is surrounded by peritoneum and has a mesentery, which allows considerable mobility. At its junction with the rectum, the sigmoid colon becomes fixed to the posterior pelvic wall.

The rectum begins near the middle of the sacrum and follows the curvature of the sacrum and coccyx onto the pelvic floor. The levator ani muscle supports the rectum on the pelvic floor. The rectum penetrates the levator ani muscle to become the anal canal. In the female, the peritoneum over the anterior surface of the rectum extends to the surface of the uterus and forms the **rectouterine pouch.** Inferior to the rectouterine pouch, the rectum is related anteriorly to the vagina. In the male, the upper portion of the rectum is separated from the urinary bladder by peritoneum, which forms the **rectovesical pouch.** Inferior to this, the rectum is related anteriorly to the urinary bladder, the seminal vesicles, and the prostate without the intervening peritoneum.

Urinary Organs

The upper half of each **ureter** is located in the abdomen, but the lower half enters the pelvis. The ureter crosses over the pelvic brim near the bifurcation of the common iliac artery. As it enters the pelvis, the ureter is anterior to the internal iliac artery and follows a course similar to that of the vessel. Retroperitoneally located and closely adherent to the peritoneum over it, the ureter descends along the lateral pelvic wall to a point near the ischial spine, where it turns medially to enter the urinary bladder on its posterior surface.

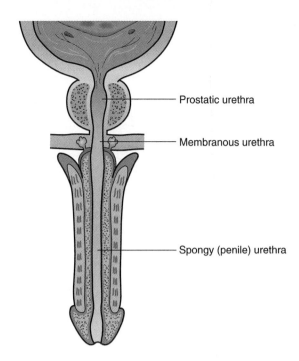

Prostatic urethra

Membranous urethra

Spongy (penile) urethra

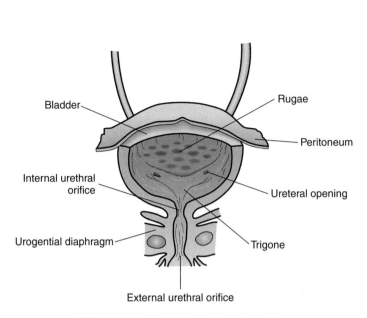

Bladder

Rugae

Peritoneum

Internal urethral orifice

Ureteral opening

Urogential diaphragm

Trigone

External urethral orifice

FIG. 6-7 Urinary bladder and female urethra.

FIG. 6-8 Three regions of the male urethra.

The **urinary bladder** is a distensible, muscular organ that, when empty, lies entirely within the true pelvis. As it fills, the bladder may extend into the abdomen. In the female, the urinary bladder rests on the pelvic floor posterior to the symphysis pubis. In the male, the prostate gland is between the urinary bladder and the pelvic floor. The superior surface is covered by peritoneum and is related to the sigmoid colon and coils of the ileum. In the female, the peritoneum reflects from the superior surface of the bladder onto the anterior wall of the uterus to form the **vesicouterine** pouch. In the male, the peritoneum reflects from the superior surface of the bladder over the ductus deferens and the seminal vesicles onto the rectum to form the **rectovesical** pouch. Held in place by peritoneal ligaments, the bladder is relatively movable except in the inferior neck region where it is firmly anchored. In the female, the neck is attached to the pelvic diaphragm. In the male, the neck rests on the prostate gland. Urine is conveyed from the bladder to the exterior through the urethra.

Internally, the mucosal lining of the bladder is arranged in irregular folds, which allow for expansion. The oblique openings of the two ureters, which convey urine from the kidneys to the bladder, are in the base of the bladder. These two openings plus the **internal urethral orifice** form a triangular region, called the **trigone,** in the base. This is illustrated in Fig. 6-7. The trigone is the region of the bladder that is most sensitive to pain.

The **female urethra,** illustrated with the urinary bladder in Fig. 6-7, is a short, muscular tube about 4 cm long that conveys urine from the bladder to the exterior. The external urethral orifice opens into the vestibule just anterior to the vagina. About five times as long as the female

urethra, the **male urethra** opens to the exterior at the tip of the glans penis. For descriptive purposes, it may be divided into three regions. The **prostatic urethra** passes through the substance of the prostate gland, and the ejaculatory duct and ducts from the prostate gland open into this portion. The **membranous urethra,** the shortest and narrowest portion, penetrates the urogenital diaphragm to enter the penis. The final portion is the **penile** or **spongy urethra.** This is the longest part, extending the full length of the corpus spongiosum of the penis. The ducts of the bulbourethral glands open into the proximal region of the spongy urethra. Fig. 6-8 illustrates the three parts of the male urethra.

Female Reproductive Organs

The female reproductive organs that are located within the pelvic cavity are the ovaries, uterine tubes, uterus, and a portion of the vagina. These are illustrated in Fig. 6-9.

To visualize the relationships of these organs and their peritoneal ligaments, it is necessary to understand the nature of the primary peritoneal fold in the female pelvis. The peritoneum projects upward in a fold over the midline uterus and then drapes from the uterine tubes that extend laterally from the uterus. To visualize this, imagine an individual standing with arms outstretched at the sides with a sheet draped over the head and arms. The sheet illustrates the peritoneum, the body represents the uterus, and the arms portray the uterine tubes. This large fold of peritoneum, called the **broad ligament,** divides the pelvic cavity into two compartments. One compartment contains the urinary bladder and the other compartment contains the rectum.

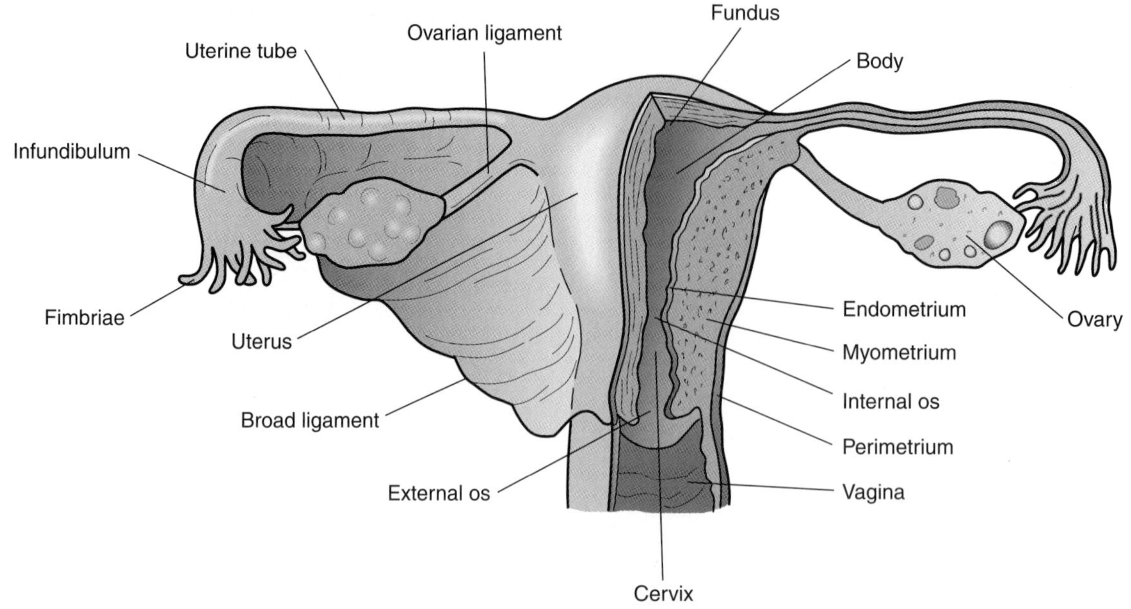

FIG. 6-9 Internal female reproductive organs.

A girl is born with about a quarter of a million primary oocytes, each capable of developing into a mature ovum. This multitude of potential ova is contained in a pair of **ovaries.** Each ovary is a small, solid, oval structure about 3 cm long. It resembles an almond in size and shape. After menopause the ovaries gradually become smaller.

Each ovary is located in an ovarian fossa, a shallow depression in the lateral wall of the pelvis, on either side of the uterus. Three peritoneal ligaments loosely anchor the ovary in place. The **mesovarium** attaches the ovary to the posterior layer of the broad ligament of the uterus. The **ovarian ligament,** a cord-like thickening in the broad ligament, attaches the ovary to the lateral wall of the uterus. An extension of the broad ligament, the **suspensory ligament,** carries the ovarian vessels and attaches the ovary to the lateral pelvic wall. The position of the ovaries varies considerably, especially during pregnancy when they are moved upward by the expanding uterus. Loops of intestine may also displace the ovaries.

The outer ovarian tissue is granulated in appearance because of the presence of the numerous ovarian follicles. Each month an ovarian follicle matures into a Graafian follicle. At ovulation, the mature follicle ruptures to release an oocyte, with some surrounding follicular cells, into the peritoneal cavity.

The two slender **uterine tubes,** also called **fallopian tubes** or **oviducts,** are about 10 or 12 cm long. They are in the upper border of the broad ligament and extend from the upper lateral angle of the uterus to the region of the ovary. The lumen of the tube is continuous with the cavity of the uterus. Near the ovary, the tube expands to form a funnel-shaped **infundibulum,** which is edged with finger-like extensions called **fimbriae.**

The ovary and the uterine tube are not directly connected; however, some of the fimbriae may touch the ovary. The ovulated oocyte is swept into the tube by a current set up in the peritoneal fluid by the beating motion of the fimbriae. Once inside the tube, the oocyte is propelled by the cilia that line the tube and by the contraction of smooth muscle in the walls. Passage through the uterine tube takes about 3 days.

Fertilization, if it occurs, usually takes place while the oocyte is moving through the uterine tube. The fertilized ovum, or zygote, continues the passage into the uterus for implantation and subsequent development. Occasionally something interferes with the passage into the uterus and implantation occurs in the uterine tube. This results in an ectopic tubal pregnancy. The uterine tube cannot expand sufficiently to accommodate the growing embryo, consequently it is likely to rupture. This may result in a severe, life-threatening hemorrhage that necessitates immediate surgery to control the bleeding.

The proximal end of each uterine tube opens into the uterine cavity. The infundibular, or distal, end opens into the peritoneal cavity. These openings in the uterine tubes permit communication between the external environment and the peritoneal cavity and provide a pathway for pathogens to enter the abdominopelvic cavity.

The **uterus,** a hollow muscular organ shaped somewhat like a pear, functions to receive the embryo that results from a fertilized egg and to sustain its life during development. Although its size and shape change greatly during pregnancy, the typical, nonpregnant, premenopausal uterus is about 7 or 8 cm long and 5 cm across at its widest part. It is located in the anterior portion of the pelvic cavity, above the vagina. The uterus is usually tilted forward relative to

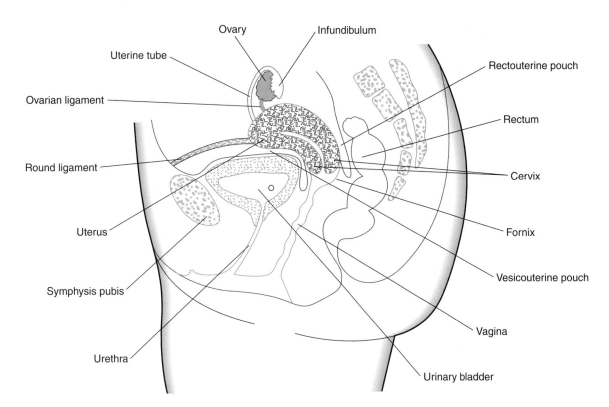

FIG. 6-10 Relationships of the uterus.

the vagina (anteverted) and is bent forward over the upper surface of the urinary bladder (anteflexed). Occasionally, the uterus tilts posteriorly in a retroverted position.

The wall of the uterus is relatively thick and is composed of three layers. The lining, called the **endometrium,** is a special type of mucous membrane that is covered with columnar epithelium and contains numerous glands. It also contains blood vessels and connective tissue. The middle layer, or **myometrium,** is a thick layer of interlaced smooth muscle fibers. Contraction of the myometrium helps expel the fetus from the uterus during childbirth. A layer of serous peritoneum, called the **perimetrium,** covers the outside of the uterus. The perimetrium is continuous with the broad ligament.

The upper two thirds of the uterus, called the **body,** has a bulging superior surface known as the **fundus.** When the uterus is anteverted and anteflexed, the fundus is directed anteriorly. The **uterine tubes,** or oviducts, enter the uterus at its broadest part, between the fundus and the body. The lower one third of the uterus is a tubular **cervix** that extends downward into the upper portion of the **vagina.** The opening of the cervix into the vagina is called the **external os.** When the uterus is in its normal anteflexed position, it is bent forward on its own axis so that the body is at an angle to the cervix. Fig. 6-10 illustrates some of the relationships of the uterus.

Folds of peritoneum anchor and support the uterus in the pelvic cavity. Laterally the peritoneum extends from the anterior and posterior uterine surfaces to the lateral pelvic wall. This peritoneal extension is the **broad ligament,** which not only supports the uterus but also encloses the uterine tubes. A pair of **round ligaments** extend from the lateral walls of the uterus, near the uterine tubes, to the anterior pelvic wall. The round ligaments pass through the inguinal canal on each side and attach to the subcutaneous tissue of the **labia majora.** The **uterosacral ligaments** extend from the uterus to attach on the sacrum. The **lateral cervical (cardinal) ligaments** extend from the lateral walls of the cervix to the pelvic floor and primarily stabilize the cervix. Even with the support of the various ligaments, the body of the uterus is relatively mobile and its principal support is the muscles of the pelvic floor and pelvic viscera.

Peritoneum is reflected from the superior surface of the bladder onto the uterus forming the **vesicouterine** pouch. This pouch, or space, is usually empty but may contain a loop of small intestine. The peritoneum continues over the surface of the uterus as the perimetrium, then it is reflected onto the rectum. This forms the **rectouterine** pouch, or pouch of Douglas. The vesicouterine and rectouterine spaces are sometimes called cul-de-sacs.

The **vagina** plays a key role both in the beginning and in the end of the reproductive process. In addition to receiving the erect male penis during coitus, it functions as the birth canal during parturition, or childbirth. The vagina is a muscular tube that is 10 to 15 cm long and extends from the cervix of the uterus to the vestibule on the exterior. It is situated between the urethra and bladder anteriorly and the rectum posteriorly.

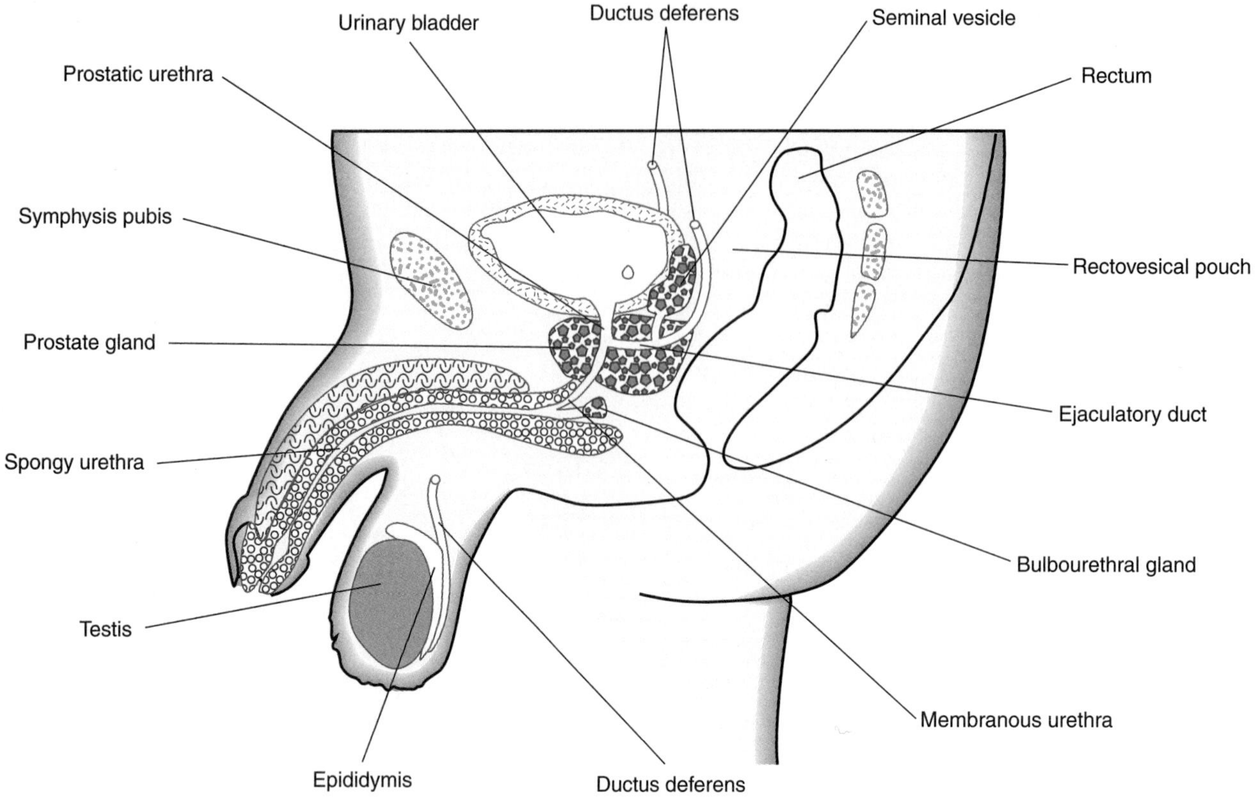

Urinary bladder

Ductus deferens

Seminal vesicle

Rectum

Prostatic urethra

Symphysis pubis

Rectovesical pouch

Prostate gland

Ejaculatory duct

Spongy urethra

Bulbourethral gland

Testis

Membranous urethra

Epididymis

Ductus deferens

FIG. 6-11 Relationships of the male reproductive organs.

The cervix of the uterus projects into the vagina at an angle, which makes the anterior wall of the vagina shorter than the posterior wall. The vagina forms recesses, or spaces, around the cervix, which are called **fornices** (singular, **fornix**). The posterior fornix is longer than the anterior fornix because of the angle at which the cervix enters the vagina. The posterior fornix is related to the rectouterine pouch of the peritoneum, consequently, instruments inserted into the vagina may penetrate the peritoneum of the rectouterine pouch with subsequent hemorrhage and peritonitis.

The muscular walls of the vagina are lined with stratified squamous epithelium that is arranged in transverse folds, called **rugae,** which allow for expansion during coitus and parturition.

Male Reproductive Organs

The male genital organs include the testes within the scrotum, the ductus deferens, the ejaculatory duct, the seminal vesicles, the prostate, the bulbourethral glands, and the penis. All of these are located within the pelvic cavity except for the testes and penis. The penis is discussed with the male external genitalia. The testes are included in this section. The anatomical relationships of the male reproductive organs are illustrated in Fig. 6-11.

The primary reproductive organs of the male are the paired **testes,** which are illustrated in Fig. 6-12. These

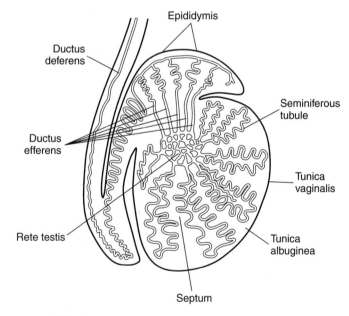

Epididymis

Ductus deferens

Seminiferous tubule

Ductus efferens

Tunica vaginalis

Tunica albuginea

Rete testis

Septum

FIG. 6-12 Sagittal section of a testis and epididymis.

ovoid structures are suspended in a sac of skin called the *scrotum.* Each testis is covered by a tough fibrous connective tissue, the **tunica albuginea.** Extensions of the tunica albuginea project inward, dividing each testis into about 300 lobules. Each lobule contains one to three tightly coiled **seminiferous tubules.** Spermatogenesis, the production of sperm, takes palce within the seminiferous tubules.

In addition to the tunica albuginea, the testes are covered by a thin serous sac, the **tunica vaginalis,** which is derived from peritoneum. Because this is a serous membrane, it has two layers: a parietal layer, which lines the scrotum, and a visceral layer, which covers the testes. The testes develop in the lumbar region of the abdomen and usually descend into the scrotum through the inguinal canal shortly before birth. An extension or diverticulum of peritoneum precedes the testes during the descent into the scrotum. This peritoneum becomes the tunica vaginalis. It is important that the testes descend into the scrotum because spermatoza cannot survive the warmer temperatures of the abdominal cavity.

The **epididymis** is a flattened, tightly coiled, tubular structure on the posterior surface of each testis. The spermatids that are produced by spermatogenesis in the seminiferous tubules pass through efferent ducts into the epididymis for maturation and storage. The epididymis is continuous with the ductus deferens, which transports sperm to the ejaculatory duct.

The **scrotum** is a saclike structure that contains the testes, their coverings, or tunics, and the epididymis. The scrotum consists of a layer of skin, which covers a thin layer of connective tissue that is interspersed with smooth muscle fibers, called the **dartos muscle.** Contraction of the dartos muscle gives a wrinkled appearance to the scrotum. Internally, the scrotum is divided by a **median raphe,** or septum, into two compartments, each containing a testis that is suspended by the **spermatic cord.** Each **ductus deferens** is a thick-walled, muscular tube that is a continuation of the epididymis. Beginning in the tail of the epididymis at the inferior border of the testis, the ductus deferens ascends in the spermatic cord and passes through the inguinal canal. As the ductus deferens enters the pelvis, it crosses over the external iliac vessels. From the inguinal canal, the ductus deferens descends retroperitoneally along the lateral wall of the pelvis, then it crosses the ureter to pass between the ureter and the bladder. The ductus deferens descends posterior to the bladder and medial to the ureter and the seminal vesicles. The terminal portion, near the base of the bladder, is joined by the duct from the seminal vesicles to form the **ejaculatory duct,** which opens into the prostatic urethra.

A **spermatic cord** extends from each testis to the inguinal canal on the same side. Structures passing to and from the testis make up the contents of the spermatic cord. This includes the ductus deferens, the testicular artery, a venous plexus (pampiniform plexus), lymph vessels, nerves, and connective tissue. This bundle of structures is surrounded by connective tissue and muscle fibers to make a cord that suspends the testis in the scrotum. The **cremaster muscle,** derived from the internal oblique muscle of the abdomen, extends through the spermatic cord to the testes. The muscle functions with the dartos muscle to alter the position of the testes to maintain optimum temperature for the production and maturation of spermatozoa.

The **seminal vesicles** are paired accessory glands that consist of coiled tubes that appear to be twisted to form small pouches or vesicles. The glands are located between the posterior surface of the bladder and the rectum. The duct of each seminal vesicle joins with the associated ductus deferens to form an **ejaculatory duct,** which opens into the prostatic urethra. The secretion of the seminal vesicles has a high fructose content that provides an energy source for the sperm.

The largest accessory gland of the male reproductive system is the **prostate.** It is composed partially of glandular parenchyma and partially of connective tissue stroma. Located inferior to the bladder, this chestnut-shaped gland surrounds the prostatic urethra. About 20 to 30 small prostatic ducts empty into the urethra. The secretion of the prostate gland aids in the motility and fertility of the sperm. Because of its close relationship to the urethra, hypertrophy of the prostate frequently interferes with the passage of urine. Subsequent problems related to the stasis of urine may then develop. Surgery may be indicated if urination becomes too difficult or impossible.

Each **bulbourethral gland,** also known as a Cowper's gland, is about 1 cm in diameter. The glands, one on either side of the urethra, are located posterior and lateral to the membranous urethra. Their relatively long ducts pass through the membranous urethra to empty into the proximal portion of the spongy urethra. In response to sexual stimulation, the bulbourethral glands secrete a small amount of an alkaline, mucoid substance that neutralizes the acidity of the spongy urethra and lubricates the tip of the penis.

PERINEUM AND EXTERNAL GENITALIA

The **perineum** is the region between the thighs that overlies (is superficial to) the pelvic diaphragm. In anatomical position, it is a narrow region that extends from the pubic arch anteriorly to the coccyx posteriorly. When the thighs are abducted, it is a diamond-shaped area bounded laterally by the inferior pubic ramus, the ischial ramus, and the ischial tuberosity. For descriptive purposes, it is conveniently divided into a posterior **anal region** and an anterior **urogenital region** by drawing a line between the ischial tuberosities as illustrated in Fig. 6-13. The posterior anal region contains the anus and the anterior urogenital region contains the external genitalia. In the female, the region between the vagina and anus is called the **clinical perineum.** During childbirth, the clinical perineum may be surgically cut to avoid excessive stretching and tearing of the tissues as the fetal head emerges.

Muscles of the Perineum

The muscles of the perineum are illustrated in Figs. 6-14 and 6-15. The muscles found in the anal region are the **levator ani** and the **sphincter ani.** The levator ani muscles

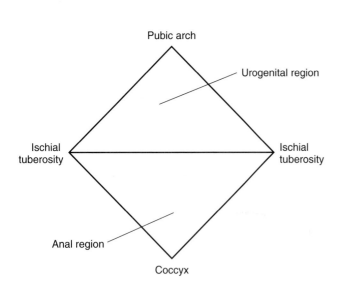

FIG. 6-13 Regions of the perineum.

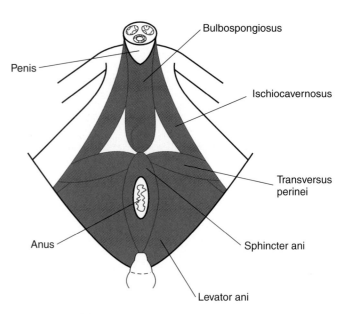

FIG. 6-15 Muscles in the male perineum.

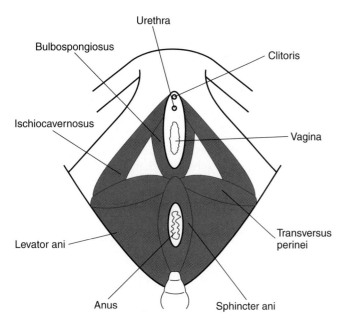

FIG. 6-14 Muscles in the female perineum.

have been described previously as primary muscles of the pelvic diaphragm. The sphincter ani muscle surrounds the opening of the anal canal, the **anus.** The musculature of the urogenital region consists of the **bulbospongiosus, ischiocavernosus,** and **transversus perinei** muscles. The muscles are the same in both sexes, however the arrangement differs. Fig. 6-14 illustrates the arrangement in the female and Fig. 6-15 shows the arrangement in the male. The **transversus perinei** muscles are horizontal, arising on the ischial tuberosities and passing medially to insert on the central perineal tendon. In other words, they pass along the line dividing the perineum into the urogenital and anal regions. The **ischiocavernosus** muscles also arise on the ischial tuberosities but pass forward to insert on the pubic

arch and the crus of the penis in the male or the clitoris in the female. The **bulbospongiosus** muscle is in the median line of the urogenital region. In the female, the two parts of this muscle are separated by the urethra and vagina. In the male, the fibers of the two muscles unite in the midline and encircle the corpus spongiosum of the penis.

External Female Genitalia

The external accessory structures of the female genital system are closely associated with the perineum. The term **vulva,** or **pudendum,** is a collective term referring to all the female external genitalia, which includes the mons pubis, the labia majora, the labia minora, the vestibule, the clitoris, and the vestibular glands. These are illustrated in Fig. 6-16.

The **mons pubis** is a subcutaneous pad of fatty tissue that is covered with skin and forms a rounded elevation anterior to the symphysis pubis. During puberty, the mons pubis becomes covered with coarse pubic hairs.

Passing posteriorly from the mons pubis, the **labia majora** are large folds of skin that are filled with subcutaneous fat. The skin on the lateral surface has sweat glands, sebaceous or oil glands, and, after puberty, is covered by pubic hair. Embryologically, the labia majora are homologous with the scrotum in the male. This means they have a similar structure and are derived from the same undifferentiated tissue. The labia majora are the lateral margins of the vulva.

The **labia minora** are two thin, delicate folds of skin that are located between the labia majora. Although devoid of fat and hair, the labia minora are richly supplied with blood vessels, nerves, and sebaceous glands. The labia minora lie on either side of the urethra and the vaginal openings, and enclose the vestibule. Anteriorly, the folds of the labia minora unite to form a prepuce over the clitoris.

The **clitoris,** which is homologous to the penis in the male, is located posterior and inferior to the mons pubis and

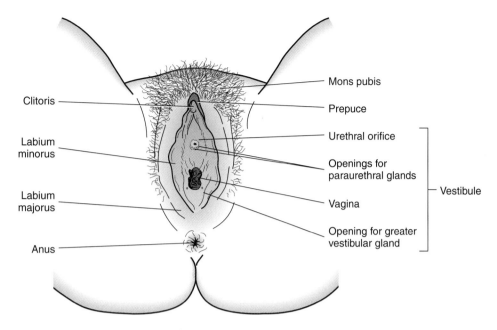

FIG. 6-16 Female external genitalia.

is between the anterior ends of the labia minora. Although only 2 to 3 cm in length, it is composed of two columns of erectile corpora cavernosa and is anchored to the os coxae by two crura. Like the male penis, it is capable of enlargement when stimulated.

The **vestibule** is the narrow cleft between the two labia minora. The clitoris is at the anterior end of the vestibule and posterior to the clitoris, the urethra opens into the anterior portion of the vestibule. The vaginal orifice is posterior to the urethra. Two elongated masses of corpus spongiosum lie along the lateral margins of the vestibule, deep to the bulbospongiosus muscle, to form the bulb of the vestibule. Vestibular glands, so named because they are located within the vestibule, include the **paraurethral glands** and the greater vestibular glands. The paraurethral glands, homologous to the prostate gland of the male, are located on the either side of the external urethral orifice and secrete mucus for lubrication. The **greater vestibular glands,** also called *Bartholin's glands,* are homologous to the bulbourethral glands of the male and are located on either side of the vaginal orifice. They secrete a mucoid substance for lubrication. Normally, vestibular glands are not palpable, but they may become enlarged and irritating when they are infected.

External Male Genitalia

External structures of the male reproductive system include the scrotum and the penis. The scrotum was discussed with the testes. The penis is described here and illustrated in Fig. 6-17.

The **penis** is a copulatory organ that is used to introduce spermatozoa into the vagina of the female. It is cylindric in shape and is divided into a root and a body. Structurally, the penis consists of three cylindric masses of erectile tissue,

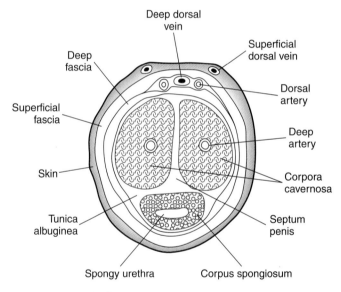

FIG. 6-17 Structure of the penis.

each surrounded by a connective tissue tunica albuginea. The two dorsal cylinders of erectile tissue are the **corpora cavernosa** and the smaller midventral cylinder, which encircles the spongy urethra, is the **corpus spongiosum.** Distally, the corpus spongiosum expands to form the **glans penis.**

The **root** of the penis is the attached portion and consists of a bulb and two crura. The **bulb** is the expanded proximal end of the corpus spongiosum. It is anchored to the tissue of the urogenital diaphragm in the pelvic floor and is enclosed by the bulbospongiosus muscle of the perineum. The two **crura** are the tapered proximal ends of the corpora cavernosa that diverge to attach to the ischiopubic rami.

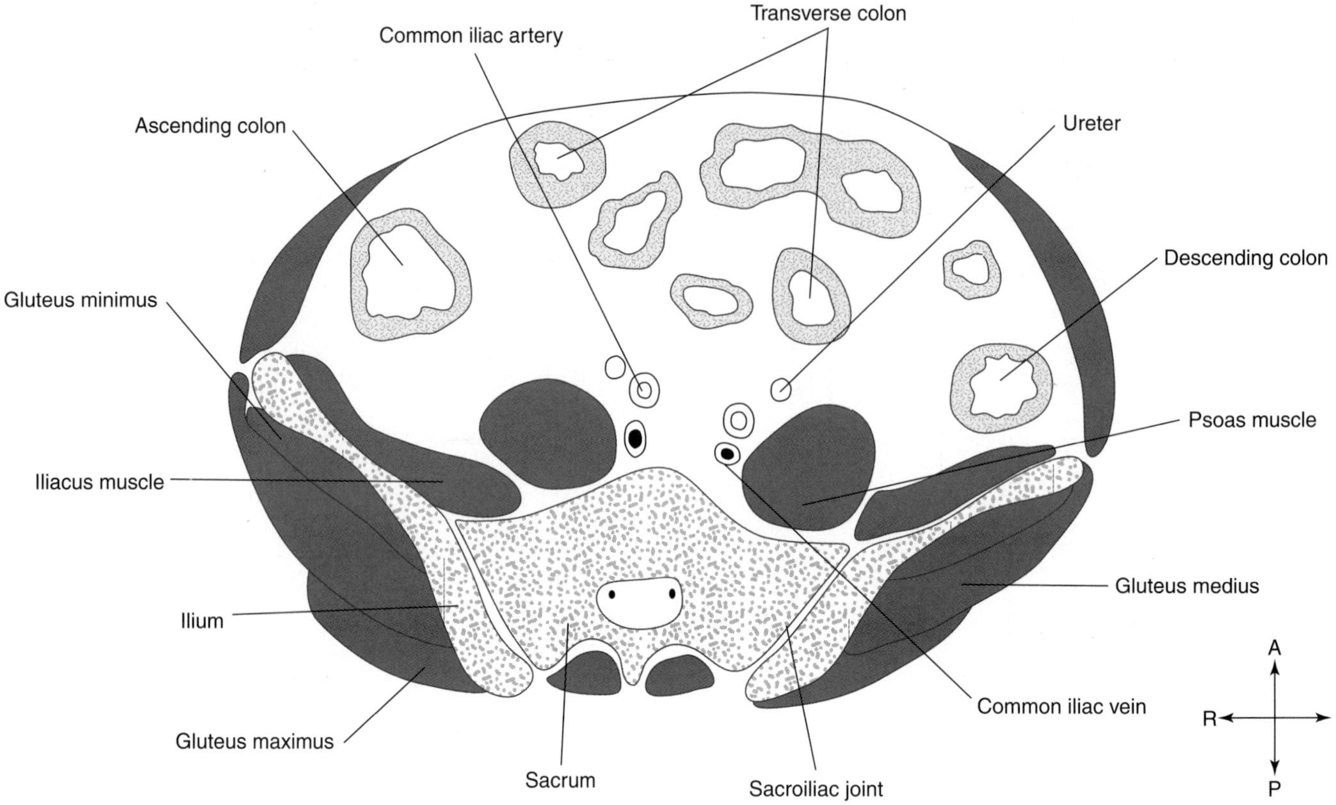

FIG. 6-18 Transverse section through the sacroiliac joint.

The ischiocavernosus muscle of the perineum envelops the crura.

The **body** of the penis is the free portion that is pendulous in the flaccid condition. The three cylindric columns of erectile tissue are surrounded by connective tissue fascia and skin. Facing anteriorly when flaccid, the dorsum of the penis is continuous with the anterior abdominal wall. The ventral, or urethral, aspect faces posteriorly in the flaccid condition and anteriorly when erect. The **glans penis,** at the distal end of the body, is corpus spongiosum and has the opening for the urethra. The skin covering the body of the penis continues over the glans penis as the **prepuce.** The prepuce, or foreskin, may be removed shortly after birth in a surgical procedure called *circumcision.*

During sexual stimulation, parasympathetic reflexes cause dilation of the arteries that supply the penis and the sinuses of the erectile tissue fill with blood. At the same time, the pressure of the dilated arteries and the filled sinuses compresses the veins leaving the penis so that the blood is retained. These vascular changes result in an erection. The penis returns to its flaccid state when the arteries constrict and pressure on the veins is reduced.

Sectional Anatomy of the Pelvis

For convenience, this discussion of the sectional anatomy of the pelvis will include the false pelvis. In other words,

transverse sections will begin with the iliac crest. In these more superior sections of the false pelvis, the organs seen will be familiar, because they are continuous with those studied in the abdomen.

SECTIONS OF THE FEMALE PELVIS

Transverse Section Through the Sacroiliac Joint

A line through the most superior point of the two iliac crests usually intersects the body of the fourth lumbar vertebra. This is the level of the aortic bifurcation into the **right** and **left common iliac arteries.** Inferior to this, at level L5, the two **common iliac veins** join to form the inferior vena cava. Fig. 6-18 illustrates a section through the sacroiliac joint. Common iliac arteries and common iliac veins are present at this level. The lower portions of the **ascending colon** and the **cecum** are located in the right iliac fossa. The smaller **descending colon** is in the left iliac fossa.

Because of the variable nature of the **transverse colon** it is impossible to state specifically when it will or will not be seen. It drapes inferiorly and anteriorly between the right and left colic flexures. In some individuals it is pendulous and extends down into the pelvis. Transverse sections through the false pelvis of these individuals show two regions of the transverse colon. One region is on the right side as the transverse colon descends and the other on the left as it ascends toward the left colic (splenic) flexure. More com-

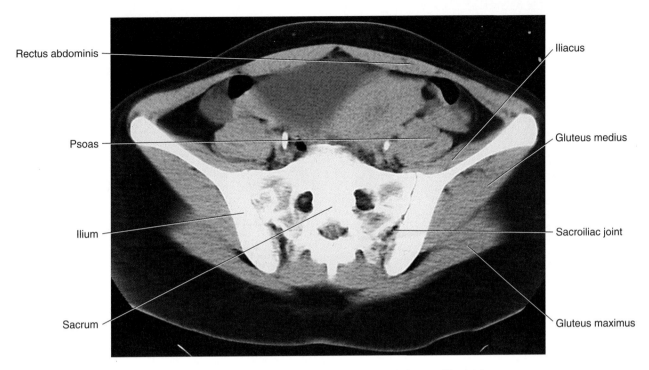

FIG. 6-19 CT image of a transverse section through the sacroiliac joint.

monly sections at this level are inferior to the transverse colon.

As in the abdomen, the **psoas muscles** are on either side of the vertebral column. The **ureters** descend anterior to the psoas muscle. The **iliacus muscle** lines the iliac fossa and the **gluteal muscle** originate on the lateral surface of the ilium. The computed tomographic image in Fig. 6-19 is near the same level as Fig. 6-18 and illustrates many of the same structures.

Transverse Section Through the Lower Part of the Sacrum

The relationships of structures at this level, primarily muscles, are illustrated in Fig. 6-20. The fibers of the psoas and iliacus muscles merge to form the **iliopsoas muscle.** Observe the close relationship of the **femoral nerve** to this muscle. All three gluteal muscles are evident lateral and posterior to the ilium. The **gluteus maximus** is the most superficial and **gluteus minimus** is the deepest, next to the ilium. The **piriformis muscle** is in the **greater sciatic foramen** (notch) between the ilium and sacrum. The **obturator internus** muscle, which lines the cavity of the true pelvis, is medial to the ilium. The common iliac vessels generally have bifurcated at this level with **external iliac vessels** associated with the iliopsoas muscles as they proceed to the upper thigh region. The **ureter** is more closely associated with the **internal iliac vessels** in the true pelvis. The computed tomographic image in Fig. 6-21 is near this level and shows many of the same structures.

Transverse Section Through the Uterus

Fig. 6-22 illustrates a transverse section through the **uterus.** This section shows the **broad ligament** that extends from the uterus to the lateral pelvic wall. **Ovaries** are attached to the posterior portion of the broad ligament by the mesovarium, and the **uterine tube** is in the upper margin of the ligament but may be difficult to see. The space between the uterus and rectum is the **rectouterine pouch** (of Douglas), which may contain loops of bowel. The **obturator internus** muscle originates on the inner surface of the ilium and covers most of the lateral wall of the true pelvis.

Transverse Section Through the Urinary Bladder

Fig. 6-23 illustrates a transverse section through the superior surface of the urinary bladder. This shows the **ureters** posterior to the bladder as they are about to penetrate the bladder wall. The **cervix** is interposed between the bladder and rectum. The **obturator internus** and **levator ani** muscles form the lateral walls and floor of the pelvic cavity. Anteriorly, the **pectineus** muscle originates on the pubis. The computed tomographic image in Fig. 6-24 is near this level and illustrates some of the same structures.

Midsagittal Section Through the Female Pelvis

Fig. 6-25 is a line drawing that illustrates a midsagittal section through the female pelvis. Posteriorly, the **rectum** follows the curvature of the sacrum. Anteriorly, the **urinary bladder** is in a position immediately posterior to the symphysis pubis. The **fundus** and **body** of the uterus are

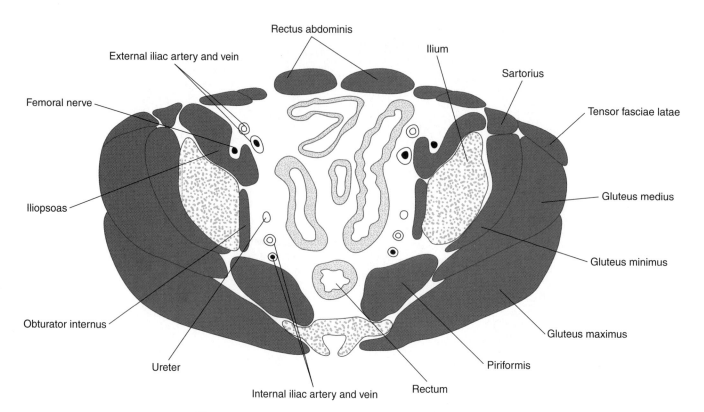

FIG. 6-20 Transverse section through the lower part of the sacrum.

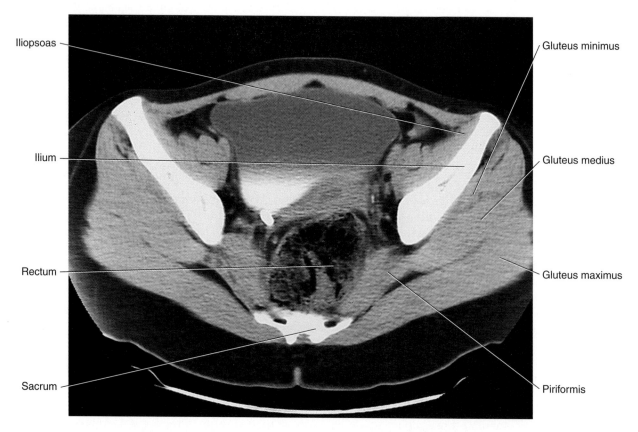

FIG. 6-21 CT image of a transverse section through the lower part of the sacrum.

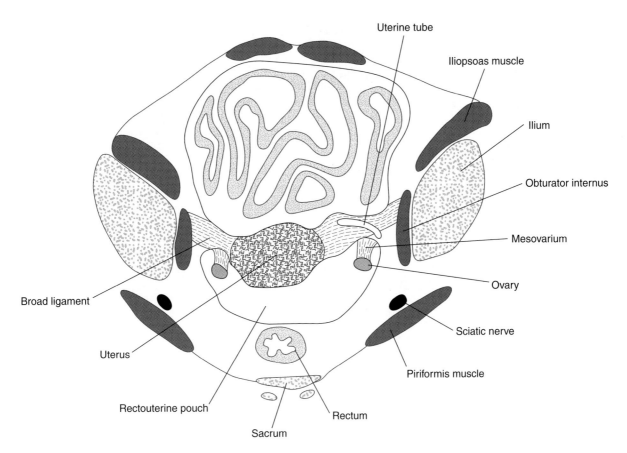

FIG. 6-22 Transverse section through the uterus.

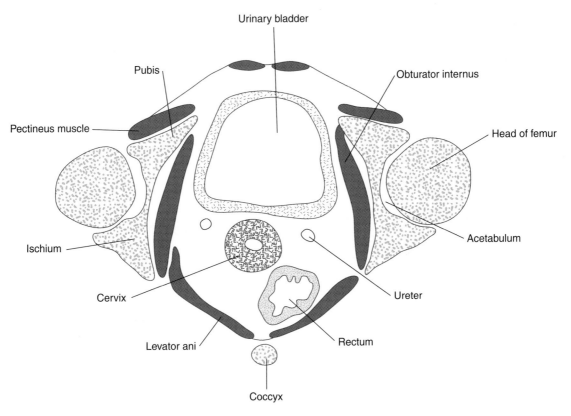

FIG. 6-23 Transverse section through the urinary bladder.

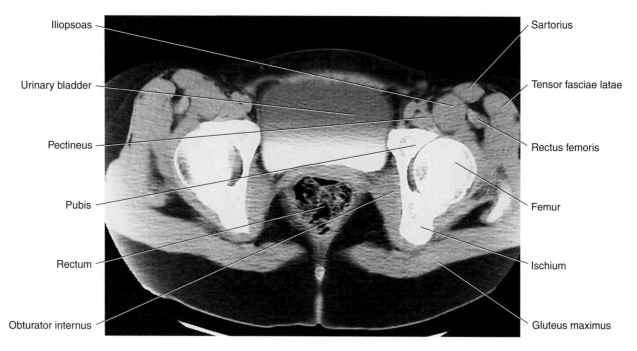

FIG. 6-24 CT image of a transverse section through the urinary bladder.

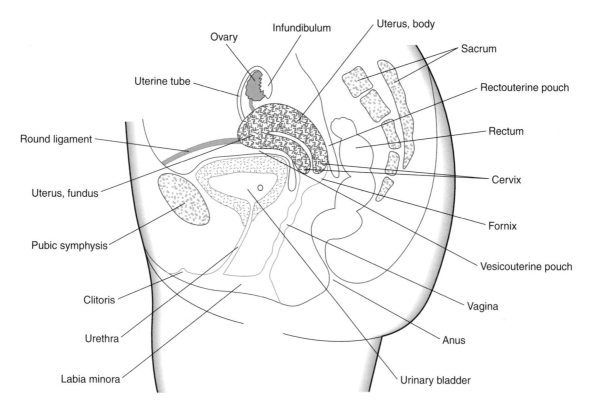

FIG. 6-25 Midsagittal section through the female pelvis.

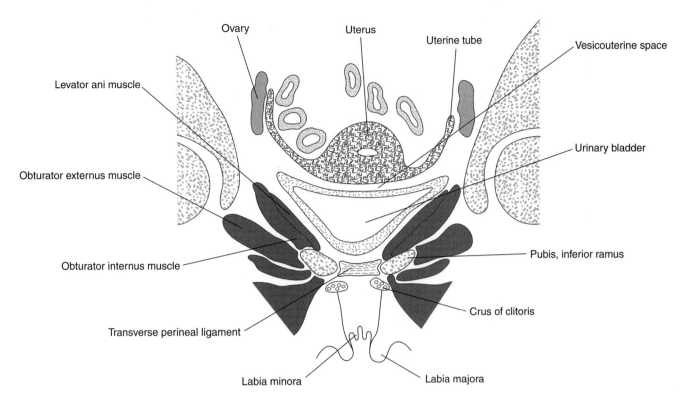

FIG. 6-26 Coronal section through the female pelvis.

anteverted over the superior surface of the bladder and are anteflexed with the **cervix.** The peritoneum forms two cul-de-sacs related to the uterus which are nicely illustrated in midsagittal sections. Posteriorly, the **rectouterine pouch** extends between the rectum and uterus, then as the peritoneum continues from the fundus of the uterus to the superior surface of the bladder, it forms the **vesicouterine pouch.** The **vagina** slants posteriorly as it ascends to the cervix of the uterus where the vagina surrounds the cervix to form the **fornices.** The **posterior fornix** is longer than the anterior fornix. The **urethra** extends from the bladder and through the urogenital diaphragm to open into the **vestibule,** anterior to the vaginal orifice and posterior to the **clitoris.** The **labia minora** form the lateral margins of the vestibule.

Coronal Section Through the Body of the Uterus

Fig. 6-26 illustrates a coronal section through the anterior part of the pelvis showing the **body** of the uterus and the **urinary bladder.** Uterine tubes extend from the uterus toward the lateral pelvic wall. The urinary bladder is inferior to the uterus and separated from it by the **vesicouterine** space. **Obturator internus** muscles form the lateral walls of the cavity and the hammock-like **levator ani** muscles form the pelvic floor. Two **crura** of the clitoris, composed of corpus cavernosum, are associated with the ischiopubis ramus. **Labia majora,** homologous to the scrotum in the male, en-

close the smaller **labia minora,** which form the lateral margins of the vestibule.

Sections of the Male Pelvis

Transverse Section Through the Seminal Vesicles

Fig. 6-27 is a line drawing that illustrates the relationships of the **ureters, seminal vesicles,** and **ductus deferens.** The ureters are shown as they penetrate the wall of the bladder. The **seminal vesicles** are glandular structures between the rectum and urinary bladder. The **ductus deferens** are medial to both the ureters and seminal vesicles. The space between the bladder and rectum is the **rectovesicle** space, a peritoneal cul-de-sac in the male. Anteriorly, between the iliopsoas and pectineus muscles, the femoral triangle contains the femoral artery, vein, and nerve. The spermatic cord, anterior and medial to the margin of the pectineus muscle, contains the testicular artery, ductus deferens, and pampiniform venous plexus.

Transverse Section Through the Prostate Gland

The **prostate gland** is inferior to the bladder and posterior to the symphysis pubis. It surrounds the **prostatic urethra** as shown in Fig. 6-28. A **prostatic venous plexus** surrounds the gland. The **rectum** is posterior to the prostate. Because the prostate rests on the curved pelvic floor, a portion of the

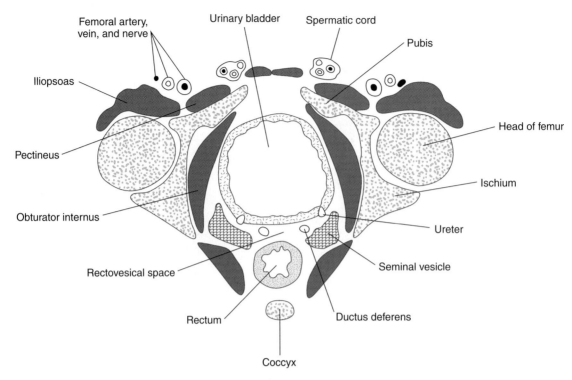

Femoral artery, vein, and nerve
Urinary bladder
Spermatic cord
Pubis
Iliopsoas
Pectineus
Head of femur
Obturator internus
Ischium
Ureter
Rectovesical space
Seminal vesicle
Rectum
Ductus deferens
Coccyx

FIG. 6-27 Transverse section through the seminal vesicles.

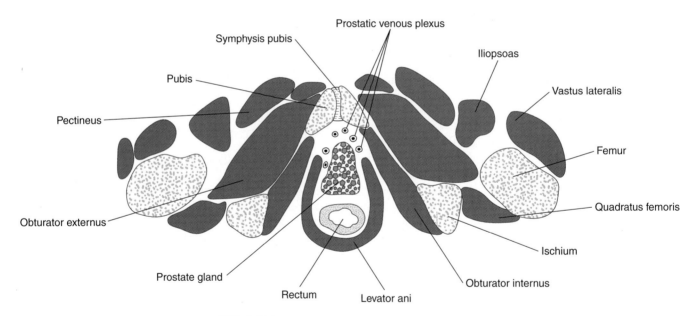

Prostatic venous plexus
Symphysis pubis
Iliopsoas
Pubis
Vastus lateralis
Pectineus
Femur
Obturator externus
Quadratus femoris
Prostate gland
Ischium
Rectum
Levator ani
Obturator internus

FIG. 6-28 Transverse section through the prostate gland.

floor, specifically the **levator ani** muscle, is evident. The pelvic walls are lined with the **obturator internus** muscle.

Transverse Section Through the Root of the Penis

The line drawing in Fig. 6-29 illustrates the root of the penis which consists of a bulb and two crura. The **bulb** portion of the root is **corpus spongiosum** and surrounds the urethra. The **transverse perinei muscle** extends horizontally between the two ischila rami with the bulb anterior and the anal canal posterior to the muscle. The **bulbospon-** giosus muscle is associated with the bulb of the penis. Lateral to the bulb, the two **crura** of **corpus cavernosum** diverge to attach to the ischial rami. The **ischiocavernosus muscle** is related to the crura.

Midsagittal Section of the Male Pelvis

Midsagittal sections of the male pelvis show the typical relationships of the male reproductive organs that were discussed previously and illustrated by Fig. 6-11. Refer to this figure while reviewing the relationships discussed in this

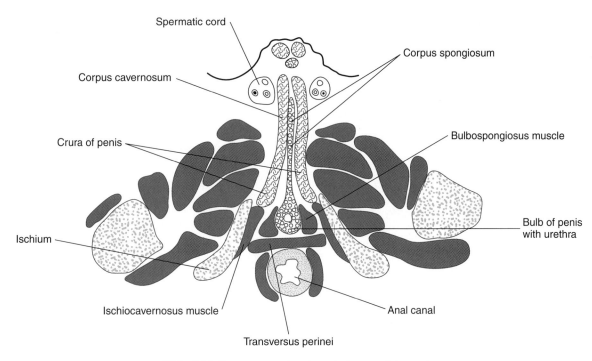

FIG. 6-29 Transverse section through the root of the penis.

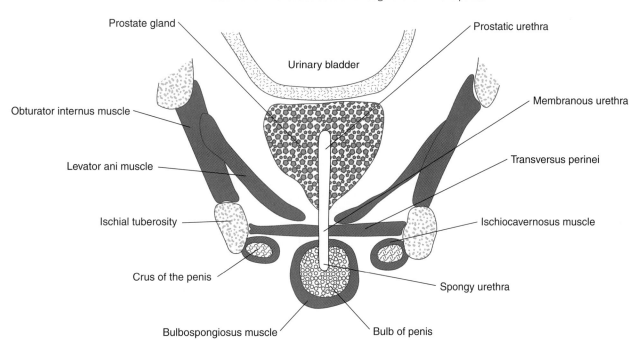

FIG. 6-30 Coronal section through the prostate gland and the root of the penis.

paragraph. This shows how the rectum follows the curvature of the sacrum. The peritoneum continues down the posterior wall then curves over the seminal vesicles and urinary bladder. The seminal vesicles are between the bladder and rectum just inferior to the peritoneal rectovesicle pouch. Posterior to the symphysis pubis, the urinary bladder rests on the pelvic floor. The duct from the seminal vesicles joins the ductus deferens to form the ejaculatory duct, which penetrates the prostate gland to empty into the prostatic urethra. The urethra continues through the urogenital diaphragm as the membranous urethra then enters the

corpus spongiosum of the penis to become the penile or spongy urethra. The duct from the bulbourethral gland empties into the spongy urethra.

Coronal Section Through the Prostate Gland and the Root of the Penis

The line drawing in Fig. 6-30 and the magnetic resonance image in Fig. 6-31 illustrate a coronal section of the male pelvis through the prostate gland and root of the penis. **Obturator internus muscles** line the pelvic wall and fill the

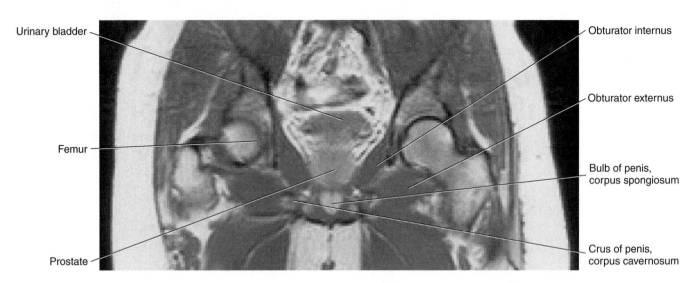

Urinary bladder

Femur

Prostate

Obturator internus

Obturator externus

Bulb of penis, corpus spongiosum

Crus of penis, corpus cavernosum

FIG. 6-31 MRI of a coronal section through the prostate gland and the root of the penis.

space of the obturator foramen. **Levator ani muscles** form the hammock-shaped pelvic floor and the **transverse perineal muscle** extends between the two ischial tuberosities. The **prostate gland,** inferior to the **urinary bladder,** rests on the pelvic floor. It encircles the **prostatic urethra.** The urethra continues through the muscle and fascia of the **urogenital diaphragm** as the **membranous urethra** and then penetrates the corpus spongiosum in the bulb of the penis to become the **spongy urethra.** The components of the root of the penis, the bulb and the two crura, are also represented. The **bulb,** which consists of **corpus spongiosum,** is surrounded by the **bulbospongiosus muscle** and anchored to perineal membrane. It encircles the spongy urethra. The two **crura** of **corpus cavernosum** are surrounded by **ischiocavernosus muscle** and are anchored to the ischial tuberosities.

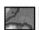

Pathology

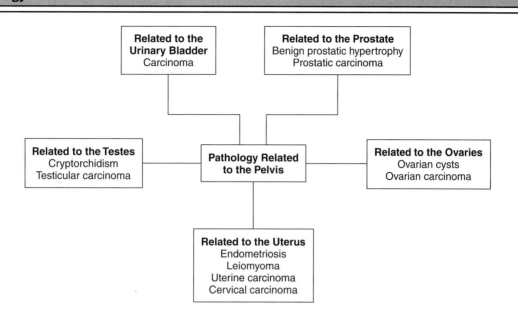

Related to the Urinary Bladder
Carcinoma

Related to the Prostate
Benign prostatic hypertrophy
Prostatic carcinoma

Related to the Testes
Cryptorchidism
Testicular carcinoma

Pathology Related to the Pelvis

Related to the Ovaries
Ovarian cysts
Ovarian carcinoma

Related to the Uterus
Endometriosis
Leiomyoma
Uterine carcinoma
Cervical carcinoma

Bladder Carcinoma

Bladder carcinoma occurs in the transitional epithelium of the mucosa, or lining, of the urinary bladder. The incidence of bladder carcinoma in males is three times the incidence in females and it usually appears after the age of 50. Smoking is the most significant risk factor. Excessive coffee drinking and exposure to certain industrial chemicals have also been implicated as possible risk factors.

Benign Prostatic Hypertrophy

Benign prostatic hypertrophy is a nonmalignant hyperplasia of the prostate gland and is common in men over the age of 50. Because the prostate surrounds the urethra, the enlargement may obstruct the flow of urine from the bladder.

Prostatic Carcinoma

Carcinoma of the glandular tissue in the prostate ranks third in the leading causes of cancer in men. Early detection is important because metastasis soon involves the regional lymph nodes, bones, and lungs.

Cryptorchidism

Cryptorchidism is the failure of one or both of the testes to descend into the scrotum. During prenatal development, the testes first appear in the abdomen. About the seventh month, they descend into the groin area, then pass through the inguinal canal into the scrotum. If this does not occur in a normal manner, cryptorchidism results. Viable sperm are not produced if the testes do not completely descend; consequently, if both testes are involved and untreated, sterility results.

Testicular Carcinoma

The incidence of malignant tumors of the testes is fairly uncommon; however, they usually occur at a relatively young age, between the ages of 18 and 40. There are two primary groups, seminoma and teratoma. The seminoma appear to arise from the seminiferous tubules of the testes and are quite radiosensitive, which makes the prognosis good with early detection. The teratoma appear to arise from primitive germ cells and are associated with a poor prognosis. Both types are malignant and metastasize through the lymphatic and blood vessels.

Ovarian Cysts

Numerous types of benign cysts may occur in the ovary, including cysts in the ovarian follicles, corpus luteum, and glandular tissue. The most common is a cystadenoma, a cyst originating from the glandular tissue. Polycystic ovaries consist of enlarged ovaries with numerous small cysts and characterized by amenorrhea and sterility. Fibroid cysts arise from unfertilized ova and often contain hair, fat, and possibly even bone and teeth.

Serous carcinoma from the surface epithelium of the ovary is the most common type of ovarian cancer. Although ovarian carcinomas are less common than other carcinomas of the female reproductive system, they are usually asymptomatic until late in the development of the disease, which greatly reduces the chance for a cure. These malignant tumors readily invade their capsule and release tumor cells all around the pelvis and abdomen.

Endometriosis

Endometriosis is a condition in which an area of endometrial tissue grows outside the uterus. The cause is unknown but it is thought to be due to retrograde menstruation or hormonal disturbances. The symptoms vary but may include pelvic pain, dysmenorrhea, and infertility.

Leiomyoma

The most common benign tumor in women is the leiomyoma, also referred to as a *fibroid tumor*. It develops from the smooth muscle layer of the uterus and grows during the reproductive years, then typically shrinks after menopause. The tumors may be small or large, single or numerous. Symptoms

Continued

Pathology—cont'd

Leiomyoma—cont'd

and treatment vary with the severity of the disease. A small tumor may be asymptomatic and require no treatment. Large tumors may put pressure on the bladder causing frequent urination, compress the rectum resulting in obstruction and constipation, and cause infertility.

Uterine Cancer

Adenocarcinoma of the uterus is one of the most common malignancies in the female reproductive system, usually occurring in postmenopausal women. It usually arises from the basal cells of the epithelial lining, the endometrium, and may cause postmenopausal bleeding. Uterine cancer may be de-

tected by dysplasia of the epithelial cells in a Pap smear. It then progresses to carcinoma in situ and finally to an invasive malignant carcinoma. With early detection, before the carcinoma becomes invasive, the prognosis is good and the cure rate is fairly high.

Cervical Carcinoma

Cervical carcinoma arises from epithelial tissue around the neck of the uterus. The most common symptom is vaginal bleeding. The treatment and prognosis for survival depend on the stage of the disease when it is diagnosed. With regular gynecologic examinations with Pap smear analysis, leading to early detection, the prognosis is good.

· REVIEW QUESTIONS ·

1. What is the difference between the true pelvis and the false pelvis?
2. What feature marks the posterior portion of the pelvic brim?
3. What are the three bones that make up an os coxa?
4. What is the large opening that is surrounded by the three bones of the os coxa?
5. What two muscles form the wall of the false pelvis?
6. What are the two principal muscles that make up the wall of the true pelvis?
7. What is the larger and more important muscle of the pelvic diaphragm?
8. What is the principal artery that supplies blood to the pelvis, including the wall and contents?
9. What branch of the sacral plexus innervates the perineum and external genitalia?
10. What is the name of the peritoneal space that is anterior to the rectum in males? In females?
11. What is the name of the peritoneal space that is inferior to the uterus?
12. What structure is between the urinary bladder and the pelvic floor in males?
13. What are the three parts of the male urethra and where are they located?
14. What are the three peritoneal ligaments that are attached to the ovaries?
15. What are the four peritoneal ligaments that are attached to the uterus?
16. What are the three parts of the uterus and which part projects into the vagina?
17. Describe the normal position of the uterus.
18. What is the relationship of the epididymis to the testes?
19. What are the components of the spermatic cord?
20. Name and state the location of three glands associated with the male reproductive system.
21. Name two muscles in the anal region of the perineum and three muscles in the urogenital region.
22. What are two types of vestibular glands in the female, where are they located, and what are they homologous to in the male?
23. What are the two components of the root of the penis, what is their composition, where are they attached, and what muscle is associated with each one?
24. What are the three columns of erectile tissue in the penis? What is their relative location? Which one contains the urethra?

· CHAPTER QUIZ ·

Name the following:

1. The feature on the pubic bones that marks the pelvic brim.
2. The pelvic wall muscle that closes the greater sciatic notch.
3. The larger muscle of the pelvic diaphragm.
4. The muscle that lines the lateral wall of the true pelvis.
5. The triangular-shaped region that is outlined by the openings of the two ureters and the urethra.
6. The large fold of peritoneum that extends from the sides of the uterus.
7. The vaginal space around the cervix of the uterus.
8. The extension of the internal oblique muscle that is found in the spermatic cord.
9. The male accessory gland that is between the posterior surface of the urinary bladder and the rectum.
10. The female accessory gland that is homologous to the male prostate.

True/False

1. The urogenital diaphragm is superficial to the pelvic diaphragm.
2. Sperm pass from the epididymis into the ejaculatory duct.
3. Ovaries are usually displaced inferiorly during pregnancy.
4. The uterus is normally retroverted and anteflexed.
5. There are two dorsal columns of corpus spongiosum in the body of the penis.
6. The crura of the penis are associated with the ischiocavernosus muscle.
7. The psoas muscle is more medial than the iliacus muscle.
8. The sciatic nerve is associated with the iliopsoas muscle.
9. Both males and females have an ischiocavernosus muscle, but only males have a bulbospongiosus muscle.
10. The prostate gland is between the urinary bladder and the pelvic diaphragm.

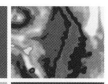

CHAPTER SEVEN

The Vertebral Column and Spinal Cord | 7

OBJECTIVES

Upon completion of this chapter, the student should be able to do the following:
- Describe the general structure of vertebrae and identify the structural components on a diagram.
- State the characteristics that distinguish cervical vertebrae from other types.
- Distinguish the first two cervical vertebrae from other cervical vertebrae and state their specific names.
- Identify the characteristic features that distinguish thoracic vertebrae from other vertebrae.
- Identify the characteristic features that distinguish lumbar vertebrae from other vertebrae.
- Describe the structural features of the sacrum and coccyx.
- Discuss the composition and purpose of intervertebral discs.
- Identify the curvatures of the vertebral column and state the direction of the curvatures.
- Identify three types of abnormal curvatures of the vertebral column.
- Describe and state the location of the following ligaments associated with the vertebral column: anterior and posterior longitudinal ligaments, ligamenta flava, interspinous ligaments, supraspinous ligaments, ligamentum nuchae, and intertransverse ligaments.
- Identify the muscles in the superficial, intermediate, and deep layers of the intrinsic back muscles.
- Describe the meninges of the spinal cord.
- Identify the structural features of the spinal cord in longitudinal and cross-sectional views.
- Name the five groups of spinal nerves and state the number of nerves in each group.
- Distinguish between dorsal and ventral nerve roots and state the components of each.
- Describe the location, components, and functions of the four major nerve plexuses and name the principal nerves that emerge from each plexus.
- Describe the vasculature of the spinal cord.

Vertebral Column

The vertebral column is a bony structure composed of individual vertebrae and the fibrocartilaginous pads, called intervertebral discs, that are between the vertebrae. The column supports the body weight, helps to maintain posture, and protects the spinal cord.

STRUCTURE OF VERTEBRAE

General Structure

All vertebrae have a common structural pattern (Fig. 7-1), although variations exist between them. The thick, anterior, weight-bearing portion is the **body,** or **centrum.** The posterior, curved portion is the **vertebral arch.** Together, the body and vertebral arch surround a central opening, the **vertebral foramen.** When the vertebrae are stacked together, the vertebral foramina make a vertebral canal that contains and protects the spinal cord. The vertebral arch is formed by the transverse processes, the spinous process, the pedicles, the laminae, and the superior and inferior articular processes. **Transverse processes** project laterally from the vertebral arch, and in the posterior midline is a **spinous process.** These processes are places for muscle attachment. The spinous processes can be felt as bony projections along the midline of the back. The portion of the vertebral arch adjacent to the body, between the body and the transverse process, is the **pedicle.** A concave surface on the upper and lower margins of the pedicles is called the **vertebral notch.** When the superior and inferior vertebral notches of adjacent vertebrae meet, they form **intervertebral foramina,** which transmit spinal nerves and blood vessels. The portion between the transverse process and the spinous process is the **lamina. Superior** and **inferior articular processes**

project superiorly and inferiorly, respectively, from the vertebral arch. The superior articular process of one vertebra articulates with the inferior articular process of the preceding vertebra in the column. Fig. 7-2 is a radiograph of cervical vertebrae demonstrating some of these features.

Cervical Vertebrae

The seven cervical vertebrae are designated C1 through C7. In general, the cervical vertebrae, shown in Fig. 7-3, can be distinguished from other vertebrae because the cervicals have **transverse foramina** in the transverse processes, which allow passage of the vertebral arteries as they ascend through the neck to the brain. Also, the spinous processes of cervical vertebrae are forked, or bifid. The exception to this is the seventh cervical vertebra (C7), which has a long spinous process that is typically not bifid. The C7 spinous process is easily palpable at the base of the neck.

The first two cervical vertebrae are modified and have no disc between them. The **atlas** (C1), illustrated in Fig. 7-4, has no body, no spinous process, and short transverse processes. It is a ring that consists of an anterior arch, a posterior arch, and two large lateral masses that have large articular facets. The superior facets articulate with the occipital condyles on the occipital bone and the inferior facets articulate with the vertebra below. The **axis** (C2), shown in Fig. 7-5, has a **dens,** or **odontoid process,** which projects upward from the vertebral body like a tooth. The odontoid process acts as a pivot for rotation of the atlas.

Thoracic Vertebrae

The 12 thoracic vertebrae are designated T1 through T12. These can be distinguished from other vertebrae by the **costal facets,** located on the bodies and transverse processes, for articulation with the ribs. The head of the rib articulates with the vertebral body and the tubercle of the rib articulates with the transverse process. They also have long, pointed spinous processes. These features are illustrated in Fig. 7-6.

Lumbar Vertebrae

The five lumbar vertebrae, designated L1 through L5, make up the part of the vertebral column in the small of the back. The lumbar vertebrae, shown in Fig. 7-7, have large, heavy bodies because they support most of the body weight and have many back muscles attached to them. They also have short, blunt spinous processes.

Sacrum and Coccyx

The sacral region of the vertebral column, illustrated in Fig. 7-8, consists of five vertebrae that fuse to form the sacrum. The transverse processes of the vertebrae fuse to form the **lateral masses (ala),** which articulate with the pelvic girdle laterally at the **sacroiliac joints.** Located within the lateral

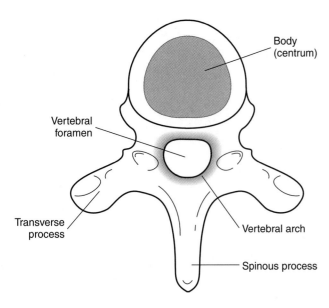

FIG. 7-1 General features of vertebrae.

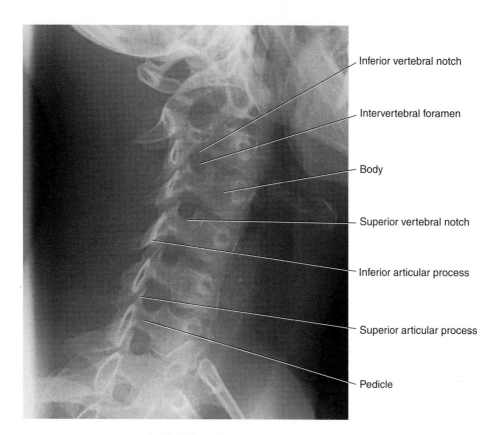

Inferior vertebral notch

Intervertebral foramen

Body

Superior vertebral notch

Inferior articular process

Superior articular process

Pedicle

FIG. 7-2 Radiograph of cervical vertebrae.

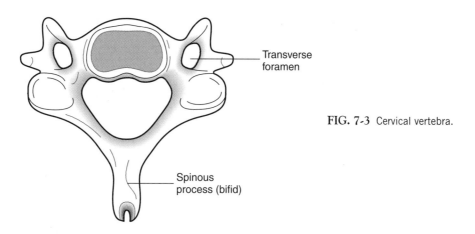

Transverse foramen

Spinous process (bifid)

FIG. 7-3 Cervical vertebra.

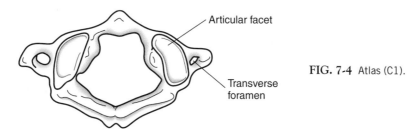

Articular facet

Transverse foramen

FIG. 7-4 Atlas (C1).

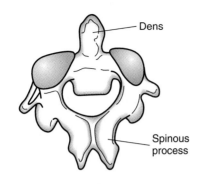

FIG. 7-5 Axis (C2).

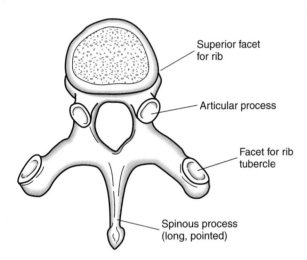

FIG. 7-6 Thoracic vertebra.

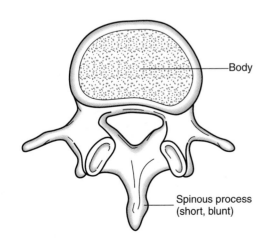

FIG. 7-7 Lumbar vertebra.

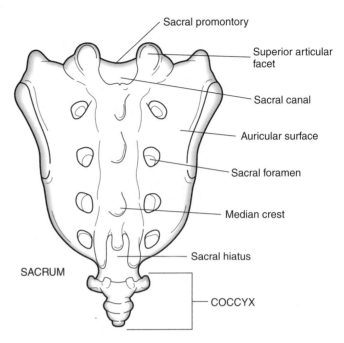

FIG. 7-8 Sacrum and coccyx.

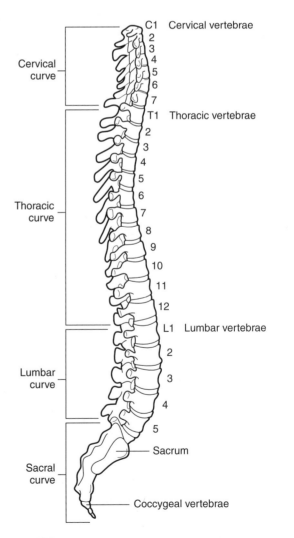

FIG. 7-9 Curvatures of the vertebral column.

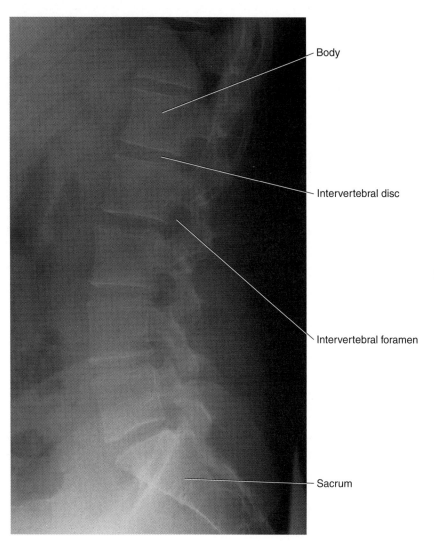

Body

Intervertebral disc

Intervertebral foramen

Sacrum

FIG. 7-10 Radiograph of the lumbar curvature.

masses, **sacral foramina** allow for passage of nerves. The first sacral segment has a prominent ridge, called the **sacral promontory,** on the visceral surface. The region inferior to this landmark is the true pelvic cavity. The spinous process of the S5 segment is absent, leaving an opening called the **sacral hiatus.**

The coccyx, or tailbone, is the most inferior region of the vertebral column. There are four (the number varies from three to five) separate small bones in the child, but these fuse to form a single bone in the adult. Several muscles have some point of attachment on the coccyx.

INTERVERTEBRAL DISCS

The intervertebral discs, located between the vertebral bodies, are fibrocartilaginous pads classified as symphysis joints. They are designed for strength. In addition to the discs, the vertebral bodies are joined by ligaments. Each disc consists of a soft central core, called the **nucleus pulposus,** and a firm outer ring, called the **anulus fibrosus.** The nucleus pulposus acts as a shock absorber and a ball-bearing during flexion, extension, and lateral bending of the vertebral column. The anulus fibrosus is composed of rings of fibrocartilage

that run obliquely from one vertebra to another to form strong bonds between the vertebrae. The intervertebral discs are thickest in the cervical and lumbar regions, which provides greater flexibility in these regions. As people get older, the nucleus pulposus may become thinner, which accounts for some of the loss of height that occurs as a result of aging. Changes also may occur in the anulus fibrosus that permit the nucleus pulposus to protrude through the outer ring, causing a herniated disc. The protrusion may compress an adjacent spinal nerve, causing pain in the lower back and/or leg.

CURVATURE OF THE VERTEBRAL COLUMN

Normally, when viewed from the side, as illustrated in Fig. 7-9, the vertebral column has four curvatures. These curvatures increase strength, resilience, and flexibility of the vertebral column. The thoracic and sacral curvatures are concave anteriorly (convex posteriorly) and are present at birth. The cervical and lumbar curvatures are convex anteriorly (concave posteriorly). The cervical curvature develops when the baby holds its head erect and the lumbar curvature develops when the child begins to stand. Fig. 7-10 is

TABLE 7-1   *Ligaments of the Vertebral Column*

Ligament	Description and Location
Anterior longitudinal ligament	Extends from C1 to sacrum; attached to anterior surface of vertebral bodies and discs; prevents hyperextension
Posterior longitudinal ligament	Extends from C1 to sacrum; narrow band that is attached to posterior edges of vertebral bodies and discs; located within vertebral canal; prevents hyperflexion
Ligamenta flava	Short bands that connect laminae of adjacent vertebrae on each side of spinous process; help maintain normal curvature of column
Interspinous ligaments	Short bands that connect the margins of adjacent spinous processes in thoracic and lumbar regions
Supraspinous ligaments	Short bands that connect the tips of adjacent spinous processes in thoracic and lumbar regions
Intertransverse ligaments	Short bands that connect adjacent transverse processes; poorly developed except in lumbar region
Ligamentum nuchae	Combination of interspinous and supraspinous ligaments in the cervical region

a radiograph of the lumbar spine that shows the anteriorly convex curvature. Several types of abnormal variations occur in the curvatures of the vertebral column. Some of these are congenital, whereas others may be due to poor posture, disease, or unequal muscle pull on the column. Scoliosis is an abnormal lateral curvature that most commonly occurs in the thoracic region. If untreated it may become severe and result in breathing difficulties. Kyphosis is an exaggerated dorsal curvature in the thoracic region. It is frequently seen in older individuals as a result of osteoporosis. It also may be due to a bone deformity known as *rickets*. Lordosis is an exaggerated lumbar curvature. This may occur temporarily in pregnant women when they throw back their shoulders and accentuate their lumbar curvature in an attempt to maintain their center of gravity.

LIGAMENTS OF THE VERTEBRAL COLUMN

The vertebral column is held in place by straplike ligaments. The major supporting ligaments are the **anterior** and **posterior longitudinal ligaments.** The anterior longitudinal ligament begins at C1 and extends downward along the entire anterior surface of the vertebral bodies to the sacrum. It is strongly attached to the bony vertebral bodies and to the discs to maintain stability of the joints and to prevent hyperextension (bending too far backward). The posterior longitudinal ligament is a narrow ligamentous band that runs inside the vertebral canal, along the posterior surface of the vertebral bodies, for the entire length of the vertebral column. It is somewhat weaker than the anterior longitudinal ligament. The ligament is attached to the intervertebral discs and the posterior edges of the vertebral bodies. The posterior longitudinal ligament tends to prevent hyperflexion (bending too far forward) of the vertebral column. **Ligamenta flava** are short bands of yellow elastic fibers that are located on each side of the spinous process. These ligaments connect the laminae of adjacent vertebrae and help to maintain the normal curvature of the vertebral column.

The margins of adjacent spinous processes from C7 to the sacrum are joined by **interspinous ligaments. Supraspinous ligaments** join the tips of the spinous processes in the same region. From C7 upward to the occipital bone, the interspinous and supraspinous ligaments are represented by the **ligamentum nuchae. Intertransverse ligaments** connect adjacent transverse processes. These consist of a few scattered ligamentous fibers, except in the lumbar region where they are membranous. The ligaments associated with the vertebral column are summarized in Table 7-1.

MUSCLES ASSOCIATED WITH THE VERTEBRAL COLUMN

The muscles associated with the back are arranged in three layers. The superficial and intermediate layers are extrinsic muscles and are concerned with respiration and movement of the limbs. These muscles, described in other portions of this book, include the trapezius, the latissimus dorsi, the levator scapulae, the rhomboids, and the serratus posterior. The deep muscle layer includes the true back muscles. These are the intrinsic muscles and they are concerned with the maintenance of posture and movements of the vertebral column. The intrinsic muscles are summarized in Table 7-2.

The deep layer of muscles associated with the vertebral column, which are the intrinsic back muscles, is further subdivided into superficial, intermediate, and deep layers. The superficial layer includes the **splenius capitis** and the **splenius cervicis.** The fibers of these muscles run superolaterally, with their origin on the ligamentum nuchae and spinous processes of vertebrae C7 to T6. The insertion of the splenius capitis is on the mastoid process of the temporal bone and the adjacent portion of the occipital bone, whereas the splenius cervicis fibers insert on the transverse processes of C2 to C4. As a group, these muscles pull the head posteriorly (extend the head). If the muscles on one side act alone, they bend or rotate the neck to turn the face to the same side.

TABLE 7-2 *Intrinsic Muscles Associated With the Vertebral Column*

Muscle	Origin	Insertion	Function	Description
Superficial Layer				
Splenius capitis	Ligamentum nuchae and spinous processes of C7 to T6	Mastoid process of temporal bone and adjacent occipital bone	Extend the head; rotate neck if one side contracts	Superficial intrinsic muscle in the neck
Splenius cervicis	Ligamentum nuchae and spinous processes of C7 to T6	Transverse processes of C2 to C4	Extend the head; rotate neck if one side contracts	Superficial intrinsic muscle in the neck
Intermediate Layer				
Iliocostalis	Iliac crests and ribs	Angles of ribs and transverse processes of C4 to C6	Extend vertebral column to maintain posture; if one side contracts, column bends to that side	Most lateral column of the erector spinae muscle group
Longissimus	Transverse processes of lumbar through cervical vertebrae	Transverse processes of thoracic and cervical vertebrae, ribs superior to origin, and mastoid process of temporal bone	Extend vertebral column; if one side contracts, column bends to that side	Intermediate column of erector spinae muscle group
Spinalis	Spinous processes of upper lumbar and lower thoracic vertebrae	Spinous processes of upper thoracic and cervical vertebrae	Extend vertebral column	Most medial column of erector spinae muscle group
Deep Layer				
Semispinalis	Transverse processes of C7 to T12	Occipital bone, spinous processes of cervical and thoracic vertebrae	Extend vertebral column	Composite muscle of deep layer; extends from thoracic region to head; part of the transversospinal group
Multifidus	Transverse processes of vertebrae	Spinous processes of preceding vertebrae	Stabilize vertebral column and rotate to opposite side	Short muscle bundles that pass superiorly over two to five vertebrae and then insert; part of the transversospinal group
Rotatores	Transverse processes of vertebrae	Spinous process of vertebra immediately superior to origin	Extend, rotate, and stabilize the vertebral column	Shortest muscles in the transversospinal group
Interspinales	Spinous processes of vertebrae	Spinous process of vertebra immediately superior to origin	Extend vertebral column	Insignificant muscle; well developed only in cervical region
Intertransversarius	Transverse processes of vertebrae	Transverse process of vertebra immediately superior to origin	Laterally bends vertebral column	Insignificant muscle; well developed only in cervical region

The largest muscle mass associated with the vertebral column is in the intermediate layer of intrinsic muscles. As a group, these muscles are the **erector spinae,** and, with both sides working together, they extend the vertebral column to maintain posture. The erector spinae are arranged in three longitudinal columns with their fibers parallel to the long axis of the body. The most lateral column is the **iliocostalis,** the intermediate column is the **longissimus,** and the most medial column is the **spinalis.**

When the mass of erector spinae muscles is removed, the deep layer, consisting of several small muscles, is visible in the space between the spinous processes and the transverse

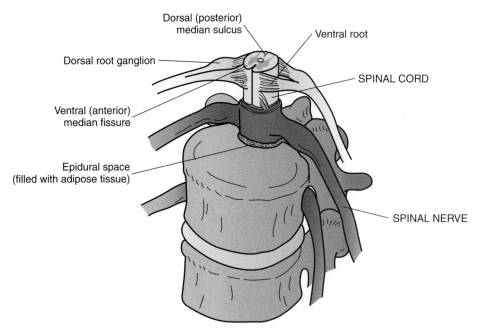

Dorsal (posterior) median sulcus

Ventral root

Dorsal root ganglion

SPINAL CORD

Ventral (anterior) median fissure

Epidural space (filled with adipose tissue)

SPINAL NERVE

FIG. 7-11 Epidural space of the spinal cord.

processes. Collectively, these muscles are called **transversospinal muscles** and their fibers run obliquely in a superomedial direction, from transverse processes to spinous processes above. The transversospinal muscles include the **semispinalis,** the **multifidus,** and the **rotatores.** They act synergistically with other intrinsic muscles. In addition to the transversospinal muscles, small, rather insignificant muscle fibers run between the spinous processes of adjacent vertebrae **(interspinales)** and between the transverse processes of adjacent vertebrae **(intertransversarius).** These are usually well developed only in the cervical region.

Spinal Cord

The spinal cord is a part of the central nervous system. It is located within the vertebral canal of the vertebral column. Like the brain, it is protected by bone, cerebrospinal fluid, and meninges. The spinal cord has two main functions. It is a conduction pathway for impulses going to and from the brain, and it serves as a reflex center.

Meninges

The three layers of meninges that surround the spinal cord are the same as those that surround the brain: the dura mater, the arachnoid, and the pia mater. These have been described in Chapter 2. Unlike the dura mater around the brain, the dura mater of the spinal cord consists of a single layer and is separated from the vertebral bones by an epidural space, which is filled with loose connective tissue and adipose tissue. This is illustrated in Fig. 7-11. The spinal cord terminates at vertebral level L1, but the meninges extend beyond

the end of the cord, down to the upper part of the sacrum. From there, a fibrous cord of pia mater, the **filum terminale,** extends down to the coccyx, where it is anchored. Cerebrospinal fluid circulates in the subarachnoid space between the arachnoid and pia mater. The subarachnoid space beyond the end of the spinal cord, between the end of the cord and the termination of the dura mater and arachnoid at the sacrum, provides a region for withdrawing cerebrospinal fluid with little danger of damage to the spinal cord.

Structure of the Spinal Cord

The spinal cord, illustrated in Fig. 7-12, begins as a continuation of the medulla oblongata, the inferior portion of the brainstem, at the level of the foramen magnum, and continues downward for a distance of about 43 to 46 cm until it terminates at the level of the first lumbar vertebrae. Distally, at L1, the spinal cord terminates in a triangular, or cone-shaped, region called the **conus medullaris.** The spinal cord is divided in 31 segments with each segment giving rise to a pair of spinal nerves: eight cervical segments (C1 through C8), 12 thoracic segments (T1 through T12), five lumbar segments (L1 through L5), five sacral segments (S1 through S5), and one coccygeal segment. The spinal cord segments do not correspond directly with the vertebral levels. This is illustrated in Fig. 7-13. At the distal end of the cord, many spinal nerves extend beyond the conus medullaris to form a collection that resembles a horse's tail. This is the **cauda equina.** The cord has two enlarged sections, one in the cervical region and one in the lumbar region. The **cervical enlargement** includes the C4 to the T1 segments of the cord and extends from approximately the C3 to the C7 vertebral bodies. It gives rise to the nerves that supply the upper ex-

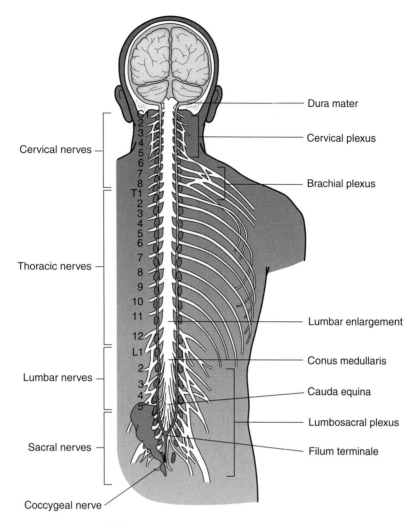

FIG. 7-12 Gross anatomy of the spinal cord.

tremity. The **lumbosacral enlargement** includes the L2 to the S3 segments of the cord and extends from approximately the T11 to the L1 vertebral bodies. Nerves from this enlargement supply the lower extremity.

In cross section, illustrated in Fig. 7-14, the spinal cord appears oval in shape. A narrow, deep, **dorsal (posterior) median sulcus** and a shallower, but wider, **ventral (anterior) median fissure** partially divide the cord into right and left halves. Peripheral white matter surrounds a core of gray matter that resembles a butterfly or the letter H in shape. Each side of the gray matter is divided into **dorsal, lateral,** and **ventral horns.** These contain the terminal portions of sensory neuron axons, entire interneurons, and the dendrites and cell bodies of motor neurons. The central connecting bar between the two large areas of gray matter is the **gray commissure.** This surrounds the **central canal,** which contains cerebrospinal fluid. The gray matter divides the surrounding white matter into three regions on each side. These regions are the **dorsal, lateral,** and **ventral funiculi,** or **columns.** The white matter contains longitudinal bundles of myelinated nerve fibers, called **nerve tracts.**

SPINAL NERVES

Thirty-one pairs of spinal nerves emerge laterally from the spinal cord. Each pair of nerves corresponds to a segment of the cord and they are named accordingly. This means there are **eight cervical nerves** (C1 through C8), **12 thoracic nerves** (T1 through T12), **five lumbar nerves** (L1 through L5), **five sacral nerves** (S1 through S5), and **one coccygeal nerve** (Co).

Spinal Nerve Roots

Each spinal nerve is connected to the spinal cord by a **dorsal root** and a **ventral root** (see Figs. 7-11 and 7-14). The dorsal root can be recognized by an enlargement, the **dorsal root ganglion,** which contains the cell bodies of afferent (sensory) neurons that are transmitting impulses from the periphery of the body to the central nervous system. The cell bodies of efferent (motor) neurons are in the ventral horns of the gray matter. The dorsal root has only sensory fibers and the ventral root has only motor fibers. The two roots join to form the spinal nerve just before the nerve leaves the vertebral

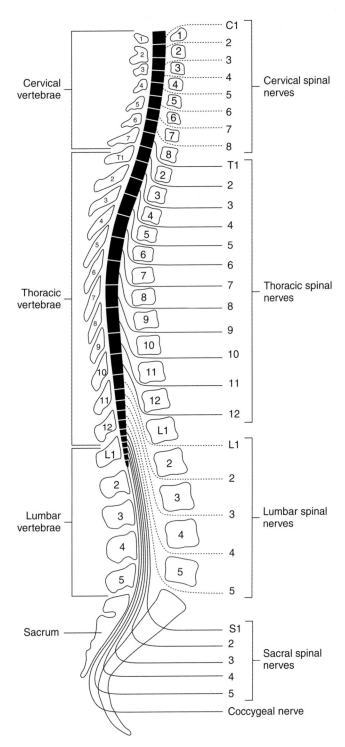

FIG. 7-13 Relationship of spinal cord segments to vertebral bodies.

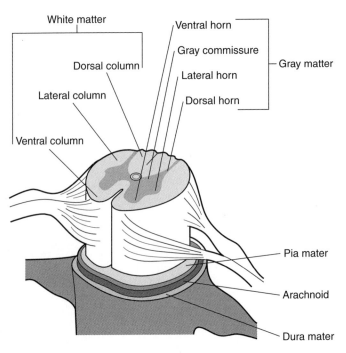

FIG. 7-14 Cross section of the spinal cord.

Nerve Plexuses

Immediately after leaving the vertebral column, each spinal nerve divides into **dorsal** and **ventral rami.** Each ramus con-column through the corresponding intervertebral foramen. Because all spinal nerves have both afferent (sensory) and efferent (motor) components, they are all mixed nerves.

tains both sensory and motor fibers. The dorsal rami supply the skin and muscles of the posterior portion of the body trunk. In the thoracic region, the ventral rami of nerves T2 through T12 go directly to the thoracic wall where they are called **intercostal nerves.** In other regions, the ventral rami form complex networks called **plexuses,** which supply the skin and muscles of the extremities. In the plexus, the fibers are sorted and recombined so that the fibers associated with a particular body part are together even though they may originate from different regions of the cord. The four major nerve plexuses are the cervical, brachial, lumbar, and sacral, which are described below and summarized in Table 7-3.

The **cervical plexus,** located deep in the neck and under the sternocleidomastoid muscle, arises from the ventral rami of spinal nerves C1 through C4. It supplies the skin and muscles of the neck and shoulder. One of the important nerves that emerges from the plexus is the phrenic nerve, which supplies the diaphragm. Trauma in the cervical region may damage the phrenic nerve and result in paralysis of the diaphragm.

The **brachial plexus** is located deep to the clavicle, between the neck and axilla. It runs between the anterior and middle scalene muscles. Ventral rami of spinal nerves C5 through C8 and T1 form this plexus. Five major nerves and several smaller nerves emerge from the brachial plexus to supply the skin and muscles of the upper extremity. The larger nerves are the musculocutaneous, ulnar, median, radial, and axillary.

The **lumbar plexus** is formed within the psoas major muscle by the ventral rami of the first four lumbar nerves. In about 50% of people, the ventral ramus of T12 also contributes. The nerves from the lumbar plexus innervate the

TABLE 7-3 *Spinal Nerve Plexuses*

Plexus	Location	Spinal Nerves Involved	Region Supplied	Major Nerves Leaving Plexus
Cervical	Deep in the neck; under the sternocleidomastoid muscle	C1 through C4	Skin and muscles of the neck and shoulder; diaphragm	Phrenic
Brachial	Deep to the clavicle, between neck and axilla; between anterior and middle scalene muscles	C5 through C8 and T1	Skin and muscles of the upper extremity	Musculocutaneous Ulnar Median Radial Axillary
Lumbar	Within psoas major muscle	T12 and L1 through L4	Skin and muscles of lower abdominopelvic region, buttocks, and anterior thighs	Femoral Obturator
Sacral	Within the true pelvis where it is associated with the anterior surface of the piriformis muscle	L4, L5, and S1 through S4	Pelvic diaphragm, external genitalia, posterior thigh, leg, and foot	Sciatic Pudendal

skin and muscles of the lower abdominopelvic region, the buttocks, and the anterior thighs. The largest and most important branches that emerge from the lumbar plexus are the femoral and the obturator nerves.

The **sacral plexus** is located in the true pelvis, where it is closely associated with the anterior surface of the piriformis muscle. Branches from this plexus innervate the pelvic diaphragm, the external genitalia, the posterior thigh, and the leg and foot. Important nerves that emerge from the sacral plexus are the pudendal and sciatic, which is the largest nerve in the body. The sacral plexus is formed by the ventral rami of spinal nerves L4 and L5 and by the ventral rami of S1 through S4. Note that L4 contributes to both the lumbar plexus and the sacral plexus. The lumbar and sacral plexuses are closely related and are sometimes collectively referred to as the **lumbosacral plexus.**

VASCULATURE OF THE SPINAL CORD

The arterial blood supply for the spinal cord comes from three longitudinal vessels, a single **anterior spinal artery** and two **posterior spinal arteries.** The anterior spinal artery runs the entire length of the cord in the ventral (anterior) median fissure. It is formed by two small branches of the vertebral arteries and it supplies the anterior two thirds of the spinal cord. The posterior spinal arteries also arise as

branches of the vertebral arteries and are adjacent to the dorsal roots of spinal nerves. These arteries anastomose freely with each other and supply the posterior one third of the spinal cord. The blood from the vertebral arteries that enters the anterior and posterior spinal arteries is sufficient only for the cervical segments of the cord. Blood for the remaining segments comes from the numerous **radicular arteries** that contribute blood to the anterior and posterior spinal arteries. Radicular arteries arise as branches of the **segmental arteries,** which are formed by the parietal branches of the thoracic and abdominal aorta, particularly the intercostal and lumbar arteries. The radicular arteries enter the vertebral canal through the intervertebral foramina and provide the blood supply for the vertebrae and meninges in addition to contributing blood to the spinal arteries.

Spinal veins have a distribution similar to that of the spinal arteries. The veins are arranged longitudinally and anastomose freely with each other. Within the vertebral canal is a plexus of veins that surrounds the spinal dura. The vertebral venous plexus and the anterior and posterior spinal veins drain into intervertebral veins, which then empty into the vertebral veins, ascending lumbar veins, and the azygous venous system. The arteries and veins of the spinal cord are difficult to visualize in cross-sectional images because of their small size.

· REVIEW QUESTIONS ·

1. What parts of a vertebra make up the vertebral arch?
2. What are the unique features that distinguish each type of vertebra from all the other types?
3. What portion of the vertebral column articulates with the os coxae?
4. What is the most inferior region of the vertebral column?
5. In what two regions of the vertebral column are the intervertebral discs the thickest?
6. What are the two parts of an intervertebral disc and which is the inner portion?
7. Which two curvatures of the vertebral column are present at birth?
8. What is the purpose or advantage of the curvatures in the vertebral column?
9. What is the difference between ligamenta flava and the ligamentum nuchae?
10. What are the three columns of erector spinae muscles and what is their sequence from lateral to medial?
11. What is the collective term for the deep layer of intrinsic back muscles?
12. How long is the spinal cord? Inferior to the termination of the spinal cord, what is present in the vertebral canal?
13. What is in the epidural space around the spinal cord?
14. Where are the two enlargements of the spinal cord located?
15. What type of tissue is in the dorsal, lateral, and ventral horns of the spinal cord?
16. How many segments are in the spinal cord? How many spinal nerves emerge from the spinal cord?
17. How many nerves are in each of the five groups, or categories, of spinal nerves?
18. What is the difference in composition between dorsal and ventral roots of spinal nerves?
19. Name four nerve plexuses and at least one nerve that emerges from each plexus.
20. Name the longitudinal vessels that provide the arterial blood supply for the spinal cord and state where each one is located.

· CHAPTER QUIZ ·

Name the Following:

1. The portion of a vertebra that is between the transverse process and the spinous process
2. The portions, or features, of vertebrae that form the intervertebral foramina
3. The portion of the sacrum that articulates with the pelvic girdle
4. The outer ring of an intervertebral disc
5. An exaggerated dorsal curvature in the thoracic region
6. The strongest major supporting ligament of the vertebral column
7. The two muscles in the superficial layer of intrinsic back muscles
8. The triangular terminal portion of the spinal cord
9. The spinal cord enlargement that gives rise to nerves that supply impulses to the upper extremity
10. The spinal nerve root that contains only motor fibers

True/False:

1. The body and vertebral arch of a vertebra surround the vertebral foramen.
2. The atlas has a dens or odontoid process.
3. With a herniated disc, the anulus fibrosus protrudes through the nucleus pulposus.
4. Lordosis is an exaggerated lumbar curvature.
5. Ligamenta flava are short bands of yellow elastic fibers that connect the laminae of adjacent vertebrae.
6. The filum terminale is a fibrous cord of pia mater that anchors the spinal cord to the coccyx.
7. The anterior spinal artery is located in the ventral median fissure.
8. In the spinal cord, the gray matter is peripherally located and the white matter is more central.
9. The phrenic nerve that innervates the diaphragm originates from the brachial plexus.
10. The largest nerve in the body originates in the sacral plexus.

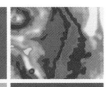

CHAPTER EIGHT

Upper Extremity | 8

OBJECTIVES

Upon completion of this chapter, the student should be able to do the following:
- Identify the bones that make up the pectoral girdle.
- Describe the location and the functions of three groups of muscles that are associated with the attachment of the pectoral girdle and the upper extremity to the trunk of the body.
- Describe the boundaries and contents of the axilla.
- Identify the skeletal, muscular, vascular, and neural components of the arm.
- Identify the structural components of the arm in transverse sections through the proximal and distal regions.
- Describe the boundaries and contents of the cubital fossa and identify its components in a transverse section.
- Identify the skeletal, muscular, vascular, and neural components of the forearm.
- Identify the structural components of the forearm in transverse sections through the proximal and distal regions.
- Name and locate the eight bones in the wrist and discuss the structure and significance of the carpal tunnel.
- Describe the structure of the shoulder joint and discuss the anatomical relationships of its components.
- Identify structural components of the shoulder joint in transverse sections through the humeral head and the glenoid fossa.
- Describe the structure of the elbow joint and discuss the anatomical relationships of its components, including the humeroulnar, humeroradial, and radioulnar articulations.
- Identify the structural components of the elbow joint in sagittal sections through the humerus and the ulna, through the humerus and the radius, and in a transverse section through the radius and the ulna.

The upper extremity consists of the arm, forearm, wrist, hand, and fingers. The arm has a single bone, the humerus. Two bones, the radius on the lateral side and the ulna on the medial side, form the framework of the forearm. The wrist, or carpus, consists of eight small bones that are collectively called carpals. The hand has five bones that are known as the metacarpals, and distal to these are 14 phalanges that form the fingers. These bones are covered with muscle, fascia, and skin.

ATTACHMENT OF THE UPPER EXTREMITY TO THE TRUNK

The scapula and the clavicle make up the **pectoral girdle,** which provides the connection between the upper extremity and the axial skeleton. The bones of the pectoral girdle are illustrated in Fig. 8-1. Muscles anchor the upper extremity and the pectoral girdle to the trunk of the body. These muscles can be divided into three groups.

One group extends from the trunk to the scapula. The muscles in this group can, in appropriate combinations, move the scapula upward, downward, forward, backward, clockwise, or counterclockwise. These actions assist in movement of the shoulder.

A second group of muscles extends between the scapula and the humerus. These muscles move the arm at the glenohumeral (shoulder) joint. The muscles and tendons that extend over the shoulder strengthen and stabilize the joint.

A third group attaches the humerus to the trunk. This group, which includes the pectoralis major and the latissimus dorsi, adducts the arm. Table 8-1 summarizes the muscles associated with the trunk, the scapula, and the humerus.

AXILLA

The space at the junction of the arm and the thorax, between the upper limb and the chest wall, is called the **axilla.** The anterior wall of the axilla is formed by the **pectoralis major** and the **pectoralis minor** muscles. Predominant structures in the posterior wall are the **scapula** and the **subscapularis** muscle. Medially, the axilla is delineated by the **ribs,** the **intercostal muscles,** and the **serratus anterior** muscle. The narrow lateral wall is formed by the head of the **humerus;** specifically, it is formed by the **intertubercular (bicipital) groove,** where the anterior and posterior walls converge. The long head of the biceps brachii muscle is located in the intertubercular groove. The short head of the biceps brachii muscle and the coracobrachialis muscle are closely associated in this same region. The boundaries of the axilla are illustrated in Fig. 8-2.

The axilla functions as a passageway for vessels and nerves that pass between the root of the neck and the arm. The vessels in this region include the axillary artery and vein, together with their branches. The nerves, which are all branches of the brachial plexus, innervate the arm. The axilla also contains numerous lymph nodes, which are drained by axillary lymph vessels that pass through this region. The lymph nodes are of particular significance because of their frequent involvement in breast cancer.

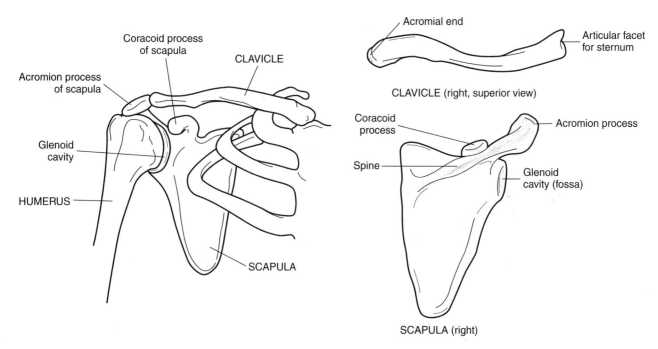

FIG. 8-1 Components of the pectoral girdle.

TABLE 8-1   *Muscles Associated with Trunk, Scapula, and Humerus*

Muscle	Origin	Insertion	Action	Innervation
Extend from Trunk to Scapula				
Trapezius	Thoracic vertebrae	Spine of scapula	Adduct scapula	Accessory (XI)
Rhomboids	Cervical and thoracic vertebrae	Medial border and spine of scapula	Adduct scapula	Dorsal scapular
Levator scapulae	Cervical vertebrae	Medial border of scapula	Elevate scapula	Dorsal scapular
Pectoralis minor	Third to fifth ribs	Coracoid process of scapula	Pull scapula inferiorly	Medial pectoral
Serratus anterior	First eight ribs	Medial border of scapula	Rotate scapula	Long thoracic nerve
Extend from Scapula to Humerus				
Deltoid	Acromion and spine of scapula; clavicle	Deltoid tuberosity of humerus	Abduct arm	Axillary
Supraspinatus	Supraspinous fossa	Greater tubercle of humerus	Abduct arm	Suprascapular
Subscapularis	Subscapular fossa	Lesser tubercle of humerus	Medial rotation of arm	Subscapular
Infraspinatus	Infraspinous fossa	Greater tubercle of humerus	Lateral rotation of arm	Suprascapular
Teres minor	Lateral margin of scapula	Greater tubercle of humerus	Lateral rotation of arm	Axillary
Teres major	Superior lateral margin of scapula	Intertubercular groove of humerus	Adduct arm	Subscapular
Coracobrachialis	Coracoid process of scapula	Shaft of humerus	Adduct arm	Musculocutaneous
Extend from Trunk to Humerus				
Pectoralis major	Clavicle, sternum, costal cartilages	Intertubercular groove of humerus	Adduct and medially rotate humerus	Medial and lateral pectoral
Latissimus dorsi	Thoracic and lumbar vertebrae; crest of ilium	Intertubercular groove of humerus	Adduct and medially rotate humerus	Thoracodorsal

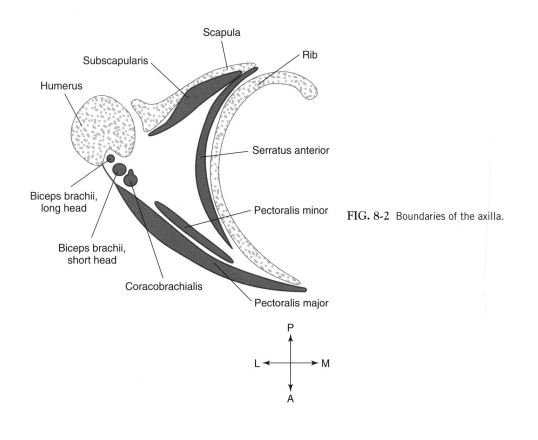

FIG. 8-2 Boundaries of the axilla.

General Anatomy of the Arm

OSSEOUS COMPONENTS

The region from the shoulder to the elbow is the arm, or brachium. The only bone in the arm is the humerus, which is the longest bone in the upper extremity. The features of the humerus are illustrated in Fig. 8-3.

MUSCULAR COMPONENTS

The muscles of the arm are arranged in anterior and posterior compartments that are separated by an intermuscular septum of fascia. The muscles of the arm are summarized in Table 8-2.

The anterior muscle compartment consists of three muscles that act as flexors and are innervated by the musculocutaneous branch of the brachial plexus. The largest of the muscles is the **biceps brachii.** As the name implies, the biceps

TABLE 8-2 *Muscles Located in the Arm*

Muscle	Origin	Insertion	Action	Innervation
Anterior Compartment				
Biceps brachii	Long head: supraglenoid tubercle Short head: coracoid process	Radius and ulna	Flex and supinate forearm	Musculocutaneous
Coracobrachialis	Coracoid process	Medial humerus	Flex and adduct shoulder	Musculocutaneous
Brachialis	Distal humerus	Ulna	Flex forearm	Musculocutaneous
Posterior Compartment				
Triceps brachii	Long head: infraglenoid tubercle Lateral head: proximal shaft of humerus Medial head: distal shaft of humerus	Olecranon process of ulna	Extend arm at elbow and stabilize shoulder	Radial

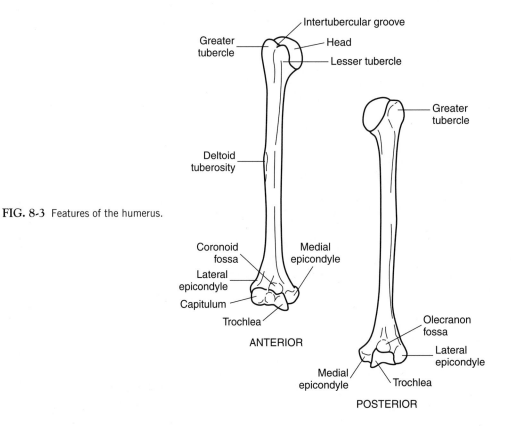

FIG. 8-3 Features of the humerus.

brachii has two heads of origin. The short head originates on the coracoid process of the scapula and the long head originates from a tubercle just above the glenoid fossa (supraglenoid tubercle). The two heads merge to form a single muscle belly that inserts on the radial tuberosity and on the ulna by way of an aponeurosis. In addition to being a flexor of the forearm at the elbow, the biceps brachii is a supinator of the forearm. The muscle originates superior to the shoulder and passes over the joint; thus it assists in stabilizing and strengthening the shoulder joint. The biceps brachii also acts as a flexor of the arm at the shoulder.

The **coracobrachialis** is a short muscle on the medial surface of the superior part of the arm. It has a common origin with the short head of the biceps brachii on the coracoid process of the scapula, and it inserts on the medial side of the humerus near the midpoint of the shaft. The coracobrachialis, along with the biceps brachii, acts as a weak flexor and adductor of the shoulder. This muscle is visible only in sections through the upper part of the arm. The coracobrachialis is the only muscle that, although predominantly located in the arm, acts on the shoulder joint.

The third muscle of the anterior compartment is the **brachialis.** This is a deep muscle, underlying the biceps brachii. It has an extensive origin along the anterior surface of the distal half of the humerus, and it terminates on the coronoid process of the ulna. The brachialis is a strong flexor of the forearm at the elbow joint. It is seen only in sections through the lower part of the arm.

The posterior compartment of the arm is occupied by a single, large muscle, the **triceps brachii.** As the name implies, this muscle has three heads of origin. The long head originates via a tendon from the infraglenoid tubercle. The lateral head attaches to the posterior surface of the proximal shaft of the humerus. The medial head is deep to both the long and the lateral heads. Its origin is on the posterior surface of the shaft of the humerus, distal to the origin of the lateral head. All three heads merge to form a single muscle belly that inserts on the olecranon process of the ulna via a single tendon. An olecranon bursa is located between the tendon and the olecranon process. The triceps brachii is a powerful extensor of the elbow. The long head spans the shoulder joint; consequently, it also helps stabilize that joint. The radial nerve innervates the triceps brachii.

Vascular Components

The primary arterial blood supply to the arm is the **brachial artery** and its branches. The brachial artery begins at the inferior border of the teres major muscle, as a continuation of the axillary artery, and it ends in the cubital fossa, where it divides into the radial and ulnar arteries. The vessel is superficial throughout its length, and it runs its course in the fascia of the medial intermuscular septum that divides the muscles into the anterior and posterior compartments. In the septum, it is associated with the basilic vein, the median nerve, and the ulnar nerve. Numerous branches supply the muscles of the arm.

One, or possibly two, **brachial veins** accompany the brachial artery. These deep veins ascend through the arm to continue as the axillary vein. In addition to the deep brachial vein, two important superficial veins are in the arm. The **cephalic vein** is in the superficial fascia, anterolateral to the biceps brachii muscle. As it courses superiorly, it passes between the deltoid and the pectoralis major muscles to empty into the axillary vein. The **basilic vein** is in the superficial fascia on the medial side of the arm. About one third of the way up the arm from the elbow, the basilic vein passes deep to the superficial fascia and continues upward to merge with the brachial vein to form the axillary vein. Both the superficial cephalic and basilic veins are frequently visible through the skin.

Nerves in the Arm

The major nerves traversing the arm are the **musculocutaneous,** the **median,** the **ulnar,** and the **radial.** A fifth nerve, the **axillary,** supplies the skin over the upper part of the arm. The nerves are all terminal branches of the **brachial plexus.** Both the median and the ulnar nerves descend the arm without giving off branches. They supply the elbow joint and the forearm. In the uppermost part of the arm, the median nerve may be either lateral or anterior to the brachial artery. About midway down the arm, the nerve crosses over the vessel to the medial side. The ulnar nerve is situated near the brachial artery in the upper half of the arm. It then penetrates the intermuscular septum and descends through the arm just anterior to the medial head of the triceps brachii. The musculocutaneous and radial nerves give off branches to supply the muscles of the arm. The musculocutaneous nerve descends between the biceps brachii and the brachialis muscles. As it descends, its branches innervate those two muscles and the coracobrachialis muscle. The radial nerve enters the arm on the medial side of the humerus, then curves around the bone, in the radial groove, to descend in the intermuscular septum on the lateral side.

Sectional Anatomy of the Arm

Transverse Sections

Section Through the Proximal Arm

Fig. 8-4 illustrates a transverse section through the upper region of the arm. The **deltoid** muscle is superficial on the lateral side of the humerus and the long head of the **biceps brachii** is anterior. The **cephalic vein** is in the superficial fascia, anterior to these two muscles. At upper levels, such as the level in Fig. 8-4, the **coracobrachialis muscle** is adjacent to the long head of the biceps brachii. The coracobrachialis has a common origin with the short head of the biceps, and at this level, the two may be indistinguishable. The **musculocutaneous nerve** enters the arm by penetrating the coracobrachialis muscle; in Fig. 8-4 this nerve is

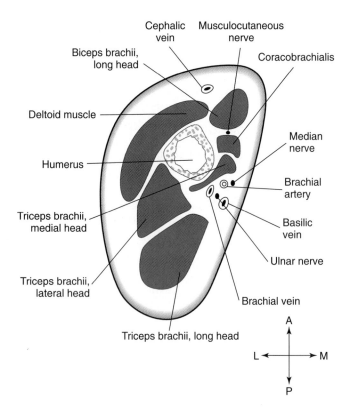

FIG. 8-4 Transverse section through the proximal portion of the arm.

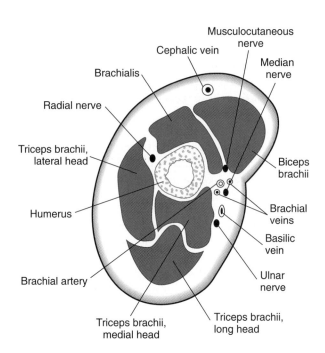

FIG. 8-5 Transverse section through the distal arm.

apparent between the coracobrachialis and the biceps brachii. The posterior compartment contains the lateral head and the long head of the **triceps brachii.** A small portion of the medial head is evident on the posterior surface of the humerus. Several vessels and nerves are apparent in the fascia of the medial intermuscular septum. The artery of note is the **brachial artery,** with the **median nerve** located anterior to it, and the **ulnar nerve** located posterior to it. The deep vein is the **brachial vein,** and the **basilic vein** is more superficial.

Section Through the Distal Arm

In the distal half of the arm, as illustrated by the line drawing in Fig. 8-5, the anterior muscle compartment includes the **biceps brachii** and the **brachialis** muscles. The brachialis is lateral and deep to the biceps brachii. The coracobrachialis muscle, seen in the proximal arm, is not evident in the lower sections, because this short muscle inserts near the middle of the humeral shaft. The posterior compartment continues to contain the **triceps brachii.** The **radial nerve** is now lateral to the shaft of the humerus, between the triceps brachii and the brachialis muscles. At this level, the **median nerve** is medial to the brachial artery. The **ulnar nerve** is closely associated with the triceps brachii on the medial side.

CUBITAL FOSSA

The cubital fossa is a triangular area on the anterior side of the elbow joint. It contains vessels and nerves that pass

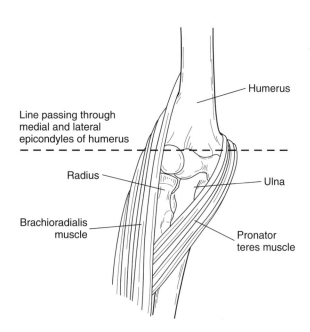

FIG. 8-6 Diagram of the boundaries of the cubital fossa.

from the arm to the forearm. The sides of the fossa are formed by the **brachioradialis muscle** laterally and the **pronator teres muscle** medially. Both of these muscles follow a somewhat oblique course; thus they meet to form the apex of a triangle. The base of the triangle is an imaginary line between the lateral and medial epicondyles of the humerus. These boundaries of the cubital fossa are illustrated by the diagram in Fig. 8-6. The floor is formed by

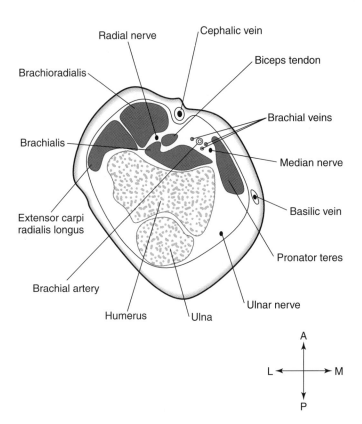

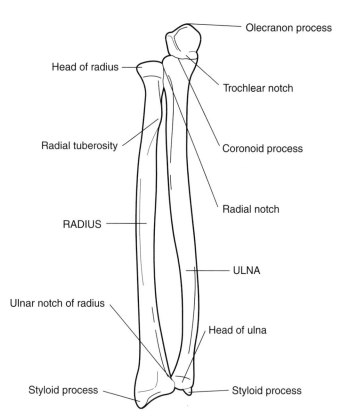

FIG. 8-7 Transverse section through the cubital fossa showing the boundaries and contents of the fossa.

FIG. 8-8 Features of the radius and the ulna.

the **brachialis** and the **supinator muscles.** The roof consists of deep fascia and a triangular sheet of tendon called the **bicipital aponeurosis.** The contents of the fossa, from medial to lateral, include the **median nerve,** the **brachial artery** with its accompanying veins, the **tendon of the biceps brachii,** and the **radial nerve.** In the distal part of the fossa, near the apex, the brachial artery branches into the radial and ulnar arteries, and the radial nerve divides into the superficial radial and posterior interosseous branches. All of these structures are embedded in fatty connective tissue within the fossa. The superficial fascia, overlying the cubital fossa, contains superficial blood vessels and nerves. One of the most significant of these is the **median cubital vein,** which connects the basilic and cephalic veins and is frequently used for venipuncture. A transverse section through the cubital fossa is illustrated in Fig. 8-7.

General Anatomy of the Forearm

OSSEOUS COMPONENTS

The forearm, or antebrachium, extends from the elbow to the wrist. The skeleton of the forearm consists of two bones, the **radius** and the **ulna.** In anatomical position, the bones are parallel, with the radius on the lateral side and the ulna on the medial side. An interosseous membrane connects the two bones and also separates the muscles of the forearm into the anterior flexor and the posterior extensor compart-

ments. Rotation of the proximal and distal radioulnar joints allows the hand to function in either the pronated or the supinated position. Some of the features of the radius and the ulna are illustrated in Fig. 8-8.

MUSCULAR COMPONENTS

In general, the muscles of the forearm act on the wrist, the hand, and the digits (Table 8-3). Exceptions to this include the brachioradialis, which flexes the elbow joint, and the pronator and supinator muscles. The radius and ulna, with an interosseous membrane between them, form a dividing line that separates the muscles into anterior and posterior compartments.

The anterior muscle compartment contains the **flexor/ pronator** group of muscles. Superficial muscles in this group arise from the medial epicondyle of the humerus by a common flexor origin. These muscles cross the elbow joint and are anterior to it; consequently, they act as weak flexors of the elbow, in addition to their function with the wrist or hand. All of the superficial muscles, except the flexor carpi ulnaris, are innervated by the median nerve. The flexor carpi ulnaris is innervated by the ulnar nerve.

The deep muscles of the anterior compartment, which include two flexor muscles and a pronator, originate from the anterior surfaces of the radius and the ulna. These are innervated by the anterior interosseous branch of the median nerve. A portion of the flexor digitorum profundus is supplied by the ulnar nerve.

TABLE 8-3 *Muscles Located in the Forearm*

Muscle	Origin	Insertion	Action	Innervation
Anterior Compartment				
Superficial Muscles				
Flexor carpi radialis	Medial epicondyle	Metacarpals, second and third	Flex hand	Median
Flexor carpi ulnaris	Medial epicondyle	Carpals: pisiform and hamate	Flex hand	Ulnar
Palmaris longus	Medial epicondyle	Flexor retinaculum	Flex hand	Median
Pronator teres	Medial epicondyle	Radius, lateral surface	Pronate hand	Median
Flexor digitorum superficialis	Medial epicondyle	Middle phalanges of fingers	Flex fingers	Median
Deep Muscles				
Flexor digitorum profundus	Ulna	Distal phalanges of fingers	Flex fingers	Median and ulnar
Flexor pollicis longus	Radius	Distal phalanx of thumb	Flex thumb	Median
Pronator quadratus	Distal ulna	Distal radius	Pronate hand	Median
Posterior Compartment				
Superficial Muscles				
Extensor carpi ulnaris	Lateral epicondyle	Fifth metacarpal	Extend hand	Radial
Extensor carpi radialis brevis	Lateral epicondyle	Third metacarpal	Extend hand	Radial
Extensor digiti minimi	Lateral epicondyle	Proximal phalanx of fifth finger	Extend fifth finger	Radial
Extensor digitorum	Lateral epicondyle	Phalanges	Extend fingers	Radial
Extensor carpi radialis longus	Lateral supracondylar ridge	Second metacarpal	Extend hand	Radial
Brachioradialis	Lateral supracondylar ridge	Styloid of radius	Flex forearm	Radial
Deep Muscles				
Extensor pollicis brevis	Radius	Proximal phalanx of thumb	Extend thumb	Radial
Extensor pollicis longus	Ulna	Distal phalanx of thumb	Extend thumb	Radial
Extensor indicis	Ulna	Phalanx of index finger	Extend index finger	Radial
Abductor pollicis longus	Radius and ulna	First metacarpal	Abduct thumb	Radial
Supinator	Lateral epicondyle	Proximal radius	Supinate hand	Radial

The posterior muscle compartment contains the **extensor/supinator** group of muscles. In addition, the brachioradialis muscle is considered to be part of this compartment. Four of the superficial extensors arise from a common origin on the lateral epicondyle of the humerus.

The brachioradialis and the extensor carpi radialis longus arise from the lateral supracondylar ridge of the humerus rather than from the common extensor origin with the other superficial muscles. The brachioradialis is a lateral muscle that inserts on the styloid process of the radius, and it flexes the elbow joint rather than acting on the wrist or hand. Four of the five deep muscles are extensors. The fifth muscle, the supinator, acts on the forearm, rather than on the hand and digits. The radial nerve and its branches innervate all the muscles of the posterior compartment.

VASCULAR COMPONENTS

The brachial artery, which is located in the arm, divides into the **radial** and the **ulnar** arteries in the cubital fossa. The radial artery, which is the smaller of the two vessels, courses distally, deep to the brachioradialis muscle. Near the wrist, it becomes more superficial and can be palpated against the anterior surface of the radius. The radial artery enters the palm and terminates in the deep palmar arch. Along its course, the radial artery gives off branches to nearby muscles.

The ulnar artery continues distally from the cubital fossa, between the superficial and deep muscle layers on the medial side of the anterior compartment. Near its origin in the cubital fossa, the ulnar artery gives off a **common interosseous branch.** This branch immediately divides into the **anterior** and **posterior interosseous arteries.** The an-

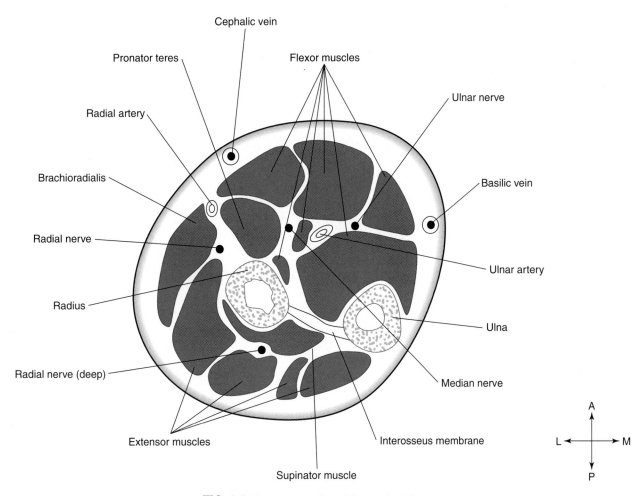

FIG. 8-9 Transverse section of the proximal forearm.

terior branch courses distally along the anterior surface of the interosseous membrane. The posterior interosseous artery enters the posterior compartment and supplies the muscles in that region. The ulnar artery terminates in superficial and deep palmar arches. Veins accompany most of the arteries.

NERVES IN THE FOREARM

The largest nerve in the forearm is the **median nerve.** It begins in the axilla as a branch of the brachial plexus and descends through the arm without dividing into branches. In the cubital region, the median nerve passes over the ulnar artery and then descends through the forearm, lateral to the ulnar artery, between the superficial and deep muscle layers in the anterior compartment. Near the wrist, the nerve becomes superficial. The median nerve supplies all of the superficial muscles in the anterior compartment, except the flexor carpi ulnaris. The anterior interosseous branch of the median nerve supplies most of the deep muscles of the anterior compartment.

The **ulnar nerve** is on the medial side of the anterior compartment. It supplies the flexor carpi ulnaris muscle. The

radial nerve descends along the lateral side of the arm and supplies muscles of the posterior compartment. In the region of the elbow, the radial nerve divides into the superficial and the deep branches. The superficial branch continues distally under the brachioradialis muscle and innervates the brachioradialis and the flexor carpi radialis muscles. The deep branch becomes the posterior interosseous nerve, which descends along the posterior surface of the interosseous membrane. This nerve supplies all the muscles of the posterior compartment, with the exception of two muscles that are supplied by the superficial branch of the radial nerve.

Sectional Anatomy of the Forearm

TRANSVERSE SECTIONS

Section Through the Proximal Forearm

Transverse sections through the upper part of the forearm show the **radius** and the **ulna,** with the **interosseous membrane** between them as illustrated in Fig. 8-9. These structures separate the muscles into anterior flexor and posterior

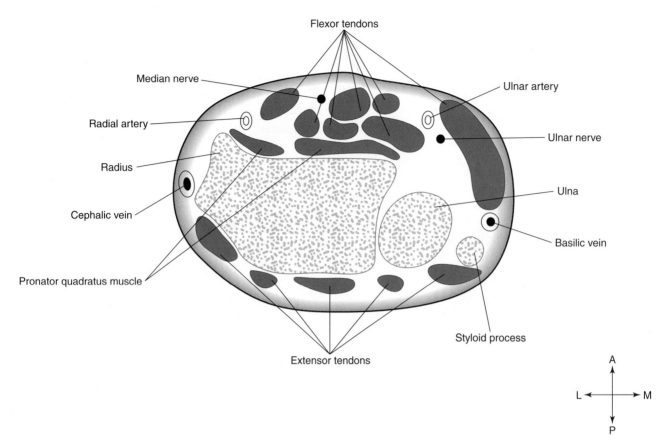

FIG. 8-10 Transverse section of the distal forearm.

extensor compartments. Within the anterior compartment, the **ulnar artery** and **ulnar nerve** are on the medial side, the **median nerve** is centrally located, and the **radial artery** is lateral and near the surface. The superficial branch of the **radial nerve** is adjacent to the brachioradialis muscle. The deep branch of the radial nerve is more posteriorly located. The medial **basilic** and the lateral **cephalic veins** are situated in the superficial fascia.

Section Through the Distal Forearm

Transverse sections through the most distal part of the forearm show little musculature, because this region consists primarily of tendons going to the hand and fingers. A transverse section through the distal radius and ulna is illustrated in Fig. 8-10. The large distal **radius** dominates this section. It articulates with the small **ulnar head** at the inferior radioulnar joint. The **styloid process** of the ulna is medial to the ulnar head. The space posterior to the osseous components is filled with tendons of the extensor muscles and with fascia. Tendons of the flexor muscles, together with arteries and nerves, fill the anterior space. The **ulnar artery** and **ulnar nerve** are anterior to the ulnar head. The **radial artery** is just anterior to the lateral side of the radius. The **median**

nerve is close to the surface, anterior to the midpoint of the radius. The superficial **cephalic** and **basilic veins** are on the lateral and medial sides, respectively.

WRIST AND CARPAL TUNNEL

The wrist, or carpus, which is illustrated in Fig. 8-11, consists of eight bones that are arranged in two irregular rows of four bones each. The proximal row, from lateral to medial, contains the scaphoid, lunate, triquetral, and pisiform. The distal row, from lateral to medial, contains the trapezium, trapezoid, capitate, and hamate. Fig. 8-12 shows a radiograph of the carpal bones.

The eight carpal bones in the wrist are tightly bound together by ligaments in such a way that they form an anterior depression, or concavity, called the *carpal groove*. A fibrous connective tissue sheet, called the **flexor retinaculum,** bridges over the carpal groove, making it into a carpal tunnel. On the medial side, the flexor retinaculum is anchored to the hook of the hamate bone. On the lateral side it attaches to the trapezium bone.

The carpal tunnel, illustrated in Fig. 8-13, is completely filled with the flexor tendons that pass from the forearm to the hand and digits. In addition to the tendons, the **median**

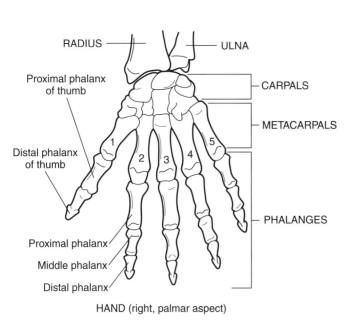

RADIUS — ULNA

Proximal phalanx of thumb

Distal phalanx of thumb

Proximal phalanx
Middle phalanx
Distal phalanx

CARPALS

METACARPALS

PHALANGES

1 2 3 4 5

HAND (right, palmar aspect)

FIG. 8-11 Bones of the wrist (carpus).

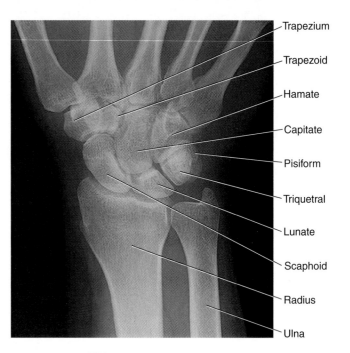

Trapezium
Trapezoid
Hamate
Capitate
Pisiform
Triquetral
Lunate
Scaphoid
Radius
Ulna

FIG. 8-12 Radiograph of the wrist.

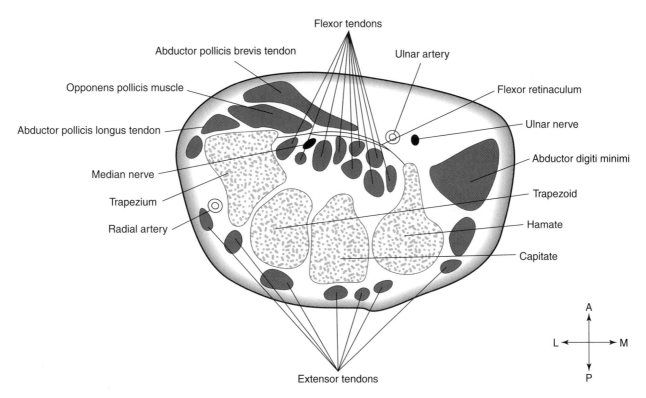

Flexor tendons
Abductor pollicis brevis tendon
Opponens pollicis muscle
Abductor pollicis longus tendon
Median nerve
Trapezium
Radial artery

Ulnar artery
Flexor retinaculum
Ulnar nerve
Abductor digiti minimi
Trapezoid
Hamate
Capitate

Extensor tendons

A
L — M
P

FIG. 8-13 Transverse section through the carpal tunnel.

nerve is just beneath the flexor retinaculum on the lateral side. At times, the tendons may compress the nerve, leading to "carpal tunnel syndrome." The **ulnar artery** and **ulnar nerve** are more medially located and are superficial to the retinaculum.

• ARTICULATIONS ASSOCIATED WITH THE UPPER EXTREMITY •

An articulation, or joint, is where two bones come together. Numerous joints in the body allow little, if any, movement. For example, the sutures in the skull are joints, but they permit no movement. The symphysis pubis and intervertebral discs permit limited movement because the fibrocartilage in these joints is somewhat flexible. Other joints, such as the shoulder, allow a wide range of motion. These are synovial joints, which are more complex in structure than other types of joints. Synovial joints are found principally in the appendicular skeleton because this is the part of the skeleton involved in movement. The other, less movable joints, are more common in the axial skeleton, where they contribute rigidity to form and structure.

Synovial joints are characterized by a **fibrous joint capsule** that is lined with a **synovial membrane.** The synovial membrane secretes **synovial fluid,** which helps lubricate the joint. The ends of the bones comprising the joint are covered with a layer of hyaline cartilage called the **articular cartilage.** The synovial membrane lines all aspects of the joint, except over the articular cartilage. Fig. 8-14 illustrates the structure of a "typical" synovial joint. In addition to the components common to all synovial joints, some have additional features, such as articular discs and intracapsular ligaments. Frequently, the fibrous capsule itself is thickened in places, forming a type of ligament.

It is impossible and unnecessary in this chapter to describe all the synovial joints found in the body. The few presented here have been selected because of their interest and/or importance in imaging.

Description of the Shoulder Joint

The shoulder joint is a ball-and-socket joint in which the rounded head of the humerus articulates with the shallow concavity of the glenoid fossa of the scapula. It is given several names, each reflecting the osseous components of the joint. It may be called the **humeral,** the **glenohumeral,** or the **humeroscapular joint.** The shoulder joint offers a wide range of motion, but this is at the expense of stability. In other words, stability has been sacrificed for mobility. Although three ligaments help to support the joint, most of the support for the joint comes from the strong muscle tendons that pass over it. For this reason, the shoulder is easily dislocated in young children before muscular strength is developed.

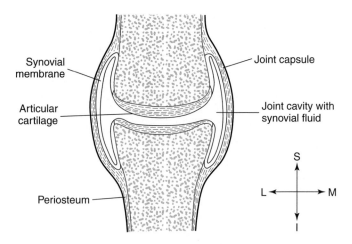

FIG. 8-14 Diagram of a "typical" synovial joint.

ARTICULAR SURFACES AND THE JOINT CAPSULE

The shallow **glenoid fossa** is deepened by a fibrocartilage rim called the **glenoid labrum.** The joint capsule extends from the glenoid labrum to the anatomical neck of the humerus. The capsule is somewhat thin and loose, which contributes to the flexibility of the joint. An arch over the joint protects it from above and helps prevent superior displacement. The arch is formed by the **acromion** and the **coracoid processes of the scapula** and by the **coracoacromial ligament** between them. The **deltoid muscle** covers the joint. The osseous components of the pectoral girdle and the shoulder joint are illustrated by the radiograph in Fig. 8-15.

CAPSULAR LIGAMENTS OF THE SHOULDER

Three ligaments, illustrated in Fig. 8-16, help to reinforce the joint capsule. The **transverse humeral ligament** thickens the joint capsule between the greater and the lesser tubercles of the humerus. This ligament holds the tendon from the long head of the biceps in place. The **coracohumeral ligament** strengthens the superior part of the capsule. This ligament extends from the coracoid process of the scapula to the anatomical neck of the humerus, near the greater tubercle. The **glenohumeral ligament** consists of three slight thickenings on the anterior side of the capsule. These thickenings extend from the margin of the glenoid fossa to the anatomical neck and lesser tubercle of the humerus. The glenohumeral ligaments may be indistinct or absent entirely. The coracoacromial ligament, shown in Fig. 8-16, completes the arch over the shoulder.

MUSCULAR SUPPORT FOR THE SHOULDER

The primary support for the shoulder joint comes from the muscles surrounding it. Four of these muscles, the **supraspinatus,** the **infraspinatus,** the **subscapularis,** and the **teres minor,** are collectively known as the **rotator cuff mus-**

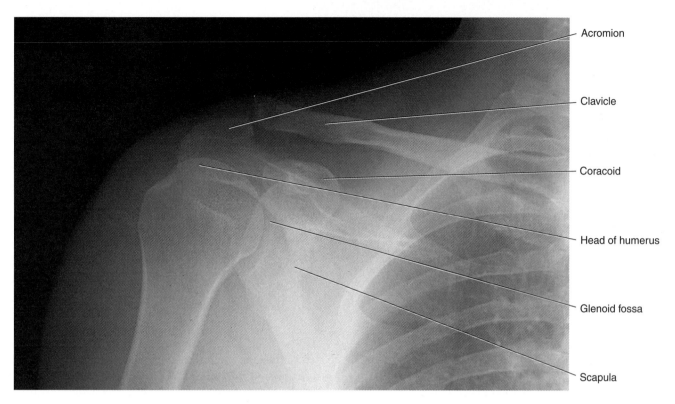

FIG. 8-15 Radiograph of the shoulder.

Acromion
Clavicle
Coracoid
Head of humerus
Glenoid fossa
Scapula

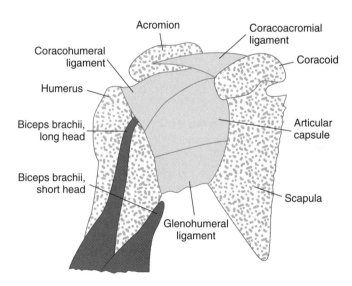

FIG. 8-16 Anterior surface view of the humeroscapular joint showing the joint capsule and reinforcing ligaments.

Acromion
Coracoacromial ligament
Coracohumeral ligament
Coracoid
Humerus
Biceps brachii, long head
Articular capsule
Biceps brachii, short head
Scapula
Glenohumeral ligament

cles. These muscles, associated with the scapula, pull the head of the humerus upward and medially into the glenoid fossa. The tendon of the long head of the biceps brachii muscle also helps hold the humeral head in place. This tendon attaches to the supraglenoid tubercle of the scapula, passes over the head of the humerus within the joint capsule, and descends along the intertubercular groove. Little support exists for the shoulder joint inferiorly; consequently, most dislocations are in that direction.

Bursae

Several bursae are associated with the shoulder. Bursae are synovial membrane sacs filled with synovial fluid. They are found where tendons cross bones, ligaments, or other tendons. Bursae act as cushions to reduce the friction between the moving parts. Four of the shoulder bursae are the **subdeltoid,** the **subacromial,** the **subscapularis,** and the **subcoracoid.** The subacromial bursa is illustrated in Fig. 8-17, which represents a coronal view of the shoulder.

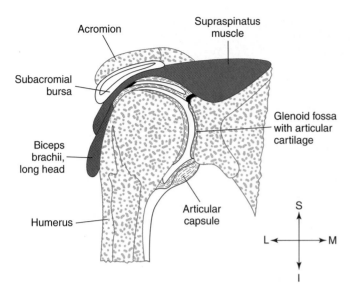

FIG. 8-17 Subacromial bursa in a coronal view of the shoulder joint.

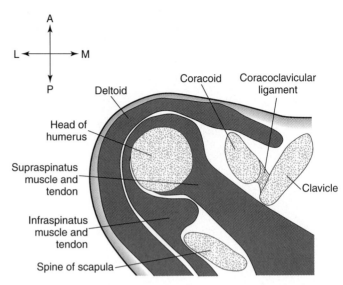

FIG. 8-18 Transverse section of the shoulder joint through the humeral head.

Sectional Anatomy of the Shoulder Joint

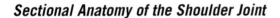

There are relatively few components to look for when examining the sectional anatomy of the shoulder. The osseous elements are the humerus and scapula, with its acromion, spine, coracoid, and glenoid. Superiorly, the clavicle is seen as it contributes to the coracoclavicular articulation. The muscular elements are the rotator cuff muscles and tendons of the biceps brachii. The deltoid muscle covers the joint anteriorly, laterally, and posteriorly. Representative sections showing the osseous/muscular components are illustrated in Figs. 8-18 and 8-19.

TRANSVERSE SECTIONS

Section Through the Humeral Head

Fig. 8-18 illustrates a transverse section through the superior portion of the head of the humerus. The **coracoid of the scapula** and the **clavicle** are close together, separated only by the coracoclavicular ligament. The other osseous component, the **spine of the scapula,** is situated more posteriorly. The muscular components at this level are the **infraspinatus, supraspinatus,** and the **deltoid** muscles. The supraspinatus muscle occupies the space between the coracoid and the spine, with its tendon extending to the greater tubercle of the humeral head. The infraspinatus is evident posterior to the spine, actually in the infraspinous fossa. The tendon of this muscle also extends to the greater tubercle of the humeral head, but it is more posterior. The deltoid encloses the joint on the anterior, lateral, and posterior sides.

Section Through the Glenoid

In transverse sections through the glenoid, the **glenoid labrum** appears at the edges of the glenoid. The **tendon for**

the **supraspinatus muscle** occupies the space between the **coracoid** and the head of the humerus. The **tendon for the** long head of the **biceps brachii** is in the bicipital groove of the humerus. The **supraspinatus** and the **infraspinatus muscles** are associated with the spine of the scapula. The **deltoid muscle** continues to enclose the joint anteriorly, laterally, and posteriorly. These features are illustrated in Fig. 8-19.

CORONAL SECTION

Section Through the Shoulder

The MRI in Fig. 8-20 is similar to the line drawing in Fig. 8-17 and shows a coronal view of the shoulder. This view shows the head of the humerus and the acromion and glenoid of the scapula. The glenoid labrum is around the periphery of the glenoid and deepens the fossa. The muscular components include the deltoid, supraspinatus, and subscapularis muscles. The trapezius muscle is present, but it does not contribute to the shoulder joint.

Description of the Elbow Joint

The joint capsule at the elbow encloses three separate articulations. Two of the articulations are uniaxial hinge joints that allow flexion and extension of the forearm. The third is a pivot joint that permits pronation and supination of the forearm. These articulations are illustrated by the radiographs in Figs. 8-21 and 8-22.

HUMEROULNAR ARTICULATION

On the medial side, the **trochlear notch of the ulna** articulates with the **trochlea of the humerus** forming the humeroulnar joint. This is a uniaxial hinge joint that permits

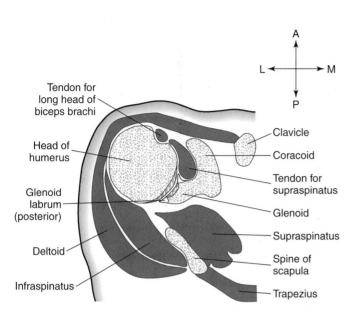

FIG. 8-19 Transverse section of the shoulder joint through the glenoid fossa.

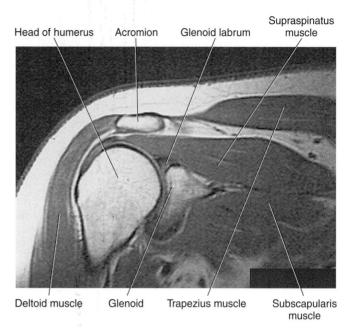

FIG. 8-20 MRI showing a coronal view of the shoulder.

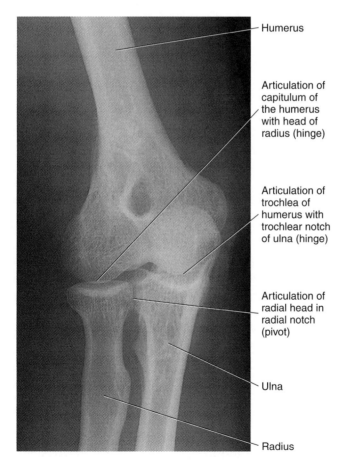

FIG. 8-21 Radiograph of the elbow in an extended position showing the relationship among the humerus, the radius, and the ulna.

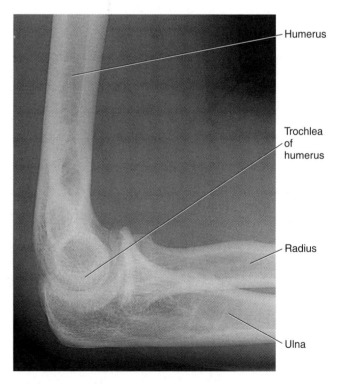

FIG. 8-22 Radiograph of the elbow in a flexed position showing the relationship among the osseous components.

flexion and extension. On the distal posterior surface of the humerus is a deep concavity called the **olecranon fossa,** which accomodates the **olecranon process of the ulna.** On the distal anterior surface of the humerus is a shallow depression called the **coronoid fossa,** which accommodates the **coronoid process of the ulna.**

HUMERORADIAL ARTICULATION

The humeroradial articulation is on the lateral side of the elbow. The articulating surfaces are the **head of the radius** and the **capitulum of the humerus.** This is also a uniaxial hinge joint that permits flexion and extension. The humeroulnar and the humeroradial articulations make up what is commonly called the *elbow joint.*

RADIOULNAR ARTICULATION

The third articulation, enclosed within the elbow joint capsule, is between the **head of the radius** and the **radial notch of the ulna.** This is the proximal radioulnar joint. It is a pivot joint, which allows rotation of the radius. The **annular ligament** wraps around the head of the radius and attaches to the anterior and posterior margins of the radial notch to help hold the radial head in place.

JOINT CAPSULE OF THE ELBOW

The fibrous joint capsule of the elbow is relatively weak anteriorly and posteriorly, but it is strengthened laterally and medially by collateral ligament. Proximally, the fibrous capsule is attached to the superior margins of the radial and coronoid fossae on the anterior surface, and to the olecranon fossa posteriorly. The distal attachments are to the margins of the trochlear notch, the coronoid process, and the annular ligament. The **lateral (radial) collateral** and **medial (ulnar) collateral ligaments** strengthen the joint capsule on the sides. Stability of the joint depends on these two ligaments.

MUSCULAR ACTION ON THE ELBOW

The primary flexor of the forearm at the elbow is the **brachialis muscle.** The **biceps brachii** is also an important flexor when resistance to movement occurs. Flexion is limited by the presence of the collateral ligaments, the tension in the antagonistic muscles, and the opposing surfaces of the arm and forearm. The principal extensor muscle acting on the elbow is the **triceps brachii.** Extension is limited by the collateral ligaments, the tension in the antagonistic muscles, and the olecranon process of the ulna in the olecranon fossa of the humerus.

Sectional Anatomy of the Elbow Joint

The musculoskeletal features of the elbow are probably best illustrated by sagittal sections through the humeroulnar and

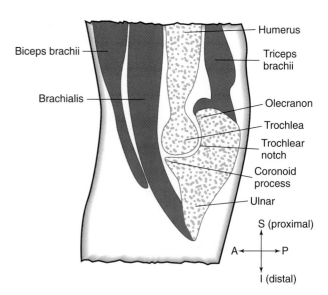

FIG. 8-23 Sagittal section through the medial portion of the elbow showing the articulation of the humerus and the ulna.

humeroradial articulations and by a transverse section through the radioulnar articulation.

SAGITTAL SECTIONS

Section Through the Humerus and the Ulna

Fig. 8-23 illustrates the medial portion of the elbow joint. In this region, the **trochlear notch** of the ulna articulates with the **trochlea** of the humerus. The powerful flexor muscle, the **brachialis,** is on the anterior surface of the joint. The **biceps brachii,** which also acts as a flexor, is superficial to the brachialis. These muscles are opposed by the **triceps brachii,** a powerful extensor, that is located on the posterior surface of the humerus. These muscles insert on the ulna.

Section Through the Humerus and the Radius

In sagittal sections through the lateral portion of the elbow (Fig. 8-24), the **radius** and the **capitulum of the humerus** are evident. The **triceps brachii** and **brachialis** muscles are less apparent, because they insert on the ulna and only their association with the humerus is evident in lateral sections. More muscles associated with the forearm are visible in this section.

TRANSVERSE SECTION

Section Through the Radius and the Ulna

Fig. 8-25 illustrates a transverse section through the **head of the radius** as it articulates in the **radial notch of the ulna.** This is a pivot joint that allows rotation of the forearm. The **annular ligament** holds the radial head in place. The **ulnar nerve** and a branch of the **ulnar artery** are near the surface on the medial side. The extensor and flexor muscles are apparent at this level.

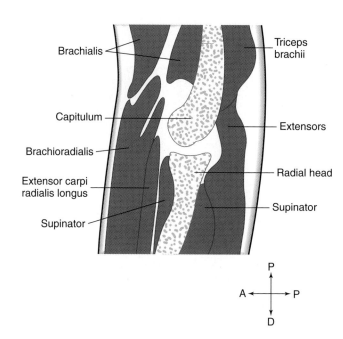

Brachialis

Triceps brachii

Capitulum

Extensors

Brachioradialis

Radial head

Extensor carpi radialis longus

Supinator

Supinator

P

A ← → P

D

FIG. 8-24 Sagittal section through the lateral portion of the elbow showing the articulation of the humerus and the radius.

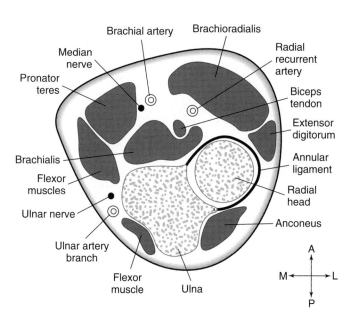

Brachial artery

Brachioradialis

Median nerve

Radial recurrent artery

Pronator teres

Biceps tendon

Extensor digitorum

Brachialis

Annular ligament

Flexor muscles

Radial head

Ulnar nerve

Anconeus

Ulnar artery branch

Flexor muscle

Ulna

A

M ← → L

P

FIG. 8-25 Transverse section through the proximal portion of the forearm showing the relationship of the head of the radius to the ulna.

Case Study

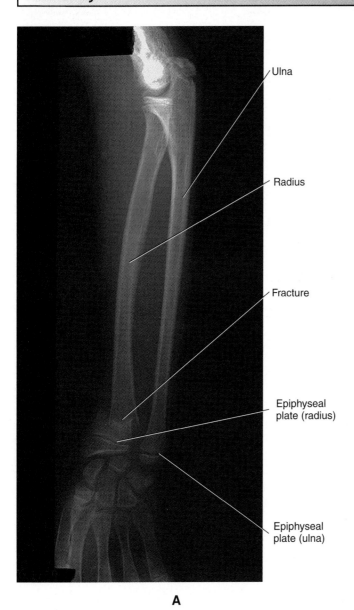

Ulna

Radius

Fracture

Epiphyseal plate (radius)

Epiphyseal plate (ulna)

A

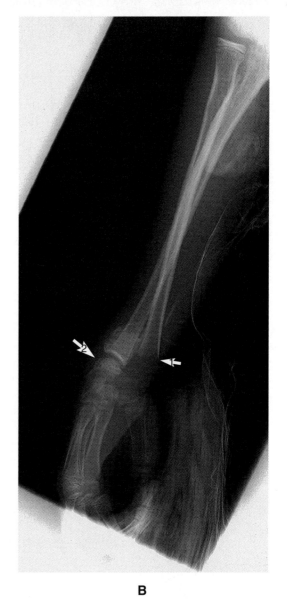

B

This is a 13-year-old male (note the epiphyseal plates at the distal ulna and proximal radius) who injured his left wrist in a bicycle accident. Radiograph A is a posteroanterior (PA) projection of the forearm that demonstrates a complete fracture of the distal radius (Colles' fracture) with the distal portion of the fracture fragment displaced laterally away from the ulna. Radiograph B is a horizontal beam lateral projection that demonstrates significant anterior-posterior displacement of the fracture fragments. Notice that the end of the proximal fragment *(arrow 1)* is projected anterior to the ulna, whereas the distal fragment *(arrow 2)* is displaced posteriorly and superimposed over the distal ulna.

· REVIEW QUESTIONS ·

1. What bones make up the pectoral girdle?
2. What muscles form the anterior boundary of the axilla?
3. What are the three muscles in the anterior compartment of the arm?
4. What are the four terminal branches of the brachial plexus that traverse the arm?
5. What are the two superficial veins found in the arm and where are they located?
6. What muscle forms the lateral boundary of the cubital fossa? What muscle forms the medial boundary?
7. List the contents of the cubital fossa in sequence from medial to lateral.
8. What significant vein is located in the superficial fascia overlying the cubital fossa?
9. What two bones are in the forearm and what are their relative positions?
10. What is the function of the muscles in the anterior compartment of the forearm? What is the function of the muscles in the posterior compartment?
11. What nerve supplies the muscles of the posterior compartment of the forearm?
12. Name the four bones in the proximal row of carpals. Name the four bones in the distal row.
13. What nerve is just underneath the flexor retinaculum and is implicated in carpal tunnel syndrome?
14. Name four features present in all synovial joints.
15. Name the three structures that form an arch over the glenohumeral joint.
16. Name the four rotator cuff muscles.
17. What ligament strengthens the superior part of the fibrous capsule around the glenohumeral joint? What ligament strengthens the anterior portion?
18. Name three different articulations that are enclosed by the fibrous capsule of the elbow. Which one is a pivot joint?
19. What muscle is the primary flexor the forearm at the elbow? What muscle is the primary extensor?
20. What is the significance of the biceps brachii in action at the elbow?

· CHAPTER QUIZ ·

Name the Following:

1. The space at the junction of the arm and the thorax
2. The tendon located in the bicipital (intertubercular) groove
3. The superficial vein on the medial side of the arm
4. The nerve plexus from which the nerves in the arm originate
5. The vein in the superficial fascia over the cubital fossa
6. The bone on the lateral side of the forearm
7. The bone with an olecranon process and a coronoid process
8. The nerve that supplies the muscles in the posterior compartment of the forearm
9. The fibrous connective tissue sheet that bridges of the carpal groove
10. The fibrocartilaginous rim around the glenoid fossa

True/False

1. The transverse humeral ligament connects the two ends of the glenoid labrum.
2. The rotator cuff muscles pull the head of the humerus upward and medially into the glenoid fossa.
3. In transverse sections through the head of the humerus, the infraspinatus muscle appears posterior (superficial) to the spine of the scapula.
4. The radioulnar articulation is a pivot joint.
5. The ulnar collateral ligament strengthens the fibrous capsule of the elbow on the lateral side.
6. The annular ligament holds the head of the radius in the radial notch of the ulna.
7. The pectoralis major and latissimus dorsi muscles extend from the trunk of the body to the scapula.
8. Muscles that extend between the scapula and the humerus tend to move the scapula.
9. The anterior muscles in the forearm are extensors and the posterior muscles are flexors.
10. The coracobrachialis muscle, located in the arm, acts primarily on the shoulder joint.

CHAPTER NINE

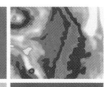

Lower Extremity | 9

OBJECTIVES

Upon completion of this chapter, the student should be able to do the following:

- Name muscles in the gluteal region and describe their anatomical relationships with other body structures.
- Identify skeletal/muscular/vascular/nerve components of the thigh and describe location/boundaries/contents of femoral triangle.
- Identify structural components of the thigh in transverse sections.
- Identify skeletal/muscular/vascular/nerve components of the leg and describe location/boundaries/contents of popliteal fossa.
- Identify structural components of the leg in transverse sections.
- Identify bones of the foot.
- Describe structure of the hip (coxal) joint and discuss the anatomical relationships of its components.
- Identify structural components of the hip (coxal) joint in transverse, sagittal, and coronal sections.
- Describe structure of the knee joint and discuss the anatomical relationships of its components.
- Identify structural components of the knee in sagittal and coronal sections.
- Describe structure of the ankle joint, including talocrural/talocalcaneal articulations and musculotendinous structures.

GENERAL ANATOMY OF THE LOWER EXTREMITY

The lower extremity consists of the thigh, the leg, and the foot. The thigh is the superior portion of the lower extremity and articulates with the axial skeleton. The single bone in the thigh is the femur. Two bones, the fibula on the lateral side and the tibia on the medial side, form the framework of the leg. The leg articulates with the thigh and the foot by hinge joints at the knee and ankle. The foot constitutes the most distal part and includes the tarsals, metatarsals, and phalanges. The lower extremity supports the weight of the body; thus some freedom of movement in the joints has been sacrificed to acquire strength and stability.

ATTACHMENT OF THE LOWER EXTREMITY TO THE TRUNK

The two os coxae (innominate bones) make up the pelvic girdle, which provides the connection between the lower extremity and the axial skeleton. Each os coxa consists of an ilium, an ischium, and a pubis. In the child, these are separate bones, each with its own ossification center, and are connected by hyaline cartilage. In the adult, when ossification is complete, the three bones are fused together into a single unit called the *os coxa*. Posteriorly, each os coxa

meets the sacrum, which is a part of the axial skeleton, at the sacroiliac joint. Each os coxa has a deep fossa, called the **acetabulum,** which articulates with the head of the femur at the hip. Numerous muscles extend over the articulation between the head of the femur and the acetabulum to strengthen the joint and to provide stability. The radiograph in Fig. 9-1 shows the os coxae and their articulation with the femur on each side.

GLUTEAL REGION

The gluteal, or buttock region, is bounded superiorly by the iliac crest and inferiorly by the lower margin of the gluteus maximus muscle, which is marked by a crease or groove just below the gluteal fold. It is an intermediate region that is continuous with the lower trunk above and with the posterior surface of the thigh below. It is included here because the muscles appear in sections through the upper thigh and hip. The muscles of the gluteal region are summarized in Table 9-1.

The **tensor fasciae latae** is the most lateral muscle in the gluteal region. It originates on the iliac crest and inserts on the iliotibial tract, which continues down the side of the leg and attaches to the lateral condyle of the tibia. The tensor fasciae latae flexes the thigh, but it also helps to extend the leg at the knee by putting tension on the fascia lata. The muscle is innervated by the superior gluteal nerve.

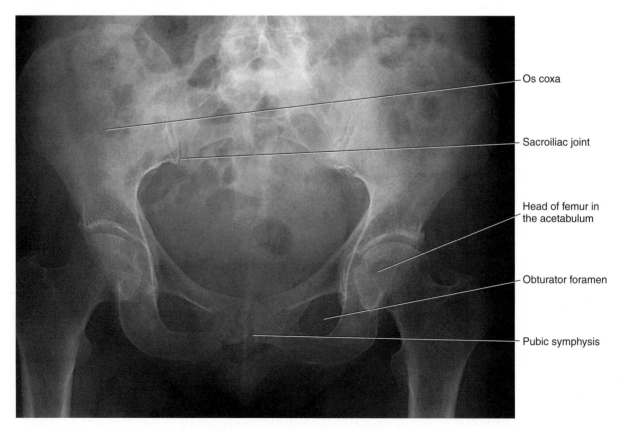

Os coxa

Sacroiliac joint

Head of femur in the acetabulum

Obturator foramen

Pubic symphysis

FIG. 9-1 Radiograph of the pelvic girdle.

The three gluteus muscles account for the bulk and contour of the region. These muscles act on the hip joint to move the thigh. The largest and most superficial of the gluteus muscles is the **gluteus maximus**, which has an extensive origin on the ilium, the sacrum, and the coccyx. The fibers descend obliquely to insert on the gluteal tuberosity of the femur and on the iliotibial tract. The gluteus maximus is a powerful extensor of the thigh. The **gluteus medius** lies deep to the gluteus maximus; however, a portion of the gluteus medius usually extends more superiorly than the gluteus maximus. The gluteus medius extends from its origin on the ilium to its insertion on the greater trochanter of the femur. The **gluteus minimus** is the smallest and the deepest of the three muscles. It also extends from the external surface of the ilium to the greater trochanter of the femur, but its points of attachment are less extensive than those of the gluteus medius. Both the gluteus medius and the gluteus minimus muscles abduct and medially rotate the thigh.

The **piriformis muscle** serves as a landmark for structures that enter the gluteal region deep to the gluteus maximus. These structures are described as entering the region either above or below the piriformis muscle. The piriformis muscle originates on the anterior surface of the sacrum, passes through the greater sciatic notch, and inserts on the greater trochanter of the femur. The superior gluteal artery, which arises from the internal iliac artery in the pelvis, and the superior gluteal nerve, which arises from the sacral plexus, pass through the greater sciatic notch and enter the gluteal region superior to the piriformis. The sciatic nerve, the largest nerve in the region, enters the gluteal region through the greater sciatic notch, just inferior to the piriformis. Muscles inferior to the piriformis are the obturator internus, the gemellus, and the quadratus femoris. The inferior gluteal artery and nerve also enter the region inferior to the piriformis.

The **obturator internus** muscle is an intrapelvic muscle, but its tendon passes through the lesser sciatic notch and becomes extrapelvic in the gluteal region. The muscle originates around the margin of the obturator foramen and covers the space of the foramen. It passes through the deep gluteal region and inserts on the greater trochanter of the femur. The obturator internus is one of the deep lateral rotators of the thigh.

The **superior** and **inferior gemellus muscles** are closely associated with the obturator internus muscle and often obscure the extrapelvic portion of the obturator internus. Some anatomists consider the three muscles to be three parts of one muscle. Both the superior and inferior gemellus muscles originate from the ischium, around the margin of the lesser sciatic notch, and insert on the greater trochanter of the femur with the obturator internus tendon. The gaster, or belly, of the superior gemellus is superior to the obturator internus tendon, whereas the inferior gemellus is inferior to the tendon. Both gemellus muscles are deep lateral rotators of the thigh.

The **quadratus femoris** is the most inferior muscle in the deep gluteal region. The muscle originates on the ischial tuberosity, inserts on the greater trochanter and shaft of the femur, and with the other deep gluteal muscles, laterally rotates the thigh.

The **obturator externus muscle** is often described with the adductor group of thigh muscles because of its location. It is included with the deep gluteal muscles because it is closely related to them functionally. The obturator

TABLE 9-1 *Muscles Located in the Gluteal Region*

Muscle	Origin	Insertion	Action	Innervation
Tensor fascia latae	Iliac crest	Iliotibial tract	Flex thigh; tense fascia lata	Superior gluteal
Gluteus maximus	Ilium, sacrum, coccyx	Gluteal tuberosity; iliotibial tract	Extend thigh	Inferior gluteal
Gluteus medius	Ilium	Greater trochanter	Abduct and laterally rotate thigh	Superior gluteal
Gluteus minimus	Ilium	Greater trochanter	Abduct and laterally rotate thigh	Superior gluteal
Piriformis	Sacrum	Greater trochanter	Laterally rotate thigh	Branches from S1 and S2
Obturator externus	Margin of obturator foramen	Trochanteric fossa	Rotate thigh laterally	Obturator
Obturator internus	Margin of obturator foramen	Greater trochanter	Rotate thigh laterally	L5 and S1
Gemellus, superior and inferior	Ischium; margin of lesser sciatic notch	Obturator internus tendon; greater trochanter	Rotate thigh laterally	Sacral plexus
Quadratus femoris	Ischial tuberosity	Greater trochanter and shaft of femur	Rotate thigh laterally	L4, L5, S1

externus originates around the margin of the obturator foramen and inserts on the trochanteric fossa of the femur. It covers the space of the obturator foramen on the exterior side. The obturator externus laterally rotates the thigh.

General Anatomy of the Thigh

The thigh is the most proximal portion of the lower extremity. Anterior, posterior, and medial muscle compartments surround the femur, which is the only bone in the thigh. A neurovascular bundle accompanies each muscle compartment. The muscles are invested by deep fascia, which also projects inward to create intermuscular septa. On the lateral side of the thigh, the deep fascia is thickened to form the iliotibial tract, which extends from the ilium to the tibia. The tensor fasciae latae and gluteus maximus muscles are attached to the upper part of the iliotibial tract. Superficial fascia and skin complete the coverings of the thigh. The superficial fascia contains the great (long) saphenous vein and its tributaries. Numerous lymph nodes are located in the superficial fascia of the inguinal region near the great (long) saphenous vein. The great (long) saphenous vein penetrates the fascia to drain into the femoral vein.

OSSEOUS COMPONENTS

The only bone in the thigh is the **femur,** which is the longest and heaviest bone in the body. The proximal end of the femur consists of a rounded **head** that fits into the acetabulum of the os coxa, a slender neck that projects laterally away from the head, and the **greater and lesser trochanters,** which provide points of attachment for muscles. The distal end of the femur, at the knee joint, is broadened with two large **condyles** for articulation with the tibia in the leg. In between the two ends of the bone is a long, fairly smooth shaft. A rough ridge on the posterior surface, the **linea aspera,** provides attachment for muscles. Superiorly, the linea aspera expands and becomes the gluteal tuberosity. Some of the features of the femur are illustrated in Fig. 9-2.

MUSCULAR COMPONENTS

Some muscles in the thigh region have origins on the pelvic girdle and insertions on the femur. These muscles move the thigh by acting on the hip joint. Other muscles that are seen in sections of the thigh originate on the femur and insert on the tibia or fibula of the leg. These muscles move the leg by acting on the knee joint. Another muscle group extends from the pelvic girdle to the leg and acts on both the hip and the knee joints. The muscles of the thigh are divided into three compartments by intermuscular septa of deep fascia. The muscles within each compartment have

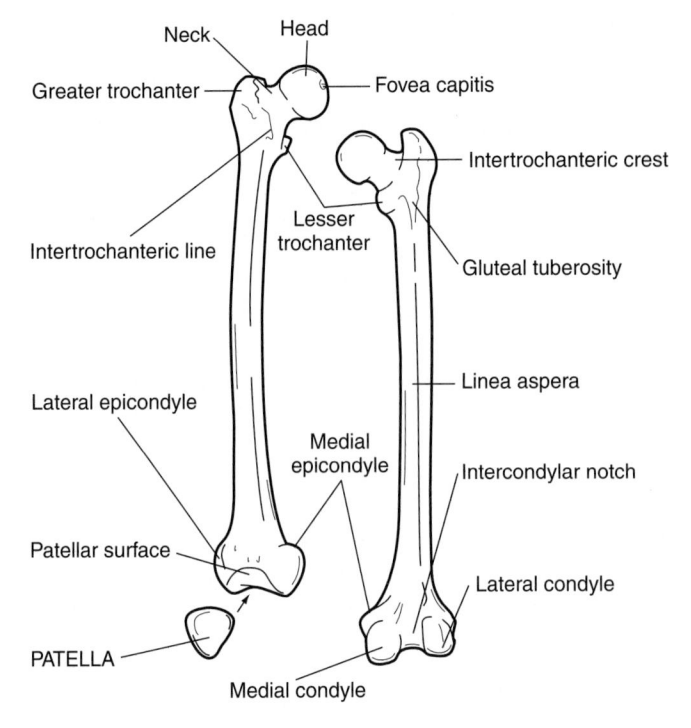

FIG. 9-2 Features of the right femur and patella.

similar functions, and each compartment has its own neurovascular bundle. The muscles of the thigh are summarized in Table 9-2.

Anterior Muscle Compartment

The largest muscle mass in the anterior muscle compartment of the thigh consists of the extensor muscle group, the **quadriceps femoris.** The compartment also contains the terminal portion of the **iliopsoas,** from the posterior abdominopelvic wall, and the **sartorius.**

The **iliopsoas** inserts on the lesser trochanter of the femur and flexes the thigh. This muscle is discussed in more detail with the musculature of the posterior abdominal wall. The **sartorius** is a long, straplike muscle that is superficial to the other anterior thigh muscles. It is the longest muscle in the body. The sartorius originates on the anterior superior iliac spine, courses obliquely across the anterior part of the thigh, and then inserts on the upper part of the medial surface of the tibia. The sartorius extends over the hip and the knee; thus it has an effect on both joints. Contraction of the sartorius causes the thigh to be flexed at the hip and the leg to be flexed at the knee. The muscle is innervated by the femoral nerve.

The **quadriceps femoris** is a group of powerful extensor muscles that occupies the major portion of the anterior compartment. As the name implies, the group comprises four muscles: namely, the **rectus femoris,** the **vastus lateralis,** the **vastus medialis,** and the **vastus intermedius.** These muscles cover the front and the sides of the femur. The rectus femoris originates on the anterior superior iliac spine with fibers that run straight down the thigh. The three vastus muscles orig-inate on the shaft of the femur. The vastus lateralis is on the lateral side, the vastus medialis on the medial side, and the vastus intermedius between the other two on the anterior portion of the shaft. These three muscles make a groove, or trough, that holds the rectus femoris. The four muscles of the quadriceps femoris have a common tendinous insertion on the superior part of the patella. The tendon continues over the patella as the patellar ligament and finally attaches to the tibial tuberosity. All four parts of the quadriceps femoris act as extensors of the leg at the knee joint and are used in climbing, walking, running, and rising from a chair. The rectus femoris extends over the hip joint; thus it also af-fects that joint by flexing the thigh. The quadriceps femoris muscles are innervated by the femoral nerve.

Medial Muscle Compartment

The main action of the muscles in the medial compartment is to adduct the thigh. All of the muscles in this compart-ment originate on either the pubis or the ischium and insert on the femur. The exception to this is the gracilis, which inserts on the tibia. The muscles in the medial compart-ment are innervated by the obturator nerve with the ex-ception of portions of the pectineus and adductor magnus, which are supplied by the femoral and sciatic nerves, re-spectively. The muscles are arranged in three levels or layers. The superficial or anterior layer consists of the pectineus, the adductor longus, and the gracilis.

The pectineus is a rectangular muscle just medial to the iliopsoas in the floor of the femoral triangle. It has its origin on the pectineal line of the pubis and inserts on the pectineal line of the femur. The adductor longus is medial to the pectineus. It originates on the body of the pubis and inserts on the middle part of the linea aspera of the femur. The most medial muscle of the anterior layer is the gracilis. It is also the longest muscle of the group; it extends down the medial side of the thigh from the pubis bone to the up-per part of the medial surface of the tibia.

The middle or intermediate layer of the thigh com-partment is occupied by the adductor brevis. This muscle also originates on the pubic bone, but it inserts on the upper part of the linea aspera of the femur. The deep or posterior layer consists of the adductor magnus. The adductor mag-nus originates on the inferior pubic ramus and the ischium and has an extensive insertion on the linea aspera and on the other aspects of the femur.

Posterior Muscle Compartment

The posterior muscle compartment consists of the ham-string muscle group. The hamstring muscles are the biceps femoris, the semitendinosus, and the semimembranosus, and all arise from the ischial tuberosity. The biceps femoris

TABLE 9-2 *Muscles Located in the Thigh*

Muscle	Origin	Insertion	Action	Innervation
Anterior Compartment				
Iliopsoas	Lumbar vertebrae and iliac fossa	Lesser trochanter	Flex thigh	Femoral
Sartorius	Anterior superior iliac spine	Superior medial tibia	Flex thigh and leg	Femoral
Quadriceps femoris				
Rectus femoris	Anterior superior iliac spine	Tibial tuberosity	Extend leg and flex thigh	Femoral
Vastus lateralis	Lateral shaft of femur	Tibial tuberosity	Extend leg	Femoral
Vastus medialis	Medial shaft of femur	Tibial tuberosity	Extend leg	Femoral
Vastus intermedius	Anterior shaft of femur	Tibial tuberosity	Extend leg	Femoral
Medial (Adductor) Compartment				
Pectineus	Pubis	Femur	Adduct thigh	Obturator and femoral
Adductor longus	Pubis	Linea aspera of femur	Adduct thigh	Obturator
Adductor brevis	Pubis	Linea aspera of femur	Adduct thigh	Obturator
Adductor magnus	Pubis	Extensive on linea aspera	Adduct thigh	Obturator and sciatic
Gracilis	Pubis	Superior medial tibia	Adduct thigh	Obturator
Posterior (Hamstring) Compartment				
Biceps femoris	Ischial tuberosity	Fibula	Flex leg at knee	Sciatic
Semitendinosus	Ischial tuberosity	Medial surface of tibia	Flex leg at knee	Sciatic
Semimembranosus	Ischial tuberosity	Medial condyle of tibia	Flex leg at knee	Sciatic

is the most lateral of the three muscles as it descends to insert on the upper part of the fibula. The middle muscle is the **semitendinosus,** which inserts on the upper part of the medial surface of the tibial shaft. The most medial of the three muscles is the **semimembranosus,** which inserts on the posteromedial surface of the medial condyle of the tibia. Near their origin on the ischial tuberosity, the tendons of the biceps femoris and the semitendinosus overlie the tendon of the semimembranosus. The hamstring muscles extend over the hip and the knee joints and, consequently, have an effect on both. These muscles extend the thigh at the hip and flex the leg at the knee. All three of the hamstring muscles are innervated by the sciatic nerve.

VASCULAR COMPONENTS

The primary blood supply to the lower limb is the **femoral artery,** which is a continuation of the external iliac artery. It begins at the midpoint of the inguinal ligament and descends in the anteromedial part of the thigh to the knee, where it continues as the popliteal artery. A **femoral vein** accompanies the femoral artery throughout the region. The **great saphenous vein** is a superficial vein that begins on the dorsal and medial side of the foot and ascends through the leg and thigh. In the upper region of the thigh it empties into the femoral vein. The great saphenous vein is the longest vein in the body.

NERVES IN THE THIGH

The **femoral nerve,** which supplies the quadriceps femoris muscle group and the sartorius, begins in the abdomen as the largest branch of the lumbar plexus. It passes under the inguinal ligament, lateral to the femoral artery and femoral vein, to enter the thigh where it divides into numerous terminal branches that supply the anterior thigh muscles.

The **sciatic nerve** is the largest nerve in the body. It begins in the pelvis as a branch of the sacral plexus, leaves the pelvis through the greater sciatic notch (foramen), enters the gluteal region inferior to the piriformis muscle, and continues into the posterior region of the thigh. The sciatic nerve is really two nerves, the **tibial** and the **common peroneal,** that are wrapped in the same connective tissue sheath. In the distal thigh, the two nerves separate and continue into the leg. The sciatic nerve and its branches supply the hamstring muscles in the posterior region of the thigh.

FEMORAL TRIANGLE

The femoral triangle is in the upper, medial part of the anterior muscle compartment of the thigh. The base of the triangle (superior margin) is formed by the inguinal ligament. The lateral margin is the medial border of the sartorius muscle and the medial margin is the lateral border of the adductor longus muscle. The iliopsoas and the pectineus muscles make up the floor of the triangle. The femoral artery

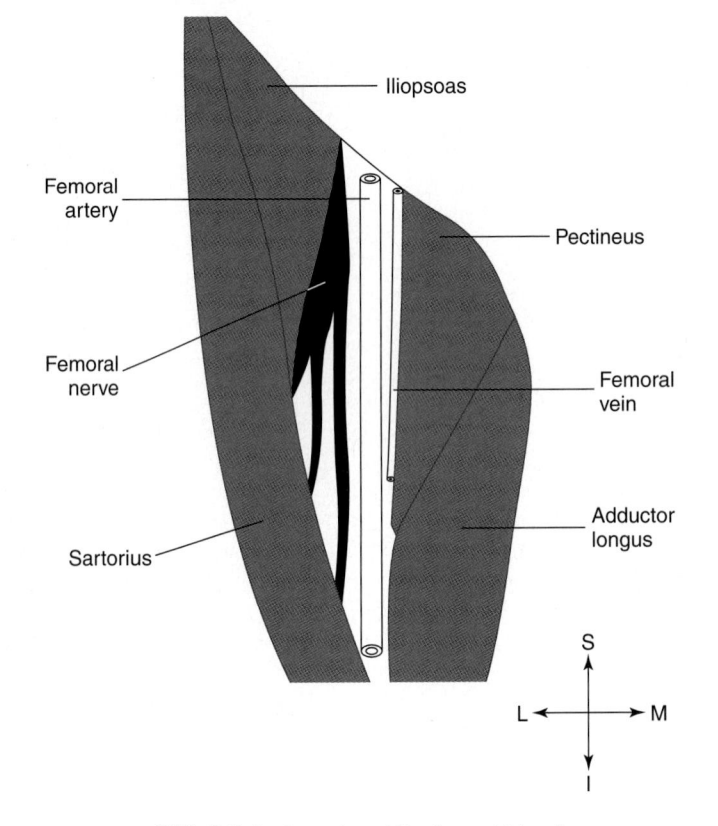

FIG. 9-3 Surface view of the femoral triangle.

and femoral vein, which are enclosed within a femoral sheath made of tough connective tissue, pass through the femoral triangle. The artery is lateral to the vein within the sheath. Fat and lymphoid tissue, also within the sheath, are medial to the artery and vein. The femoral nerve is not enclosed within the sheath, but it passes through the femoral triangle lateral to the sheath. Fig. 9-3 illustrates the components of the femoral triangle.

A subsartorial canal links the apex of the femoral triangle to the popliteal fossa. The canal is really an intermuscular groove beneath the sartorius muscle. The subsartorial canal contains connective tissue in addition to the femoral artery and vein, which are continuing their descent to the popliteal fossa.

Sectional Anatomy of the Thigh

TRANSVERSE SECTIONS

Section Through the Proximal Femur

This section, illustrated in Fig. 9-4, shows the three muscle compartments of the thigh. The anterior compartment contains the **quadriceps femoris muscle** group and the **sartorius.** Just deep to the sartorius, the **femoral artery** and **vein** descend in the subcutaneous tissue near the medial bound-

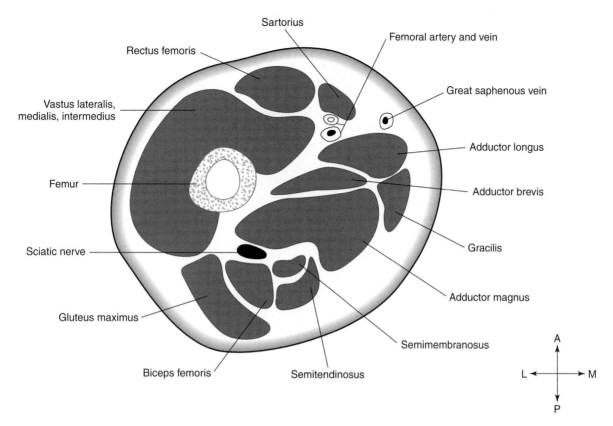

FIG. 9-4 Transverse section through the proximal portion of the femur.

ary of this compartment. The medial compartment contains the **adductor longus, adductor brevis, adductor magnus muscles,** and the **gracilis muscle,** which is more superficial than the adductors. The posterior compartment contains the **hamstrings.** At superior levels of the thigh, the **gluteus maximus** may be evident before it inserts on the iliotibial tract and gluteal tuberosity of the femur. The **sciatic nerve** supplies the posterior compartment.

Section Through the Distal Femur

The adductor muscles in the medial compartment are absent in sections through the distal femur because these muscles insert at higher levels. Only muscles that extend over the knee joint are evident. The three **vastus muscles** with the quadriceps tendon occupy the anterior compartment. In proximal regions of the femur, the sartorius is superficial in the anterior compartment. As the sartorius descends, it crosses obliquely over the thigh to insert on the medial tibia. In section through the distal thigh, the **sartorius** is next to the **gracilis** on the medial side. The three muscles of the **hamstrings** occupy the posterior compartment. The **tibial nerve,** a branch of the sciatic nerve is between the biceps femoris and semimembranosus muscles. A transverse section through the distal femur is illustrated in Fig. 9-5.

General Anatomy of the Leg

Osseous Components

The leg is the portion of the lower extremity that is between the knee and the foot. Its framework consists of two bones, the **tibia** and the **fibula.** These are illustrated in Fig. 9-6. The **tibia,** on the medial side, is the larger of the two bones and is the weight-bearing bone. The tibia articulates proximally with the condyles of the femur at the knee and distally with the talus, which is one of the tarsal bones. The distal end of the tibia is the medial malleolus. This is near the surface and can be palpated as a subcutaneous bump on the medial side of the ankle. The **fibula,** on the lateral side, is a long, slender bone that functions primarily as an attachment for muscles and to lend stability. The distal end of the fibula is the lateral malleolus, which can be palpated as a subcutaneous bump on the lateral side of the ankle. The shafts of the tibia and fibula are connected by strong, oblique, connective tissue fibers that form an **interosseous membrane.** The interosseous membrane is continuous inferiorly with the interosseous ligament, which forms the principal connection between the distal tibia and distal fibula. The inferior tibiofibular joint is strengthened also by the anterior and posterior tibiofibular ligaments. They extend from

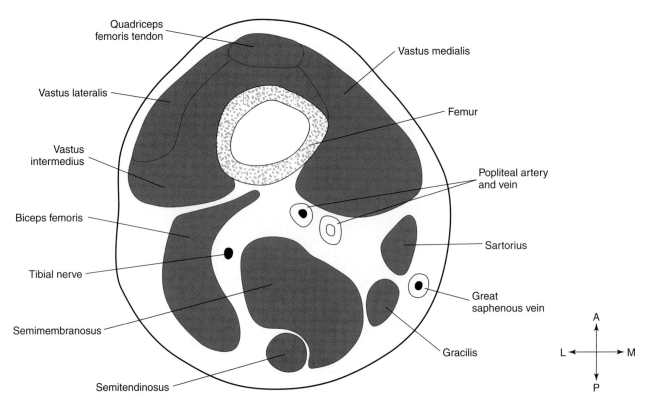

FIG. 9-5 Transverse section through the distal portion of the femur.

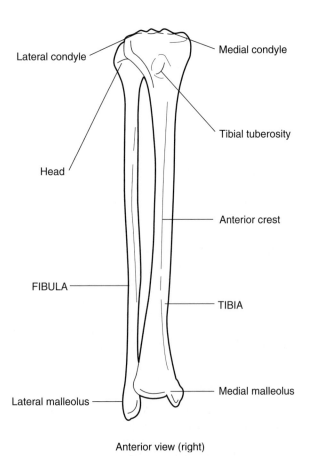

Anterior view (right)

FIG. 9-6 Features of the tibia and fibula.

the borders of the fibular notch on the tibia to the anterior and posterior surfaces of the lateral malleolus of the fibula.

MUSCULAR COMPONENTS

The muscles of the leg are divided into anterior, lateral, and posterior compartments by intermuscular septa, by the interosseous membrane, and by the tibia and fibula. A partition formed by the tibia, the fibula, and the interosseous membrane separates the anterior and posterior compartment. Intermuscular septa separate the lateral compartment from the anterior and posterior compartments. The muscles of the leg act on the foot and toes. In general, the muscles in the anterior compartment dorsiflex the foot and extend the toes. The posterior muscles plantar flex the foot and flex the toes. The lateral muscle compartment everts the foot. Inversion of the foot is accomplished by the tibialis posterior muscle in the posterior compartment. The muscles of the leg are summarized in Table 9-3.

Anterior Muscle Compartment

Located anterior to the interosseous membrane, the muscles of the anterior compartment function primarily in dorsiflexion of the foot at the ankle joint and in extension of the toes. The four muscles in the anterior compartment are the **tibialis anterior,** the **extensor digitorum longus,** the **extensor hallucis longus,** and the **peroneus tertius.** Both the tibialis anterior and the extensor digitorum longus originate

TABLE 9-3 *Muscles Located in the Leg*

Muscle	Origin	Insertion	Action	Innervation
Anterior Compartment				
Tibialis anterior	Lateral condyle of tibia	First cuneiform and metatarsal	Dorsiflex foot	Deep peroneal
Extensor digitorum longus	Lateral condyle of tibia	Phalanges of second to fifth toes	Extend toes	Deep peroneal
Extensor hallucis longus	Middle fibula	Distal phalanx of great toe	Extend great toe	Deep peroneal
Peroneus tertius	Distal fibula	Fifth metatarsal	Dorsiflex foot	Deep peroneal
Posterior Compartment				
Superficial layer				
Gastrocnemius	Lateral and medial condyles of femur	Posterior calcaneus	Plantarflex foot; flex knee	Tibial
Soleus	Tibia and fibula	Posterior calcaneus	Plantarflex foot	Tibial
Plantaris	Popliteal surface of femur	Posterior calcaneus	Plantarflex foot	Tibial
Deep layer				
Tibialis posterior	Tibia and fibula	Tarsals and metatarsals	Plantarflex and invert foot	Tibial
Flexor digitorum longus	Middle tibia	Distal phalanges of lateral four toes	Flex lateral four toes	Tibial
Flexor hallucis longus	Distal fibula	Distal phalanx of great toe	Flex great toe	Tibial
Popliteus	Lateral condyle of femur	Tibia	Medially rotate leg	Tibial
Lateral Compartment				
Peroneus longus	Lateral condyle of tibia; proximal fibula	First metatarsal	Evert and plantarflex foot	Superficial peroneal
Peroneus brevis	Distal fibula	Fifth metatarsal	Evert and plantarflex foot	Superficial peroneal

on the lateral condyle of the tibia and extend throughout the entire length of the leg. They are seen in transverse sections through the proximal leg with the tibialis anterior muscle medial to the extensor digitorum longus. The **extensor hallucis longus** and the **peroneus tertius** originate on the middle and the distal portions of the fibula and interosseous membrane. In distal sections of the leg, the sequence of these muscles, from medial to lateral, is as follows: tibialis anterior, extensor hallucis longus, extensor digitorum longus, and peroneus tertius.

Lateral Muscle Compartment

The lateral muscle compartment is separated from the other compartments by the anterior and posterior intermuscular septa and the lateral surface of the fibula. It extends from the head of the fibula to the lateral malleolus. The **peroneus longus** and **peroneus brevis** are the major muscles in the compartment. The peroneus longus is the more superficial of the two muscles. It originates on the proximal part of the fibula and on the lateral condyle of the tibia. Its tendon continues down the leg, passes behind and below the lateral malleolus, and then curves medially under the foot to at-

tach to the first metatarsal. The peroneus brevis originates on the distal half of the fibula. Its tendon also curves around the lateral malleolus, but the peroneus brevis inserts on the fifth metatarsal. Both muscles evert the foot and are weak plantarflexors at the ankle.

Posterior Muscle Compartment

Of the three muscle compartments in the leg, the posterior compartment has the largest bulk, which is due to the mass of the gastrocnemius and soleus muscles. From medial to lateral, the anterior delineation of the compartment is as follows: the tibia, the interosseous membrane, the fibula, and the posterior intermuscular septum. The posterior compartment is subdivided into superficial and deep muscles by a transverse intermuscular septum. The subdivisions of the posterior muscle compartment are illustrated in Fig. 9-7.

The principal superficial muscles of the posterior compartment are the **gastrocnemius** and the **soleus,** which form most of the contour of the calf of the leg. The gastrocnemius originates by two heads from the lateral and medial condyles of the femur. The two heads come together at the inferior margin of the popliteal fossa to form a single gaster

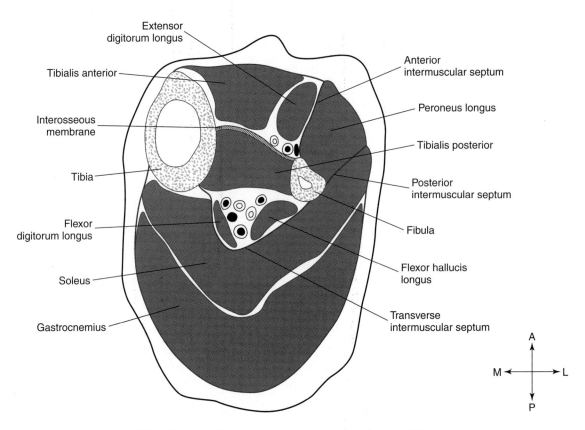

FIG. 9-7 Subdivisions of the posterior muscle compartment of the leg.

of the muscle. From the gaster, a long, tough tendon descends to insert on the posterior surface of the calcaneus. The gastrocnemius muscle is a strong plantarflexor of the foot at the ankle. Because of its origin on the femur, it is also a weak flexor of the knee. The broad, flat, fleshy soleus muscle lies deep to the gastrocnemius and is attached to the posterior surface of the tibia and fibula. The tendons of the gastrocnemius and soleus muscles join, forming a single common tendon that inserts on the posterior surface of the calcaneus. This common tendon is the **tendo calcaneus,** or **Achilles tendon.** The soleus works with the gastrocnemius in plantar flexing the joint, but it has no action on the knee. Because the gastrocnemius and soleus together have three heads of origin but a single common insertion and because they function together, they are sometimes collectively called the **triceps surae muscle.**

From medial to lateral, the deep muscles in the posterior compartment are the **flexor digitorum longus,** the **tibialis posterior,** and the **flexor hallucis longus.** The tendons of these muscles curve to the sole of the foot and insert on the tarsals, metatarsals, or phalanges. The flexor hallucis longus flexes the great toe (hallux), whereas the flexor digitorum longus flexes the lateral four toes. Both of these muscles also assist in plantar flexing the foot. A fourth deep muscle, the

popliteus, is a thin muscle in the popliteal region. It forms the floor of the popliteal fossa and acts on the knee joint to medially rotate the leg.

The small **plantaris** is a weak muscle at the superior border of the lateral head of the gastrocnemius. It has a long, thin tendon, which may become part of the Achilles tendon or may insert directly on the calcaneus. The plantaris muscle varies in size and may be absent with no apparent effect. The weak tendon may rupture during violent ankle movements and cause severe pain in the calf of the leg. Because the muscle is of little practical use in movement of the knee and ankle, its long tendon is sometimes used as a graft in reconstructive hand surgery.

VASCULAR COMPONENTS

In the superior region of the leg, the popliteal artery, which is the continuation of the femoral artery, branches into anterior and posterior tibial arteries. The **anterior tibial artery,** the smaller of the two branches, passes through the interosseous membrane and descends the leg on the anterior surface of this membrane. It supplies the muscles of the anterior compartment. The **posterior tibial artery** is the larger of the two branches. It descends through the leg on the posterior surface of the tibialis posterior muscle and

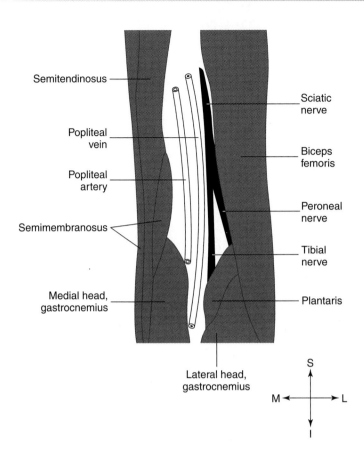

Semitendinosus

Popliteal vein

Popliteal artery

Semimembranosus

Medial head, gastrocnemius

Sciatic nerve

Biceps femoris

Peroneal nerve

Tibial nerve

Plantaris

Lateral head, gastrocnemius

FIG. 9-8 Surface view of the popliteal fossa.

POPLITEAL FOSSA

The **popliteal fossa** is the diamond-shaped, fat-filled region behind the knee joint. The vessels and nerves that continue from the thigh into the leg pass through this area. The upper two margins are formed by the diverging tendons of the **hamstring muscles.** The lateral and medial heads of the **gastrocnemius muscle** form the inferior two margins. The small **plantaris muscle** also contributes to the inferior lateral margin. The roof of the fossa consists of the deep fascia that envelops the muscles of the thigh and the leg. From superior to inferior, the floor of the fossa is formed by the popliteal surface of the femur, the capsule of the knee joint, and the popliteus muscle.

When the femoral artery and vein enter the fossa, they become the **popliteal artery** and **vein.** Lymph nodes are usually in the region of the popliteal artery. The popliteal vein is superficial to the artery. The **tibial** and **common peroneal nerves,** which are terminal branches of the sciatic nerve, also pass through the fossa. These two nerves are superficial to the popliteal vessels. The contents of the fossa are embedded in the fat. The popliteal fossa is illustrated in Fig. 9-8.

Sectional Anatomy of the Leg

TRANSVERSE SECTIONS

Section Through the Proximal Leg

The appearance of sections through the leg varies because the muscles originate and insert in different regions. A transverse section through the proximal leg, near the lower region of the popliteal fossa, shows the **lateral and medial condyles** of the tibia and the **head of the fibula.** Muscle mass is minimal at this level, especially in the anterior and lateral compartments. The two heads of the **gastrocnemius** are evident in the posterior compartment. This is illustrated in Fig. 9-9.

Section Through the Midcalf Region

At lower levels, through the shafts of the tibia and fibula in the midcalf region, more muscle mass is present and the intermuscular septa are more evident than in the proximal leg. The **tibialis anterior** and the **extensor digitorum longus muscles** are anterior to the **interosseous membrane.** The **peroneus longus** occupies most of the lateral compartment. The two heads of the **gastrocnemius** merge in the posterior compartment. The mass of the **soleus** is just beneath the gastrocnemius. The **tibialis posterior** is the most obvious deep muscle in this region. At more distal levels, near the ankle, the muscles become smaller and more tendinous. Here, the anterior tibial artery is near the surface along the anterior margin of the tibia. A transverse section through the midcalf region is illustrated in Fig. 9-10.

supplies the muscles of the posterior compartment. The **peroneal artery** is the largest and most important branch of the posterior tibial artery. It supplies the lateral muscle compartment in addition to giving off branches to some of the muscles in the posterior compartment. One or more deep veins accompany each of the arteries. The superficial **great saphenous vein,** on the medial side, and the **small saphenous vein,** on the lateral side, also ascend through the leg.

NERVES IN THE LEG

The **tibial nerve,** which is the larger terminal branch of the sciatic nerve, provides the nerve supply for all of the muscles in the posterior compartment of the leg. It descends, with the posterior tibial artery, between the soleus muscle and the posterior tibialis muscle. The **deep peroneal nerve,** one of the two terminal branches of the common peroneal nerve, accompanies the anterior tibial artery and vein as they descend the leg, anterior to the interosseous membrane. This nerve supplies the muscles of the anterior compartment. The second terminal branch of the common peroneal nerve is the **superficial peroneal nerve,** which lies anterior and lateral to the fibula and provides the nerve supply for the lateral compartment.

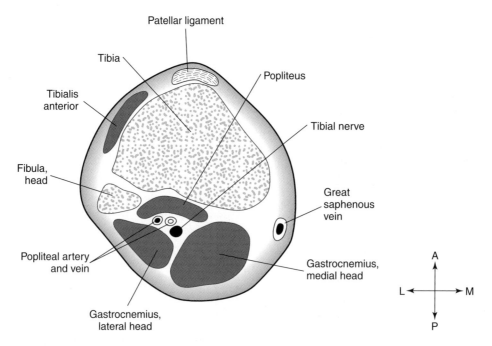

FIG. 9-9 Transverse section through the proximal portion of the leg.

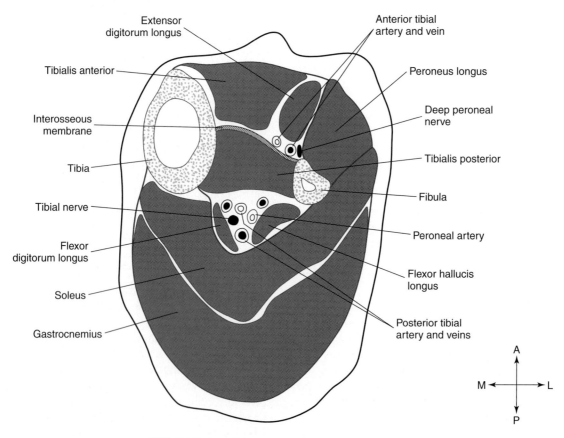

FIG. 9-10 Transverse section through the midcalf region.

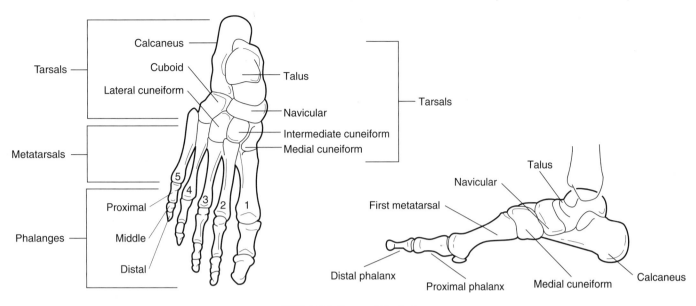

FIG. 9-11 Bones of the foot.

General Anatomy of the Foot

The foot, illustrated in Fig. 9-11, is composed of the ankle, instep, and five toes. The ankle, or **tarsus,** contains seven tarsal bones. The largest tarsal bone is the calcaneus, or heel bone. The talus, another tarsal bone, rests on top of the calcaneus and articulates with the tibia and fibula to form the talocrural joint. The articulation between the talus and calcaneus forms the talocalcanean joint. The other tarsal bones are the navicular, cuboid, and the medial, intermediate, and lateral cuneiform.

The instep of the foot, or **metatarsus,** contains five metatarsal bones, one in line with each toe. The distal ends of these bones form the ball of the foot. These bones are not named but are numbered 1 through 5 starting on the medial side. The tarsals and metatarsals, together with strong tendons and ligaments, form the arches of the foot.

The 14 bones of the toes are called **phalanges.** There are three phalanges in each toe, except for the great (or big) toe, or hallux, which has only two. The proximal phalanx of each toe articulates with a metatarsal. The distal phalanx is at the tip of the toe, under the toenail, and the middle phalanx is between the other two. The hallux does not have a middle phalanx. The radiograph in Fig. 9-12 shows some of the bones of the foot.

• ARTICULATIONS ASSOCIATED • WITH THE LOWER EXTREMITY

Description of the Hip (Coxal) Joint

The hip (coxal) joint is formed by the head of the femur articulating in the acetabulum of the os coxa (hip bone). It is a multiaxial ball-and-socket joint, which allows flexion, extension, abduction, adduction, medial and lateral rotation,

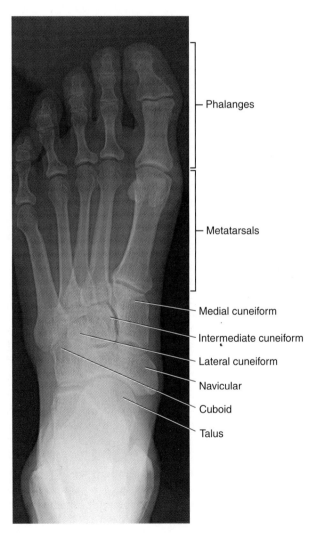

FIG. 9-12 Radiograph of the foot.

and circumduction. This joint bears the weight of the body; therefore it is strong and stable. The strength and stability of the hip are enhanced by the shape and nature of the articular surfaces, the dense joint capsule, and the capsular ligaments.

ARTICULAR SURFACES

The articular surface of the femur is the head, which represents about two thirds of a sphere. The **femoral head** is covered by articular cartilage, except at a small depression, or pit, called the **fovea capitis femoris.** The **ligamentum teres femoris** (ligament of the head of the femur) attaches to the femoral head at the fovea. The femoral head fits into the **acetabulum,** a deep cup-shaped socket in the os coxa. The shaft of the femur is displaced about 2 inches from the head by the neck. This displacement moves the femoral shaft away from the pelvis to allow more freedom of movement.

The rim of the acetabulum is incomplete at the inferior margin, leaving an **acetabular notch,** which is closed by the **transverse acetabular ligament.** The concavity of the acetabulum is further deepened by the **acetabular labrum,** which is a fibrocartilaginous rim that is attached to the bony margin of the socket. The articulating surface of the acetabulum consists of a C-shaped area covered by articular cartilage, which surrounds a centrally located, nonarticulating, **acetabular fossa.** The acetabular fossa contains a pad of fat that is covered by a synovial membrane and represents the coxal attachment of the ligamentum teres femoris. This ligament helps hold the femoral head in the acetabulum.

JOINT CAPSULE AND ASSOCIATED MUSCLES

A dense fibrous joint capsule forms a cylinder that extends from the margin of the acetabulum to the neck of the femur near the trochanters. Synovial membrane lines the fibrous joint capsule. The capsule is thickened and reinforced by the **iliofemoral, pubofemoral,** and **ischiofemoral ligaments.**

Most of the muscles associated with the hip joint function to move the thigh as well as to stabilize the joint. All of these muscles originate on some part of the pelvic girdle, and most of them insert on some part of the femur. Exceptions to this are the gracilis and sartorius muscles, which extend down to the tibia and move the knee in addition to the hip. The muscles may be divided into anterior, posterior, and medial groups. The **iliopsoas** and the **sartorius** belong to the anterior group and flex the thigh. The posterolateral group is more extensive and contains the buttock muscles and the deep lateral rotators. The buttock muscles include the **gluteus maximus,** the **gluteus medius,** and the **gluteus minimus.** The deep rotators are located directly over the posterior portion of the joint. These muscles are the **piriformis,** the **gemelli,** the **obturators,** and the **quadratus femoris.** The medial muscle group is responsible for adduction of the thigh and includes the **pectineus** and the **gracilis** in addition to the **adductor longus,** the **adductor brevis,** and the **adductor magnus.** All of the muscles associated with the hip have been described in the sections dealing with the gluteal region and the thigh.

NEUROVASCULAR STRUCTURES

The principal neurovascular structures visible in sections of the hip are the **femoral artery,** the **femoral vein,** the **femoral nerve,** and the **sciatic nerve.** The femoral vessels and the femoral nerve are closely associated with, and superficial to, the iliopsoas muscle. The sciatic nerve, a branch of the sacral plexus, is the largest peripheral nerve in the body. It begins within the pelvis, deep to the piriformis muscle. The sciatic nerve exits the pelvis through the greater sciatic notch, just inferior to the piriformis. It then descends, superficial to gemellus muscles, but deep to the gluteus maximus.

Sectional Anatomy of the Hip Joint

TRANSVERSE SECTION

Section Through the Acetabulum

Fig. 9-13 illustrates a transverse section through the upper portion of the hip. The **gluteal muscles** are clearly evident in the posterior compartment. The **piriformis muscle,** one of the deep rotators, is deep to the gluteus maximus. The piriformis is closely related to the **sciatic nerve;** they both traverse the sciatic notch. The **obturator internus,** another of the deep lateral rotators, is medial to the bones of the pelvic girdle. In the anterior muscle compartment, the **sartorius** and **tensor fasciae latae** are located superficially, with the **iliopsoas** and **rectus femoris** just deep to the sartorius. The **pectineus** is medial to the iliopsoas.

Within the **acetabulum,** the humeral head articulates at the periphery of the socket, leaving a space, the **acetabular fossa,** in the center. The **ligamentum teres femoris** attaches the femoral head to the acetabular fossa.

SAGITTAL SECTION

Section Through the Acetabulum

A sagittal section through the acetabulum, as illustrated in Fig. 9-14, shows the arrangement of the deep lateral rotators associated with the hip. The **piriformis,** at the margin of the **gluteus medius,** is the most superior of these muscles, followed by the **gemellus** and the **quadratus femoris.** The tendon for the **obturator internus** merges with the **superior** and **inferior gemelli muscles.** The **obturator externus** is deep to the **gluteus maximus** and inferior to the **piriformis.** Recall that the piriformis is a landmark for structures that are found deep to the gluteus maximus. The three layers of the **adductor muscles** in the medial compartment, as well as the **pectineus,** are evident.

CORONAL SECTION

Section (Frontal) Through the Acetabulum

Fig. 9-15 illustrates a coronal section through the acetabulum. This shows the **obturator foramen,** which is an opening between the ilium and pubis, closed off by the **obturator in-**

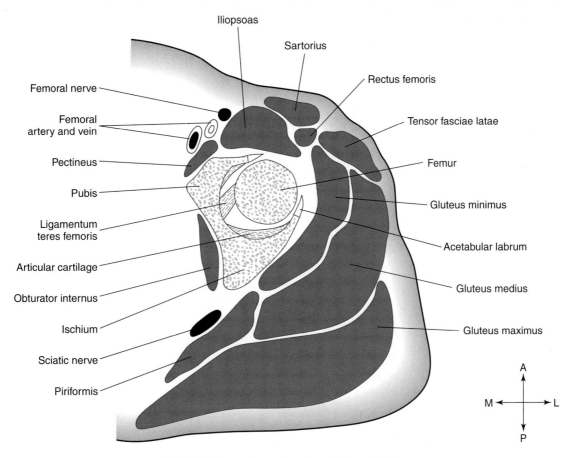

FIG. 9-13 Transverse section through the acetabulum.

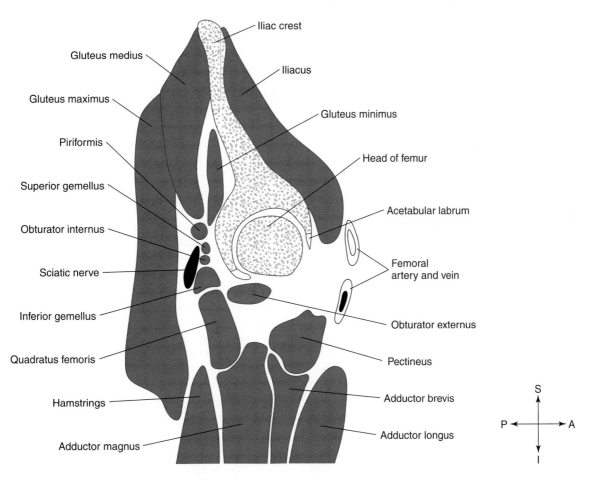

FIG. 9-14 Sagittal section through the acetabulum.

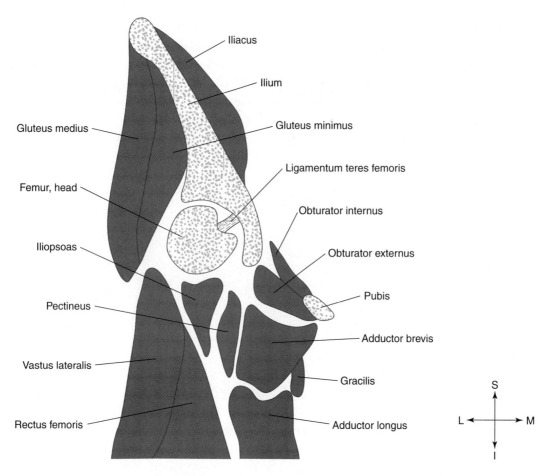

FIG. 9-15 Coronal section through the acetabulum.

ternus and **obturator externus** muscles. The lateral-to-medial sequence of the **iliopsoas, pectineus, adductor brevis,** and **gracilis** muscles is well represented. The MRI in Fig. 9-16 illustrates similar features.

Description of the Knee Joint

ARTICULAR SURFACES OF THE KNEE JOINT

The knee **(tibiofemoral)** joint is probably the most complex, yet most vulnerable, joint in the body. It is principally a hinge joint, but it also allows some gliding motion. The bony components are the **femur,** the **tibia,** and the **patella.** The large rounded condyles on the femur articulate with the rather flattened tibial plateaus. Anteriorly, the patella fits between the lateral and the medial condyles of the femur to form the patellofemoral articulation. The articulating surfaces are covered with hyaline articular cartilage. The articular surfaces of the knee joint are illustrated by the radiographs in Figs. 9-17 and 9-18.

LIGAMENTS ASSOCIATED WITH THE JOINT CAPSULE

A fibrous capsule forms a sleeve that encloses the joint. The capsule extends from a region on the femur, just proximal to

the lateral and medial condyles, down to the tibia, just distal to the articulating surfaces. The fibrous capsule is lined with a synovial membrane, which secretes a lubricating synovial fluid into the joint cavity. Numerous ligaments and tendons add stability to the joint.

Concave, fibrocartilaginous pads called **menisci** (singular, *meniscus*) are interposed between the femoral condyles and the tibial plateaus. These lateral and medial menisci make shallow sockets for the rounded condyles. Anteriorly, the two menisci are joined together by a **transverse ligament.**

The fibrous capsule is strengthened by five ligaments. These are called *external* or *extracapsular ligaments* to distinguish them from those inside the capsule. Thickenings of the capsule on the lateral and medial side form **lateral (fibular)** and **medial (tibial) collateral ligaments.** Anteriorly, the continuation of the quadriceps femoris tendon forms the **patellar ligament,** which reinforces the fibrous capsule. Posterior to the joint, in the popliteal region, the capsule is strengthened by the **oblique popliteal** and **arcuate popliteal ligaments.** The oblique popliteal ligament is a broad expansion of the semimembranosus tendon. It arises from the posterior aspect of the medial tibial condyle and attaches near the center of the capsule. The Y-shaped arcuate popliteal ligament arises from the head of the fibula, then spreads out to attach to the lateral condyle of the femur and the intercondylar area of the tibia.

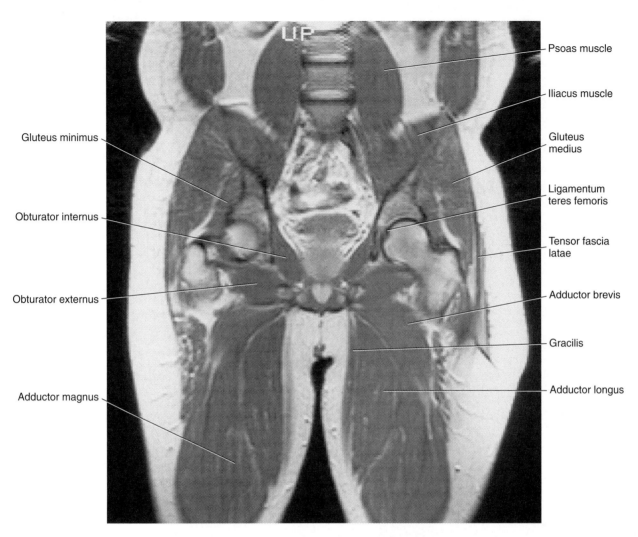

FIG. 9-16 MRI of a coronal section through the acetabulum.

Intracapsular ligaments are inside the fibrous capsule rather than external to it. The anterior and posterior cruciate ligaments are intracapsular. They are located between the lateral and medial condyles of the femur, and they attach the femur to the tibia. The **anterior cruciate ligament** extends anteriorly from the lateral condyle of the femur to a point on the anterior surface of the tibia on the medial side of the intercondylar eminence. The **posterior cruciate ligament** extends between the medial condyle of the femur and the posterior surface of the tibia. Note that the anterior cruciate ligament attaches to the anterior tibial surface and that the posterior cruciate ligament attaches to the posterior surface of the tibia.

MUSCULAR SUPPORT FOR THE KNEE JOINT

Muscles and their tendons form the major support for the knee joint. Thus proper muscle conditioning can reduce the likelihood and severity of knee injuries. Conversely, weakened muscles contribute to instability of the knee joint. The primary muscles that contribute strength to the joint include the **quadriceps femoris**, the **hamstrings**, the **sartorius**, the **gracilis**, and the **gastrocnemius.** In addition to stabilizing the knee, these muscles move the leg by their

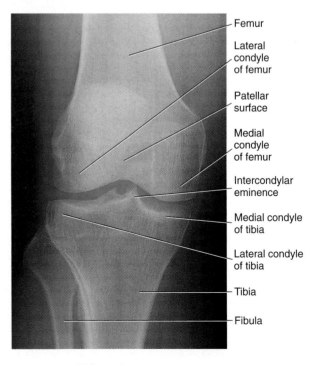

FIG. 9-17 Radiograph of the knee.

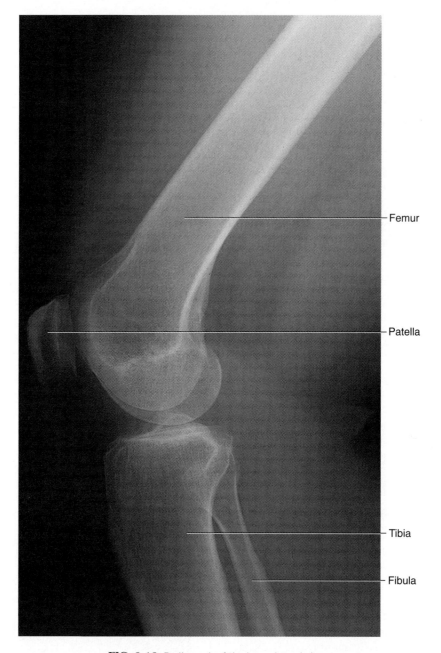

FIG. 9-18 Radiograph of the knee, lateral view.

action on the knee joint. See Tables 9-2 and 9-3 for a review of these muscles and their actions.

NEUROVASCULAR STRUCTURES ASSOCIATED WITH THE KNEE JOINT

The principal neurovascular supply to the knee comes from the vessels and nerves in the popliteal fossa, which, from medial to lateral include the **popliteal artery,** the **popliteal vein,** the **tibial nerve,** and the **common peroneal nerve.** The popliteal artery is a continuation of the femoral artery. In the popliteal fossa, it gives off several genicular arteries, which course around the bones to supply the components of the joint. The tibial and common peroneal nerves are terminal branches of the sciatic nerve.

Sectional Anatomy of the Knee Joint

SAGITTAL SECTION

Section Through the Lateral Femur and the Tibia

Fig. 9-19 illustrates a sagittal section of the knee joint. The articulation of the **lateral condyle** of the femur with the **tibia** and the **lateral meniscus** between the two bones is shown. The **patella** is anterior to the femur. The **patellar ligament** extends from the patella down to the tibial tuberosity as an extension of the quadriceps femoris tendon. Three bursae associated with the patella, two subcutaneous and one deep, are illustrated. An MRI of a similar region is shown in Fig. 9-20.

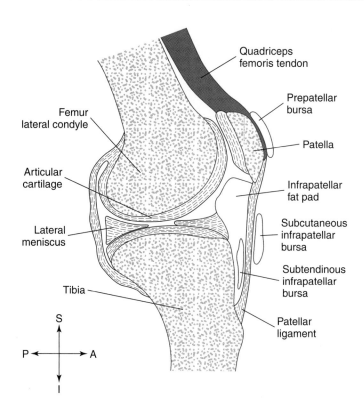

FIG. 9-19 Sagittal section through the lateral femur and tibia.

Quadriceps femoris tendon

Prepatellar bursa

Femur lateral condyle

Patella

Articular cartilage

Infrapatellar fat pad

Lateral meniscus

Subcutaneous infrapatellar bursa

Subtendinous infrapatellar bursa

Tibia

Patellar ligament

S

P ← → A

I

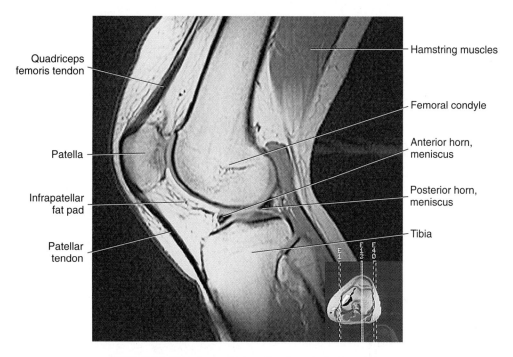

Quadriceps femoris tendon

Hamstring muscles

Femoral condyle

Patella

Anterior horn, meniscus

Infrapatellar fat pad

Posterior horn, meniscus

Patellar tendon

Tibia

FIG. 9-20 MRI of a sagittal section through the lateral femur.

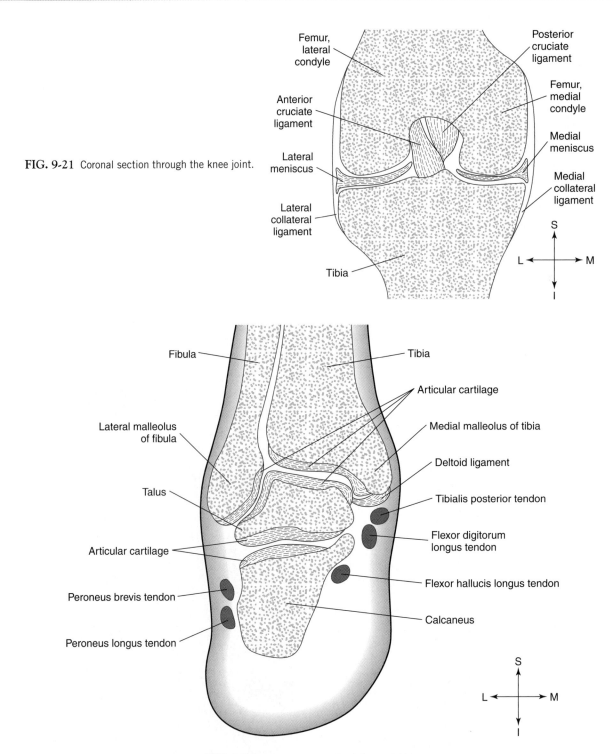

FIG. 9-21 Coronal section through the knee joint.

FIG. 9-22 Coronal section through the ankle.

CORONAL SECTION

Section (Frontal) Through the Knee Joint

A coronal (frontal) section through the knee joint, as illustrated in Fig. 9-21, shows both the **lateral** and the **medial menisci.** The joint capsule is reinforced at the sides by the **lateral** and the **medial collateral ligaments.** The intracapsular **anterior** and **posterior cruciate ligaments** are in the space between the two femoral condyles.

Description of the Ankle Joint

The ankle, or **talocrural joint,** consists of the articulation between the distal **tibia** and **fibula** of the leg and the **talus** of the tarsal bones. In addition, some attention will be given to the relationships of the talus to the **calcaneus.** The articular surfaces of the talus are shown in Fig. 9-22, which illustrates a coronal section through the ankle.

TABLE 9-4 *Ligaments of the Ankle*

Ligament Name	Origin	Insertion
Lateral (Fibular) Ligament		
Anterior talofibular	Lateral malleolus of fibula	Anterior talus
Posterior talofibular	Lateral malleolus of fibula	Posterior talus
Calcaneofibular	Lateral malleolus of fibula	Lateral surface of calcaneus
Medial (Tibial) Ligament		
(Also called *deltoid ligament*)		
Anterior tibiotalar	Medial malleolus of tibia	Anterior surface of talus
Posterior tibiotalar	Medial malleolus of tibia	Posterior surface of talus
Tibiocalcaneal	Medial malleolus of tibia	Calcaneus
Tibionavicular	Medial malleolus of tibia	Navicular bone

TALOCRURAL ARTICULATION

The talocrural joint is a hinge-type synovial joint, which permits dorsiflexion and plantarflexion of the foot. Medial and lateral movement is restricted by the medial malleolus of the tibia and the lateral malleolus of the fibula. The talus has three articular surfaces that contribute to the joint. The largest is the superior rounded surface, called the **trochlea,** which rests in the inferior concave surface of the distal tibia. Laterally and medially on the talus are facets for articulation with the malleoli of the fibula and tibia. The radiograph in Fig. 9-23 shows the three articular surfaces of the talocrural joint.

The talocrural joint is enclosed in a thin, fibrous capsule that is strengthened on the sides by ligaments. The **lateral (fibular) ligament** extends from the lateral malleolus to the talus and the calcaneus and provides lateral support. Distally, the ligament is divided into three parts, according to the area of attachment. The anterior and posterior talofibular ligaments attach to the anterior and posterior regions of the talus. The calcaneofibular ligament forms a cord that extends from the lateral malleolus to the lateral surface of the calcaneus. The ligament on the medial side is much stronger than the lateral ligament. The **medial (deltoid** or **tibial) ligament** arises from the medial malleolus and provides medial support. The fibers of the ligament fan out to form a broad base of attachment on the anterior and posterior regions of the talus, the calcaneus, and the navicular. The four individual portions of the ligament are named according to their distal attachments as the anterior and posterior tibiotalar, the tibiocalcaneal, and the tibionavicular ligaments. The ligaments of the ankle are summarized in Table 9-4.

TALOCALCANEAL ARTICULATIONS

Inferiorly, in the subtalar region, three facets of the talus articulate with the calcaneus. This **subtalar,** or **talocalcaneal, joint** has a fibrous capsule that is distinct from that of the ankle. The interosseous ligament, which is located in a

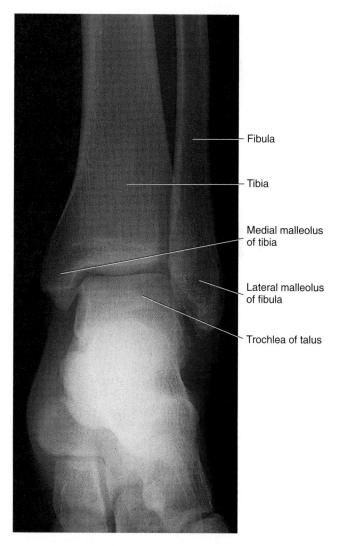

Fibula

Tibia

Medial malleolus of tibia

Lateral malleolus of fibula

Trochlea of talus

FIG. 9-23 Radiograph of the ankle showing the articulating surfaces of the talocrural joint.

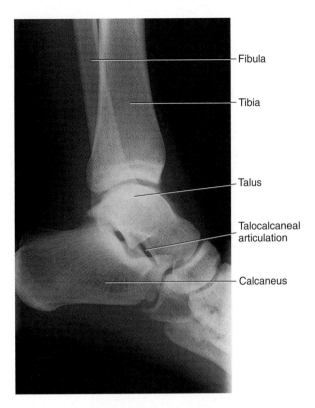

FIG. 9-24 Radiograph of the ankle showing the subtalar articulations.

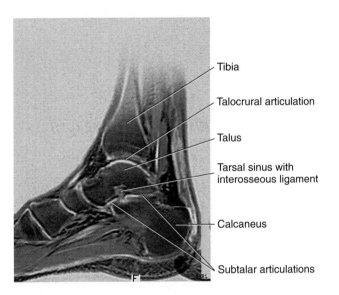

FIG. 9-25 MRI of a sagittal section through the talocrural and subtalar articulations.

space called the tarsal sinus, extends from the midtalar region to the calcaneus and provides support for the joint. The talocalcaneal joint is a gliding synovial joint that allows inversion and eversion of the foot. The radiograph in Fig. 9-24 shows the subtalar articulations. Fig. 9-25 is an MRI of a sagittal section through the talocrural and subtalar articulations.

MUSCULOTENDINOUS STRUCTURES ASSOCIATED WITH THE ANKLE

In addition to the ligaments that are summarized in Table 9-4, support for the ankle also comes from the musculotendinous structures in the region. These may be divided into medial, lateral, anterior, and posterior groups. The relationships of the musculotendinous structures of the ankle are illustrated in Fig. 9-26, which shows a transverse section just superior to the joint cavity.

The medial group includes the **tibialis posterior,** the **flexor digitorum longus,** and the **flexor hallucis longus.** The tibialis posterior is the most anterior of the three and the flexor hallucis longus is the most posterior. The **posterior tibial artery** and **tibial nerve** are located between the flexor digitorum longus and the flexor hallucis longus. Pos-

terior to the medial malleolus, the tibial nerve divides into the medial and the lateral plantar nerves.

The lateral group consists of the **peroneus longus** and the **peroneus brevis.** As the muscles descend the leg, the peroneus brevis is anterior to the peroneus longus. The two muscles follow a groove in the lateral malleolus, then curve forward under the malleolus, and extend anteriorly to the metatarsals. In the foot, the peroneus brevis is superior to the peroneus longus (see Fig. 9-22).

The anterior muscle group consists of the **tibialis anterior,** the **extensor hallucis longus,** the **extensor digitorum longus,** and the **peroneus tertius.** The tibialis anterior is the most prominent and the most medial of these muscles. The extensor digitorum longus and peroneus tertius are difficult to separate and are the most lateral muscles of the group. The **anterior tibial artery** and **deep peroneal nerve** are deep to the extensor hallucis muscle.

The **tendo calcaneus,** or Achilles tendon, constitutes the only musculotendinous structure in the posterior group. This tendon arises from the gastrocnemius and soleus muscles and attaches to the posterior surface of the calcaneus. The Achilles tendon is the thickest and strongest tendon in the body.

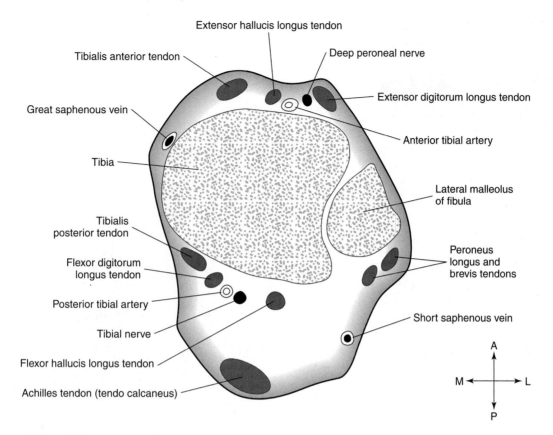

FIG. 9-26 Transverse section through the lateral malleolus of the fibula, showing the relationship of the musculotendinous structures passing through the ankle joint.

Case Study

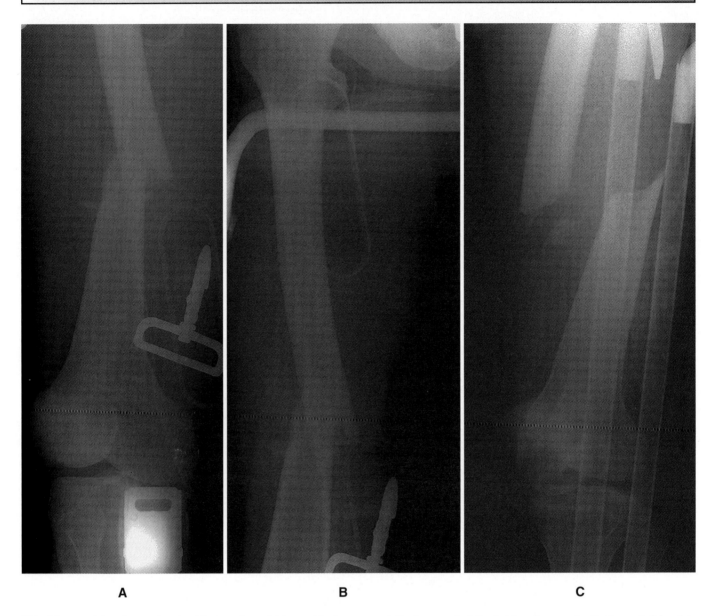

A

B

C

This 20-year-old male was involved in a motor vehicle accident. He was brought to the emergency room with extreme right leg pain. Radiographs A and B are anteroposterior (AP) projections that demonstrate a complete fracture of the femur with some lat-eral displacement of the fracture fragments. Radiograph C is a lateral projection of the fracture site that demonstrates significant anterior-posterior displacement with the distal fragment displaced posteriorly and the proximal fragment displaced anteriorly.

· REVIEW QUESTIONS ·

1. What bones make up the pelvic girdle?
2. What superficial muscle is the most lateral in the gluteal region?
3. What muscle is superior to the gemellus muscles in the deep gluteal region? What muscle is inferior to the gemellus muscles?
4. What muscles make up the quadriceps femoris muscle group? The hamstring muscle group?
5. Which muscles are located in the medial muscle compartment of the thigh?
6. What vein begins in the foot and ascends through the leg and thigh in the superficial fascia on the medial side?
7. What are the two terminal branches of the sciatic nerve?
8. What forms the lateral margin of the femoral triangle? The medial margin?
9. What is contained in the femoral triangle, from lateral to medial?
10. What two bones are in the leg and which one is lateral?
11. What three structures combine to separate the muscles of the leg into anterior and posterior compartments?
12. In general, what is the primary function of the muscles in the anterior compartment of the leg? Posterior compartment? Lateral compartment?
13. What two superficial muscles in the posterior compartment of the leg form most of the contour of the calf of the leg?
14. What nerve supplies innervation for all of the muscles in the posterior compartment of the leg? Where is it located?
15. What muscles form the margins of the popliteal fossa?
16. Name the seven tarsal bones.
17. What is the intracapsular ligament associated with the hip (coxal) joint?
18. What is the nonarticular space in the center of the acetabulum called?
19. Name the intracapsular ligaments associated with the knee joint.
20. Name the five extracapsular ligaments associated with the knee joint.
21. What portion of the talus articulates with the tibia?
22. What two ligaments reinforce the fibrous capsule of the talocrural joint?
23. What space in the talocalcaneal joint contains an interosseous ligament?
24. What is the thickest and strongest tendon in the body?

· CHAPTER QUIZ ·

Name the Following:

1. The bones that comprise the pelvic girdle
2. The most inferior muscle in the deep gluteal region
3. The two large articulating surfaces on the distal femur
4. The superficial, long, straplike muscle of the anterior thigh
5. The most lateral of the hamstring muscles
6. The nerve that supplies innervation to the sartorius and quadriceps femoris
7. The ligament that extends from the fovea capitis to the acetabular fossa
8. The most superficial muscle in the calf of the leg
9. The bone that forms a distal articulation with the tibia
10. The bone that forms a subtalar articulation with the talus

True/False

1. The muscles in the posterior muscle compartment of the thigh are collectively called the hamstring muscles.
2. From lateral to medial, the neurovascular structures in the femoral triangle are the femoral artery, the femoral nerve, and the femoral vein.
3. The tendons of the gastrocnemius muscle extend over two joints; therefore the muscle affects both the knee and the ankle.
4. The muscles in the anterior compartment function principally to dorsiflex the foot and extend the toes.
5. The transverse acetabular ligament thickens the anterior portion of the fibrous capsule of the coxal joint.
6. The oblique popliteal and arcuate popliteal ligaments are intracapsular ligaments of the knee and function to connect the femur to the tibia.
7. The fibrocartilaginous pads between the femoral condyles and the tibial plateaus are connected on the posterior margin by the transverse ligament.
8. The ankle joint is called the talocrural joint.
9. The trochlea of the talus articulates with the fibula.
10. The ligament that reinforces the fibrous capsule of the ankle on the medial side is divided four parts: the anterior tibiotalar ligament, the posterior tibiotalar ligament, the tibiocalcaneal ligament, and the tibionavicular ligament.

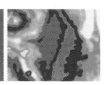

Applegate E: *The anatomy and physiology learning system*, ed 2, Philadelphia, WB Saunders, 2000.

Cahill DR, Orland MJ, Miller GM: *Atlas of human cross-sectional anatomy with CT and MR images*, ed 3, New York, Wiley-Liss, 1995.

Csillag A: *Anatomy of the living human, atlas of medical imaging*, Cologne, Germany, 1999, Konemann Verlagsgesellschaft.

Dean D, Herbener TE: *Cross-sectional human anatomy*, Philadelphia, 2000, Lippincott, Williams & Wilkins.

Ellis H, Logan B, Dixon A: *Human sectional anatomy, atlas of body sections, CT and MRI images*, ed 2, Boston, 1999, Butterworth-Heinemann.

Kelley LL, Peterson CM: *Sectional anatomy pocket guide*, St Louis, 1997, Mosby.

Marieb EN: *Human anatomy and physiology*, ed 5, San Francisco, 2000, Addison-Wesley.

Moore KL: *Clinically oriented anatomy*, ed 4, Philadelphia, 1998, Lippincott, Williams & Wilkins.

Snell RS: *Clinical anatomy for medical students*, ed 5, Philadelphia, 1995, Lippincott, Williams & Wilkins.

Spitzer VM, Whitlock DG: *Atlas of the visible human male*, Sudbury, MA, 1998, Jones & Bartlett.

Tortora GJ: *Principles of anatomy and physiology*, ed 9, San Francisco, 2000, Addison-Wesley.

Van De Graaff KM, Fox SI: *Concepts of human anatomy & physiology*, ed 5, Dubuque, 1998, McGraw-Hill.

Weir J, Abrahams PH: *Imaging atlas of human anatomy*, ed 2, St Louis, 1997, Mosby.

DATE: 05/18/07
TS2R0006 - P0020

THE UNIVERSITY OF AKRON
COMPUTER CENTER
TEST SCORING SERVICES

PAGE: 17

STUDENT ANSWER SHEET

INSTRUCTOR: DAVID WHIPPLE
SCORING METHOD USED: PERCENTAGE SCORE

DEPT CRS SEC
2760-288:001

TEST #: 02
TEST FORM: A

SOC. SEC. #	STUDENT NAME	# RIGHT	# WRONG	# OMITTED	# NOT GRADED	SCORE
279-02-3793	MANIVONG SUNGKOM	42	8	0	0	84.00

```
QUESTION #
                    1 1 1 1 1 1 1 1 1 1 2 2 2 2 2 2 2 2 2 2 3 3 3 3 3 3 3 3 3 3 4 4 4 4 4 4 4 4 4 4 5
          1 2 3 4 5 6 7 8 9 0 1 2 3 4 5 6 7 8 9 0 1 2 3 4 5 6 7 8 9 0 1 2 3 4 5 6 7 8 9 0 1 2 3 4 5 6 7 8 9 0

STUDENT   A A D D C B B A B B B C C B A D D A B E D E B B D C B D C E B A D D A B C C E A A A A C D E B A D D
ANSWER KEY        D                         C   A B D                       B   B   C
ALTERNATE
```

```
*****************************************************************************************
*** ANSWER KEY RESPONSES ARE ONLY PRINTED IF THE CORRECT ANSWER DIFFERS FROM THE STUDENT'S ***
*** ANSWER.  ALTERNATE ANSWERS WILL BE PRINTED WHENEVER THEY EXIST.                      ***
*****************************************************************************************
```

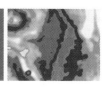

abdomen Area between the thorax and the pelvis; the belly

abdominal cavity Superior portion of the abdominopelvic cavity; contains the stomach, liver, spleen, pancreas, gallbladder, and most of the small and large intestines

abdominopelvic cavity Inferior portion of the ventral body cavity; can be subdivided into an upper abdominal cavity and a lower pelvic cavity

abducens nerve Cranial nerve VI

abduction Movement of a body part away from the axis or midline of the body or one of its parts

abscess Localized accumulation of pus

absorption Taking up of substances by the skin or other tissues of the body

acetabular labrum Rim of fibrocartilage around the margin of the acetabulum

acetabulum Cup-shaped depression on the lateral surface of the os coxae (hip bone) in which the head of the femur fits

Achilles tendon Calcaneal tendon

acidity State of being acidic; the acid content of a fluid; opposite of alkalinity

acromion process Flattened portion of bone at the lateral end of the spine of the scapula; most prominent point of the shoulder

acute Disease state with sudden onset or of short duration; opposite of chronic

adduction Movement of a body part toward the axis or midline of the body or one of its parts

adductor brevis One of the muscles that adducts the thigh; lies deep to the adductor longus but anterior to the adductor magnus

adductor longus One of the muscles that adducts the thigh; the most anterior muscle of the adductor group

adductor magnus One of the muscles that adducts the thigh; the largest and the most posterior muscle of the adductor group

adenoids Pharyngeal tonsils; enlargement of the pharyngeal tonsils as a result of chronic inflammation

adhere To stick, to bind, or to hold fast

adipose Type of connective tissue containing large quantities of fat; fatty tissue

adjoin To be in contact with or to lie next to

adrenal Gland located on top of each kidney; also called the *suprarenal gland*

afferent Carrying a nerve impulse or fluid toward an area or an organ

aggregation An accumulation or clump

ala (pl. alae) Winglike structure

alkalinity State of being alkaline or basic; the alkaline content of a fluid; opposite of acidity

alveolus Small, hollow area or cavity, e.g., the socket for a tooth or an air sac in the lungs

amylase An enzyme that splits starches into smaller molecules called *disaccharides*

anastomose Opening one into another; generally pertains to blood vessels or lymphatics

anastomosis The connection, or union, between tubular structures, e.g., in blood vessels or lymphatics

anatomy A study of the structure of the body and the relation of the parts to each other

anesthesia A partial or total loss of sensation

aneurysm A saclike bulge in a blood vessel, usually an artery, as a result of a weakening of the vessel wall

annular Relating to a ring-shaped or circular structure

antagonistic Working in opposition to each other; frequently pertains to muscle action or drugs

anteflexion A displacement that is characterized by a bending forward of the top part of an organ

anterior To the front of the body; ventral

anterolateral In front and to one side of the body

anteroposterior Directed from the front to the back

anterosuperior To the front and the superior (above) part of the body

anteversion The leaning forward (tilting) of an organ as a whole, without bending

antrum A nearly closed cavity or chamber

anulus fibrosus The fibrous outer part of the intervertebral disc

aorta The main trunk of the systemic arterial circulation

aperture A hole or opening

apex The pointed end of a conical structure

aponeurosis A white fibrous sheet composed of closely packed collagenous fibers; serves as a connection between a muscle and its attachment; a broad, flat sheet of tendon

appendage A structure attached to the body

appendicular Relating to an appendix or an appendage

aqueduct A canal or passageway, especially used for the conduction of fluid

aqueduct of Sylvius A channel through the midbrain that connects the third and fourth ventricles; also called the *cerebral aqueduct*

aqueous humor A watery, clear solution that fills the anterior cavity of the eye

arachnoid The thin cobweb-appearing layer of the meninges, located between the dura and pia mater

arbor vitae cerebelli The treelike branching arrangement of white matter in the cerebellum

arcuate artery The artery between the interlobar and the interlobular arteries in the kidney; forms an arch between the cortex and the medulla of the kidney

areola The pigmented area of skin around the nipple of the breast

artery A blood vessel that carries blood away from the heart

articular Referring to an articulation or a joint

articulate To join or to connect by means of a joint

articulation A joint; a place of contact between bones

aryepiglottic fold The membranous tissue in the larynx that attaches the arytenoid cartilage to the border of the epiglottis

arytenoid cartilages A pair of small pyramidal cartilages located in the posterior region of the larynx

ascites An accumulation of serous fluid in the peritoneal cavity

atrial Relating to an atrium, especially in the heart

atrioventricular Relating to both an atrium and a ventricle of the heart

atrium (pl. atria) The upper chambers of the heart, which receive blood from the veins

auditory Relating to the sense of hearing

auricle The external portion of the ear; also, the pouchlike projections from the atria of the heart

autonomic nervous system Division of the nervous system that transmits impulses from the brain and spinal cord to the visceral effectors, such as smooth muscles, glands, or cardiac muscle

axial Forming an axis; relating to the head, the neck, and the trunk of the body, as distinguished from the extremities

axilla (pl. axillae) The region where the arm meets the chest; commonly called the *armpit*

axillary artery Artery that arises from the subclavian artery and passes through the axilla

axon The process of a neuron that carries the nerve impulse away from the cell body; the efferent process of a neuron

azygos vein An unpaired vein that drains the thoracic wall and empties into the superior vena cava

baroreceptor Sensory nerve ending that responds to changes in blood pressure; also called *pressoreceptor*

Bartholin's glands A pair of glands, one on either side of the vaginal orifice, which open by a duct into the vestibule; also called the *greater vestibular glands*

basal ganglia Clusters of gray matter located within the white matter of each cerebral hemisphere; also called *cerebral nuclei*

basilar artery The artery that receives blood from the vertebral arteries and carries this blood into the circle of Willis at the base of the brain; located in the pontine cistern

basilic vein Superficial vein located on the medial side of the arm

biceps brachii A muscle of the arm, with two heads of origin, that flexes the forearm

bicipital groove A groove on the proximal humerus for the tendon of the long head of the biceps brachii

biconvex Having a protruding surface on both sides

bicuspid valve The left atrioventricular valve that has two cusps or flaps; also called the *mitral valve*

bifid Divided into two parts, e.g., the spinous processes of the cervical vertebrae

bifurcate To divide or separate into two parts

bile A secretion of the liver, stored in the gallbladder, that aids in the digestion of fats

bipolar Having two poles; relating to both ends of a cell

brachial Relating to the arm

brachialis muscle A muscle, located on the arm, that flexes the forearm

brachiocephalic artery The most anterior branch of the aortic arch; provides blood to the arm and the head on the right side

brachioradialis muscle A muscle, located on the arm, that flexes the forearm

brachium (pl. brachia) The arm, especially above the elbow

brainstem Portion of the brain that connects the cerebrum and spinal cord; consists of the midbrain, the pons, and the medulla oblongata

bronchial Relating to the bronchi

bronchopulmonary Relating to the bronchi and the lungs

bronchus (pl. bronchi) Either of the two branches of the trachea; further subdivides into secondary and tertiary branches and conveys air to and from the lungs

buccal Relating to the cheek or the mouth

buccinator muscle A muscle in the cheek

bulbospongiosus muscle One of the muscles of the perineum

bulbourethral glands Small, paired accessory glands of the male reproductive system; also called *Cowper's glands*

bulbus oculi The eyeball

bursa (pl. bursae) A sac, or pouch, of synovial fluid located at friction points, especially in the region of the joints

buttock One of two fleshy masses on the posterior surface of the lower trunk, formed by the gluteal muscles

calcaneofibular Relating to the calcaneus and the fibula

calcaneus One of the tarsal bones, commonly called the *heel bone*

calvaria The upper part of the skull

canaliculus (pl. canaliculi) A small channel or canal

capitulum A small rounded eminence or articular extremity of a bone; rounded surface on distal humerus that articulates with the radius; also called *capitellum*

carbohydrates A group of organic compounds composed of carbon, hydrogen, and oxygen with a 2:1 ratio of hydrogen to both carbon and oxygen; sugars, starches, cellulose

carcinoma A malignant tumor originating in epithelial cells

cardiac Relating to the heart; relating to the esophageal entrance to the stomach

carina Ridge formed at the bifurcation of the trachea into the two main stem bronchi

carotid Relating to the major arteries of the neck

carpal Relating to the bones in the wrist

cartilage A tough, nonvascular type of connective tissue

cartilaginous Consisting of cartilage

cauda equina Collection of spinal nerves that extend beyond the conus medullaris at the distal end of the spinal cord

caudal Relating to the tail

caudate nucleus One of several masses of gray matter located in the cerebrum

caval Relating to the vena cava, either superior or inferior

cavernous sinus A space, or cavity, on either side of the body and dorsum sellae of the sphenoid bone

cecum The blind pouch, or cul-de-sac, at the beginning of the large intestine, where the ileum enters

celiac trunk First major branch from the abdominal aorta; divides into the common hepatic, the left gastric, and the splenic arteries

cephalic Relating to the head; superior in position

cerebellar Relating to the cerebellum portion of the brain

cerebellomedullary cistern Subarachnoid cistern between the cerebellum and the medulla oblongata; also called the *cisterna magna*

cerebellum Portion of the brain that is below and posterior to the cerebrum and that is concerned with the coordination of movements

cerebral aqueduct A channel between the third and fourth ventricles in the brain; passes through the midbrain and contains cerebrospinal fluid; also called the *aqueduct of Sylvius*

cerebrospinal fluid A fluid that is produced by the choroid plexus of the ventricles and that circulates through the ventricles of the brain and in the subarachnoid space around the brain

cerebrum The largest part of the brain, consisting of two hemispheres

cervical Relating to the neck

cervix A neck-shaped structure; often used to denote the narrow, neck region of the uterus

chemoreceptor A nerve ending or sense organ that is sensitive to chemical stimuli

chiasma An X-shaped crossing; the optic chiasma is the X-shaped crossing of the optic nerves

chiasmatic cistern The subarachnoid space that contains cerebrospinal fluid in the region of the optic chiasma

choana (pl. choanae) A funnel-shaped opening, especially the opening of the nasal cavity into the nasopharynx; also called the *internal nares*

chordae tendineae String or chordlike structures that extend between the papillary muscles and the flaps of the atrioventricular valves in the ventricles of the heart

choroid The middle or vascular layer of the eyeball

choroid plexus Specialized vascular structures in the ventricles of the brain that produce cerebrospinal fluid

chronic Pertains to a slowly progressing disease that persists over a long period of time; opposite of acute

cilium (pl. cilia) A microscopic hairlike projection from the cell surface for cell locomotion or to move substances across the cell surface

circulus arteriosus cerebri Circle of anastomosing arteries at the base of the brain; also called the *circle of Willis*

circumcision Surgical removal of the prepuce or the foreskin from the glans penis

circumduction Circular movement of a part in which the distal end of the bone moves in a circle, whereas the proximal end remains relatively stable

circumflex Relating to arched structures

circumflex artery A branch of the left coronary artery that is located in the left artrioventricular sulcus

cistern An enclosed space or reservoir for body fluids, especially areas of the subarachnoid space that act as reservoirs for cerebrospinal fluid

cisterna ambiens The subarachnoid space at the posterior end of the corpus callosum; also called the *superior cistern* or the *cistern of the great cerebral vein*

cisterna chyli The dilatation at the beginning of the thoracic duct in the abdomen

cisterna magna Subarachnoid cistern located between the cerebellum and the medulla oblongata; also called the *cerebellomedullary cistern*

claustrum A thin layer of gray matter on the lateral margin of the external capsule of the brain

clavicle Collar bone; a bone that extends from the sternum to the acromion process of the scapula and that forms the anterior portion of the pectoral girdle

cleft palate Condition in which there is a fissure in the palate, or roof of the mouth, because the palatine processes of the two maxillae did not unite before birth

clitoris A small, erectile organ at the anterior end of the vulva in the female; homologous to the penis in the male

coccygeus muscle The smaller of the two muscles in the anal region of the pelvic floor

coccyx Three or four fused bones at the distal end of the vertebral column, commonly called the *tailbone*

cochlea The spiral cavity in the inner ear, which contains the essential organ of hearing

coitus Sexual intercourse or copulation

collateral circulation A secondary or alternate path of blood flow through anastomosing vessels

colliculus (pl. colliculi) A small round elevation, as in the midbrain

colon Portion of the large intestine that extends between the cecum and the rectum; divided into ascending, transverse, descending, and sigmoid regions

concave Characterized by having a hollow or depressed shape

concha (pl. conchae) A scroll or shell-shaped bone found in the nasal cavity; also called the *turbinate*

condyle A rounded prominence at the end of a bone for articulation with another bone

confluence of sinuses The junction of the venous sinuses in the dura mater, in the region of the internal occipital protuberance

congenital Present at birth

conjunctiva The delicate mucous membrane that lines the eyelids and that covers the exposed surface of the outer layer of the eyeball

connective tissue The most abundant tissue of the four basic tissue types; serves to bind and to support

constrict To make narrow or to reduce in size

contraction The shortening of a muscle or an increase in tension in a muscle

conus medullaris The tapered distal end of the spinal cord

convex Having a rounded or bulging surface

convoluted Twisted, coiled, or rolled

cooper's ligament Suspensory ligament of the breast

copulation Sexual intercourse, coitus

coracobrachialis A muscle that flexes and adducts the arm

coracoid process A thick, curved process at the superior border of the scapula

cornea The transparent anterior portion of the outer layer of the eyeball

corniculate cartilage A pair of small cartilages in the larynx

coronal plane Plane parallel to the long axis of the body that divides the body into anterior and posterior portions; also called the *frontal plane*

coronary arteries (left and right) First branches from the ascending aorta; located at the level of the aortic semilunar valve; supply blood to the heart wall

coronary sinus A thin-walled venous dilation on the posterior surface of the heart; drains into the right atrium

coronoid process Certain processes of bones such as the coronoid process of the mandible

corpora quadrigemina Four bodies that form the dorsal part of the midbrain

corpus (pl. corpora) Body, or main portion, of a structure

corpus callosum A large band of white fibers that connects the two cerebral hemispheres

corpus spongiosum Ventral column of erectile tissue that surrounds the urethra in the penis

corpus cavernosum Either of the two dorsal columns of erectile tissue in the penis

cortex The outer layer of an organ; the outer layer of gray matter of the cerebrum

costal Pertaining to the ribs

Cowper's gland An accessory gland of the male reproductive system; also called *bulbourethral gland*

coxa (pl. **coxae**) The hipbone, or the os coxae

cranial cavity One of the divisions of the dorsal body cavity; contains the brain

cranium The bones of the skull that enclose the brain

cremaster muscle An extension of the internal oblique muscle that is found in the spermatic cord and that contracts to elevate the testes

crest A bony ridge

cribriform plate Flat region on either side of the crista galli of the ethmoid bone, perforated by many small holes called *olfactory foramina*

cricoid cartilage Most inferior cartilage of the larynx

crista terminalis A ridge that separates the sinus venarum and pectinate regions of the right atrium

cruciate Overlapping, or crossing, such as the cruciate ligaments of the knee

crus (pl. **crura**) Derived from Latin for leg; slender, tapered portion of a muscle or organ, such as the crus of the diaphragm or the crura of the penis

cubital Relating to the forearm; cubitus refers to the elbow joint, and the cubital fossa is the depression on the anterior surface of the elbow joint

cul-de-sac A blind-ended pouch or sac

cuneiform Wedge-shaped; three of the tarsal bones

cusp A triangular piece of an atrioventricular valve in the heart; an elevation or projection on a tooth

cutaneous Pertaining to the skin

cystic duct Duct from the gallbladder

dartos Contractle tissue in the subcutaneous tissue of the scrotum

decussation Crossing over to the other side, especially in nerve tracts; if bilateral, then forms the shape of the letter X

degeneration Deterioration or breakdown of tissues

delineate To mark boundaries, to delimit

deltoid Superficial muscle over the shoulder; abducts the arm

demarcation The marking of boundaries; delimitation

detrusor muscle Smooth muscle in the wall of the urinary bladder

diaphragma sellae Extension of dura mater over the sella turcica of the sphenoid bone

diaphragmatic Relating to the diaphragm

diencephalon Portion of the brain that is surrounded by the cerebral hemispheres and that encloses the third ventricle; principal components are the thalamus and hypothalamus

digastric A muscle in the floor of the oral cavity

dilatation An enlarged or swollen area, usually used in reference to a tubular structure, opening, or cavity

dilate To expand, to enlarge, or to swell

dislocation Displacement of a part from normal position, usually used in reference to bone in joints

dissect To cut apart or to separate tissues or organs in the study of anatomy

distal Directional term for something located away from a point of reference, such as the center, the midline, the point of attachment, or the point of origin; opposite of proximal

distensible Capable of being stretched

diverge To spread apart from a common point

diverticulum (pl. **diverticula**) A pouch, or sac, protruding from the wall of a tubular organ

dopamine A compound produced in the caudate nucleus and putamen of the brain, diminished in some disease states such as parkinsonism

dorsal Directional term relating to the back or posterior surface of a structure

dorsal root ganglion An enlargement in the dorsal root of spinal nerves that contains the cell bodies of afferent neurons

dorsum The back or posterior surface of a structure

duct A tube or channel, usually for carrying secretions

duct of Wirsung Pancreatic duct

ductus arteriosus A channel or vessel between the pulmonary artery and the aorta in the fetus that allows blood to bypass the lungs in fetal circulation

ductus deferens A tube or channel that conveys sperm from the epididymis to the ejaculatory duct in the male

duodenum The first part of the small intestine

dura mater The outer, tough covering around the brain and spinal cord; the outer layer of the meninges

echogenic Tissues that produce echos

ectopic Located outside the normal place

edema Swelling caused by an abnormal accumulation of interstitial fluid

efferent Carrying a nerve impulse or fluid away from an area or an organ

ejaculatory duct The tube that transports sperm from the vas deferens to the prostatic urethra

embryo The developing human, from the time of conception to the end of the eighth week of development

eminence An elevated area or prominence, especially used in reference to regions on bones

encircle To surround

endocardium The innermost layer of the heart, composed of endothelium

endocrine A gland that secretes its hormones into the bloodstream; a ductless gland

endometrium The mucous membrane that makes up the inner layer of the uterine wall

endosteum Membranous lining of bone cavities

endothelium A thin layer of epithelial cells that lines the heart, blood vessels, and lymphatics

enunciation The formation of words

enzyme A protein, secreted by the body, that acts as a catalyst to speed up chemical reactions in the body

epicardium The visceral or innermost layer of the serous pericardium, which is in contact with the heart and forms the outermost layer of the heart wall

epicondyle Projection above or on a condyle

epicranium The scalp; structures that cover the skull, including the muscle, the aponeurosis, and the skin

epididymis A comma-shaped structure on the posterior surface of the testis; site of sperm maturation

epidural Located above or on the dura mater

epigastric region The upper, middle abdominal region, directly superior to the umbilical region

epiglottic Relating to the epiglottis

epiglottis Leaf-shaped piece of cartilage that covers the trachea during swallowing to prevent food from blocking the airway

epiploic Relating to the omentum

epiploic appendages Bodies of fat along the taeniae coli of the large intestine

epiploic foramen The opening along the right margin of the lesser omentum that allows access to the omental bursa; also called the *foramen of Winslow*

epithalamus A small area of the diencephalon above the thalamus

epithelium The nonvascular layer of cells that lines body cavities and covers the exterior surface of the body; one of the four main types of tissue in the body

equilibrium A state of balance

erectile tissue Tissue that becomes rigid when filled with blood

erector A muscle that can raise or cause a structure to become erect

erector spinae Intermediate layer of intrinsic muscles associated with the vertebral column; includes the iliocostalis, the longissimus, and the spinalis

esophagus Muscular passageway that takes food from the pharynx to the stomach

estrogens Term for female sex hormones that maintain secondary sex characteristics

ethmoid A bone resembling a sieve because of many foramina, located behind the nose

eustachian tube Tube that connects the middle ear to the nasopharynx; auditory tube

eversion The movement of turning a joint outward, e.g., eversion of the foot

evert To turn outward

excretory Relating to excretion

exocrine Glands that secrete their products to a surface via ducts

expel To force outward

extension The act of increasing the angle at a joint; opposite of flexion

extensor A muscle that increases the angle between bones at a joint

extensor carpi radialis Lateral muscle of the forearm that extends the hand

extensor carpi ulnaris Medial muscle of the forearm that extends the hand

extracapsular Located outside of a capsule

extradural Located outside of the dura mater

extrapelvic Located outside of the pelvic cavity

extremity A limb; an arm or a leg

extrinsic Located on the outside of the structure that is being acted upon

facet A very smooth bone surface for articulation with another structure

facial Relating to the face; cranial nerve VII

falciform ligament Fold of peritoneum extending from the diaphragm and the anterior abdominal wall to the surface of the liver, between the two major lobes

fallopian tube Duct that carries the ova from the ovary to the uterus; also called the uterine tube or the oviduct

falx cerebelli The triangular extension of the cranial dura mater that is located between the two lobes of the cerebellum

falx cerebri The fold of cranial dura mater that extends into the longitudinal fissure between the two cerebral hemispheres

fascia Loose connective tissue, located under the skin, or a fibrous membrane that covers and separates muscles

fauces The opening from the oral cavity into the oropharynx

femoral Relating to the femur or the thigh

femur Large bone of the thigh

fertility The ability to start or to support conception

fertilization The union of a spermatozoan with an ovum

fetal Relating to the fetus

fetus The developing offspring in the uterus from the beginning of the third month of development until birth

fibrocartilage Cartilage that contains a large number of collagenous fibers

fibromuscular Denotes a tissue that is both muscular and fibrous

fibroserous Denotes a tissue that is both serous and fibrous

fibrous Composed of fibers of connective tissue

fibula The smaller and more lateral bone of the lower leg

filtration Movement of a liquid through a filter as a result of a pressure difference

fimbriae Fingerlike projections that surround the openings of the uterine tubes

fissure A slit, cleft, or groove

flaccid Muscles without tone, flabby

flexion The act of decreasing the angle at a joint; opposite of extension

flexor A muscle that decreases the angle between bones at a joint

flexor carpi radialis Lateral muscle of the forearm that flexes the hand

flexor carpi ulnaris Medial muscle of the forearm that flexes the hand

flexure A bend or turn

foliated Resembling a leaf

follicle A mass of cells containing a cavity; a small depression in the skin from which the hair emerges

foramen (pl. foramina) A hole or opening

foramen of Magendie The medial opening in the roof of the fourth ventricle through which cerebrospinal fluid enters the subarachnoid space; also called *median aperture*

foramen magnum Large hole located in the occipital bone through which the spinal cord passes

foramen of Monro Opening from the lateral ventricle into the third ventricle; also called the *interventricular foramen*

foramina of Luschka Two lateral openings in the roof of the fourth ventricle through which cerebrospinal fluid enters the subarachnoid space; also called *lateral apertures*

fornix (pl. fornices) An arched structure, or the space caused by such a structure, e.g., the fornix of the vagina

fossa (pl. fossae) A pit or shallow depression

fovea A small depression

frenulum A small fold of mucous membrane that connects two parts and limits movement, e.g., the lingual frenulum on the underside of the tongue

frontal Relating to the forehead

frontal plane Plane parallel to the long axis of the body that divides the body into anterior and posterior portions; also called the *coronal plane*

frontalis muscle Muscle that wrinkles the forehead

fructose A simple sugar or monosaccharide

fundus The part of a hollow organ that is the farthest from, above, or opposite of its opening

galea aponeurotica The broad, flat tendon that connects the frontalis muscle with the occipitalis muscle; a part of the scalp; also called the *epicranial aponeurosis*

gallbladder An oblong sac that is located on the underside of the liver and stores bile

ganglion (pl. **ganglia**) A group of nerve cell bodies located outside the brain and spinal cord

gaster Refers to the belly

gastric Relating to the stomach

gastrocnemius Muscle of the calf that plantar flexes the foot

gastrocolic Relating to the stomach and colon or to the large intestine

gastroduodenal Relating to the stomach and the duodenum

gastroepiploic Relating to the stomach and the omentum

gastroesophageal Relating to the stomach and the esophagus

gastrohepatic Relating to the stomach and the liver

gastrointestinal Relating to the stomach and the intestines (gastroenteric)

gastrosplenic Relating to the stomach and the spleen

gemellus (pl. **gemelli**) Means twins; two muscles deep to the gluteal muscles that laterally rotate and abduct the thigh

geniohyoid One of the muscles that acts on the hyoid bone

genital Relating to reproduction

genitalia Reproductive organs

genitourinary Relating to the genital system and the urinary system; also called *urogenital*

genu Any structure that resembles a flexed knee, e.g., genu of the corpus callosum

gingiva The gum; mucous membrane that surrounds the alveolar process and the neck of the tooth

glans penis The caplike extension of the corpus spongiosum at the distal tip of the penis

glenohumeral Relating to the glenoid fossa of the scapula and to the humerus

glenoid Relating to an articular depression or socket of a joint, e.g., glenoid fossa of the scapula

glenoid labrum A rim of fibrocartilage around the margin of the glenoid fossa

globus pallidus The medial region of gray matter in the lentiform nucleus

glossopharyngeal Relating to the tongue and the pharynx

glottis Vocal apparatus in the larynx, consisting of the vocal folds and the rima glottidis between them

gluteal Relating to the buttocks

gluteus maximus The large, fleshy muscle that forms the prominent portion of the buttocks

gluteus medius The broad, thick muscle situated on the outer surface of the pelvis

gluteus minimus The smallest and deepest muscle of the three gluteal muscles

gonad Primary reproductive organ, the ovary in the female and the testes in the male

gonadal Refers to the gonad

graafian follicle A fluid-filled follicle that contains an immature ovum and its surrounding, estrogen-secreting cells; also called a *vesicular ovarian follicle*

gracilis Straplike muscle that is located on the medial surface of the thigh and that functions in adduction of the thigh

gyrus (pl. **gyri**) Rounded elevations on the surface of the brain

hallucis muscles Muscles that work on the big toe, e.g., the adductor hallucis

hallux The big toe

hamate One of the bones of the wrist (carpals)

hemidiaphragm Half or one dome of the diaphragm

hemorrhage Profuse bleeding

hepatic Relating to the liver

hepatoduodenal Relating to the liver and the duodenum

hepatogastric Relating to the liver and the stomach

hepatorenal Relating to the liver and the kidney

hernia A protrusion of an organ through an abnormal opening or weakening of the wall that usually contains it

hiatus An opening or an aperture

hilum The region where vessels and nerves enter and leave an organ

homologous Organs that are alike in structure or origin

hormones Substances that are secreted by endocrine glands and are released into the blood, causing a response in the target organ

humeral Relating to the humerus

humeroradial Relating to the humerus and the radius

humeroscapular Relating to the humerus and the scapula

humeroulnar Relating to the humerus and the ulna

humerus Bone of the upper arm

hyaline cartilage Gelatinous material with a glassy appearance found in many extracellular areas

hyoid A U-shaped bone found in the neck; serves as an anchor for the tongue

hypertrophy An increase in bulk or in size of tissue without cell division

hypochondriac region Abdominal region located superiorly and laterally, near the ribs, on either side of the epigastric region

hypogastric region The lower, middle abdominal region located directly inferior to the umbilical region

hypoglossal Located beneath the tongue

hypopharynx Below the pharynx

hypophysis Endocrine gland located under the brain; also called the *pituitary gland*

hypothalamus A portion of the diencephalon located inferior to the thalamus; also forms the floor of the third ventricle

ileocecal Relating to the ileum and the cecum

ileum The third part of the small intestine, which is connected to the colon

iliac Relating to the ilium of the os coxae

iliacus Muscle that lines the ilium of the os coxae

iliofemoral Relating to the ilium and the femur

iliopsoas Muscle that results from the joining of the iliacus and the psoas muscles, located in the upper thigh

iliotibial Relating to the ilium and the tibia

ilium The superior, broad portion of the os coxae

implantation The attaching of the fertilized ovum into the uterine wall

incisura angularis A notch, or indentation, between the body and the pylorus of the stomach

incontinence The inability to control the passage of urine or feces as a result of loss of sphincter control

incus One of three ossicles of the ear, small anvil-shaped bone of the middle ear, located between the malleus and the stapes

inferiorly Located below or inferior to another structure

infraglenoid Located below the glenoid fossa of the scapula bone

infraglottic Located below the glottis

infrahyoid Located below the hyoid bone

infraorbital Located below the orbit of the eye

infrapubic Located below the pubis

infraspinatus muscle Muscle located below the spine of the scapula

infraspinous Located below the spinous process, e.g., the infraspinous fossa located under the spine of the scapula

infrasternal Located below the sternum

infundibulum Funnel-shaped structure, e.g., the infundibulum of the pituitary gland or the infundibulum of the uterine tube

inguinal Refers to the groin

innervation Nerve or nerves that supply an area

innominate artery The first and most anterior arterial branch off the aorta; also called the *brachiocephalic artery*

inspiration The act of breathing in, inhalation

insula The hidden lobe of the brain, deep to the temporal lobe; also called the *island of Reil*

interatrial Located between the two atria

interclavicular Located between the two clavicles

intercondylar Located between two condyles

intercostal Located between adjacent ribs

intercristal Located between two crests

interiliac Located between the two ilia

intermuscular Located between muscles

interosseous Connecting or lying between bones

interpeduncular Located between the two cerebral peduncles

interposed Located between two structures

intertubercular Located between two tubercles

interventricular Located between two ventricles

interventricular foramen Opening located between a lateral ventricle and the third ventricle; also called the *foramen of Monro*

intervertebral Located between two vertebrae

intestine The portion of the gastrointestinal tract that extends from the stomach to the anus

intracapsular Located within a capsule

intracranial Located within the skull

intramuscular Located within a muscle

intrathoracic Located within the thorax

inversion Turning inside out or reversing the normal relationship between organs; turning the sole of the foot medially; the opposite of eversion

iris The colored portion of the eye, a circle of smooth muscles that controls the size of the pupil

ischiocavernosus Muscles of the perineum

ischiofemoral Relating to the ischium and the femur

ischiopubic Relating to the ischium and the pubis

ischium The lowest and most posterior portion of the ox coxae

island of Reil The hidden lobe of the brain, deep to the temporal lobe; also called the *insula*

isthmus A narrow band of tissue that connects two larger parts or a narrow passageway between two larger cavities

jejunum The middle portion of the small intestine, located between the duodenum and the ileum

jugular Relating to the neck; structures located in the neck

labia majora Two large folds of fat-filled tissue that are lateral to the labia minora

labia minora The two narrow folds of tissue that enclose or delineate the vestibule in the female

labrum A lip or an edge

laceration A jagged tear of tissues

lacerum Foramen resembling a jagged tear

lacrimal Relating to tears

lactiferous Secreting or carrying milk

lamina (pl. **laminae**) A thin layer or flat plate

laryngeal Relating to the larynx

laryngopharynx The lowest part of the pharynx, located posterior to the larynx, that leads into the esophagus

larynx Voice box, organ of voice production that contains the vocal folds

lateral Located on the side away from the middle

latissimus dorsi Broad superficial muscle of the back

lenticular nucleus, lentiform nucleus A mass of gray matter, lateral to the internal capsule, that is a part of the basal ganglia

leptomeninges Collective term relating to the arachnoid and pia mater

levator ani muscle Muscle of the pelvic floor

levator costarum muscle Muscle that raises the ribs

lienorenal Relating to the spleen and the kidney; also called *splenorenal*

ligament A band of fibrous tissue that connects bone together

ligamenta flava Short bands of elastic fibers that connect the laminae of adjacent vertebrae

ligamentum arteriosum Band of tissue that represents the remnant of the ductus arteriosus from the fetal circulation

ligamentum nuchae Supraspinous and interspinous ligaments from C7 to the occipital bone

linea alba White line, a narrow band of the anterior aponeurosis, between the two rectus abdominis muscles, in the middle of the abdomen, from the xiphoid process to the pubic symphysis

linea aspera A long ridge on the posterior surface of the femur

lingual Referring to the tongue

lobule A small lobe

longitudinal fissure Fissure of the brain that separates the cerebrum into two cerebral hemispheres

lordosis Abnormally exaggerated lumbar curve, swayback

lumbar region Abdominal region on either side of the umbilical region

lumbosacral Relating to the lumbar region of the spine and the sacrum

lumen Open space in the interior of a tubular structure

lymph Clear or yellowish fluid that is derived from the interstitial fluid and that is contained in the lymph vessels

lymphatic Relating to lymph, lymph nodes, or lymph vessels

lymphoid Referring to or resembling lymph or lymphatic tissue

malignant Refers to a disease that resists treatment and tends to be fatal; frequently pertains to tumors that have the properties of uncontrolled growth and dissemination

malleolus Projections on either side of the ankle; one is located on the tibia, the other on the fibula

malleus One of the three ear ossicles in the middle ear; the ossicle located next to the tympanic membrane and shaped like a hammer or mallet

mammary Referring to the breasts

mammillary Structures that are breast shaped and are located at the base of the hypothalamus

mandible Bone of the lower jaw

manubrium Means handle; refers to the superior part of the sternum

masseter Muscle that acts to close the jaw, a muscle of mastication

mastication The process of chewing

mastoid The projection on the temporal bone located posterior to the ear

maxilla (pl. **maxillae**) Bones that form the upper jaw

maxillary Relating to the upper jaw

meatus A channel or opening

medial Toward the middle or median plane of a body or organ

median Centrally located

mediastinal Relating to the mediastinum

mediastinum (pl. **mediastina**) The central region of the thoracic cavity

medulla The inner part of an organ

medulla oblongata Inferiormost part of the brainstem; extends from the pons to the spinal cord and is continuous with the spinal cord at the foramen magnum

melanin Dark pigment found in the skin, the hair, and the iris of the eye

meninges Membranes that cover the brain and the spinal cord

meningitis An inflammation of the meninges

meniscus (pl. **menisci**) A crescent-shaped structure; frequently refers to the pad of fibrocartilage found in certain joints, e.g., the knee

menopause The normal termination of the menstrual cycle

mesenteric Relating to the mesentery

mesentery Double layer of peritoneum that is attached to the intestines and to the body wall and that contains blood vessels and nerves

mesocolon The fold of peritoneum that attaches the colon to the posterior wall of the abdomen

mesovarium The fold of peritoneum that attaches the ovary to the posterior layer of the broad ligament

metacarpals Bones located in the hand, between the carpals and the phalanges

metastasis The transfer of disease from its starting point to a distant point

metatarsals Bones of the foot, between the tarsals and phalanges

midbrain The part of the brain that is located between the pons and the diencephalon; also called the *mesencephalon*

midsagittal The plane that divides the body into equal right and left sides

mitral valve Valve located between the left atrium and the left ventricle; also called the *bicuspid valve*

mnemonic Relating to or assisting the memory

molar A posterior tooth that grinds food

mons pubis The prominence caused by a pad of fat located over the symphysis pubis in the female

morphology The study of the form or the structure of living organisms

motility The ability to move

mucoid Resembles mucus

mucosa The mucous membrane that lines a cavity opening to the exterior; consists of epithelium and lamina propria

mucous Relating to, consisting of, or producing mucus

mucus Viscous secretions produced by specialized membranes (mucous membranes)

multiaxial Having many axes

musculature The system of muscles in the body or in a body part

myelin The fatty substance that surrounds and insulates the axon of some nerve cells

mylohyoid One of the muscles associated with the hyoid bone, located in the neck

myocardium The muscular layer of the heart

myometrium The muscular layer of the uterus

naris (pl. **nares**) One of the external openings of the nose; also called *nostril*

nasal Relating to the nose

nasolacrimal Relating to the nose and the lacrimal bones

nasopharynx The superior part of the pharynx, located above the level of the soft palate, posterior to the nasal cavity

navel Umbilicus; depressed area where the umbilical cord was attached

navicular Anterior bone of the ankle or tarsus

neural Relating to the nervous system

neurons Nerve cells; the basic functional unit of the nervous system

neurovascular Relating to the nervous and the vascular systems

neutralize To render ineffective or to make neutral

nodules Small nodes

nuchal Relating to the back or the nape of the neck

nucleus pulposus Inner, soft core of an intervertebral disc

oblique A slanting or sloping direction; deviating from the perpendicular or horizontal

obturator externus One of the muscles that closes the obturator foramen; one of the lateral rotators of the thigh

obturator internus One of the muscles that closes the obturator foramen and is part of the lateral pelvic wall; one of the lateral rotators of the thigh

occipital Relating to the back of the head

ocular Relating to the eye

oculomotor Cranial nerve III, innervates muscles that affect eye movement

odontoid Shaped like a tooth; process on the second cervical vertebra, also called the *dens*

olecranon Curved process on the ulna that forms the point of the elbow

olfactory Relating to the sense of smell; cranial nerve I

omentum (pl. **omenta**) A fold of peritoneum in the abdominal cavity, usually associated with the stomach

omohyoid One of the infrahyoid muscles

oocyte An immature cell in the ovary that, after undergoing meiosis, produces an ovum

ophthalmic Pertaining to the eye

optic Cranial nerve II; refers to the eye, vision, or properties of light

optimum Most suitable or favorable conditions

orbicularis A circular muscle

orbicularis oculi Circular muscle around the eye

orbicularis oris A circular muscle around the mouth

orbit Cavity in the skull that contains the eyeball; called the *eye socket*

orbital Relating to the orbit

organ of Corti Sensory receptors for hearing, located in the inner ear; also called the *spiral organ of Corti*

orifice An opening or aperture

oropharynx Middle portion of the pharynx, directly posterior to the oral cavity; extends from the soft palate to the hyoid bone

os Mouth or opening, such as the os of the cervix; may also refer to bone, such as os coxae

osseous Consisting of bone

ossicle A small bone; auditory ossicles are three small bones (malleus, incus, stapes) in the middle ear (see individual definitions for each ossicle)

ossification Formation of bone

ovarian Relating to the ovary

ovary Female gonad that produces ova, estrogens, and progesterone

oviduct Slender tube that extends from the uterus to the region of the ovary; also called the *uterine tube* or the *fallopian tube*

ovulation Rupture of a mature follicle in the ovary with the release of a secondary oocyte into the pelvic cavity

ovum (pl. **ova**) Female gamete or germ cell; egg cell

oxytocin Hormone produced in the hypothalamus and stored in the posterior pituitary, stimulates smooth muscle contractions in the pregnant uterus and ejection of milk from the breasts

pacemaker A structure that establishes a basic rhythmic pattern; sinoatrial node in the heart

palate Roof of the mouth, separates the oral and the nasal cavities

palatine Relating to the roof of the mouth

palmar Relating to the palm of the hand

palpate To examine by touch or by feel

palpebra (pl. **palpebrae**) Eyelid

pampiniform plexus In the male, a plexus of veins from the testicle and epididymis that is included in the spermatic cord; in the female, a plexus of ovarian veins in the broad ligament

pancreatic Relating to the pancreas

papillary muscles Conical projections of myocardium on the inner surface of the ventricles

papilledema Swelling of the optic nerve as a result of increased intracranial pressure

paranasal Located adjacent to or near the nose

parasagittal plane A vertical plane that divides the body into unequal right and left portions; does not pass through the midline

parasympathetic Refers to the part of the autonomic nervous system that is concerned with conserving and restoring energy

parathyroid gland One of four small glands embedded on the posterior surface of the thyroid gland

paraurethral glands A pair of small, mucus-secreting glands associated with the orifice of the urethra in the female; also called *Skene's glands*

parenchyma The characteristic or functional tissue of an organ or gland

parietal Pertaining to the outer wall of a body cavity

parotid Largest of the salivary glands

parturition Act of giving birth; childbirth; delivery

patella Flattened bone in front of the knee; also called the *knee cap*

pathogen Microorganism capable of causing disease

pectinate Comb shaped; region of the atria of the heart with comb-shaped muscular ridges

pectineus muscle One of the muscles that adducts and flexes the thigh

pectoral Relating to the chest or thorax

pedicle A stem or stalk; a short process that connects the body with the lamina of a vertebra

peduncle A stalk or ropelike mass of nerve fibers that connects one part of the brain to another

pelvic Relating to the pelvis

pelvis A basinlike skeletal structure that acts as an attachment for the lower extremity and contains viscera; a funnel-shaped region, such as the pelvis of the kidney

pendulous Drooping or sagging

penile Relating to the penis

penis Male copulatory organ and organ of urinary excretion

pericardium Membranous sac that encloses the heart

perineal Relating to the perineum

perineum Region bounded by the pubis, coccyx, and thighs; clinical perineum is the region between the anus and the external genitalia

periosteum Connective tissue membrane that covers bone

periphery Area away from the center; outer surface of the body

peritoneal Relating to the peritoneum

peritoneum Serous membrane of the abdominal cavity

peroneal Relating to the fibula or lateral portion of the leg

peroneus muscles A group of muscles that originate on the fibula and function to evert the foot

petrosal Relating to the petrous portion of the temporal bone

Peyer's patches Aggregated lymphatic follicles in the wall of the small intestine, especially in the ileum

phalanx (pl. **phalanges**) A bone of the finger or toe

pharyngeal Relating to the pharynx

pharynx A musculomembranous cavity or tube posterior to the nasal, oral, and laryngeal cavities

phonation Production of sound

phrenic Relating to the diaphragm

pia mater A delicate membrane, the innermost layer of meninges around the brain

piriform Pear shaped

piriformis muscle One of the muscles that laterally rotates the thigh, located in the greater sciatic notch

plantar Relating to the sole of the foot

plantar flexion Flexion at the ankle that bends the foot downward toward the sole of the foot

plantaris muscle One of the leg muscles that plantar flexes the foot

platysma A thin muscle in the superficial fascia of the anterior neck region that contracts to depress the lower jaw and to wrinkle the skin of the neck

pleura Serous membrane that covers the lungs and lines the walls of the chest cavity

pleural Relating to the pleura

plexus A network of blood vessels, lymphatic vessels, or nerves

pons Central part of the brainstem, located between the cerebral peduncles and the medulla oblongata

pontine Relating to the pons

popliteal Relating to the back of the knee

popliteus muscle A small muscle on the medial side of the back of the knee that flexes and medially rotates the leg

porta Entrance or door; the region where blood vessels, nerves, lymphatic vessels, and ducts enter and leave an organ

porta hepatis Fissure on the visceral surface of the liver through which the hepatic portal vein, the hepatic artery, and the hepatic ducts pass

posterior Nearer to or toward the back of the body; dorsal

prepuce Loose fold of skin that covers the glans penis; also called the *foreskin*

progesterone A hormone that is produced by the corpus luteum in the ovary; it functions to prepare the lining of the uterus for implantation of a fertilized ovum

prolactin A hormone that is produced in the anterior pituitary gland and that stimulates the production of milk

prolapse To fall or to slip down; the inferior displacement of an organ or part of an organ from its normal position

promontory A projection or elevation

pronate To place in a face-down position; to turn the hand so that the palm is turned downward or backward

proprioception The sense of body position and movement as a result of information received from sense receptors in the muscles and tendons

prostate An accessory gland in the male reproductive system, located inferior to the urinary bladder

proximal Located nearest the center, midline, point of attachment, or point of origin; opposite of distal

psoas muscle Large muscle mass, located on either side of the lumbar vertebrae, that flexes and medially rotates the thigh

pterygoid Wing shaped; refers to the pterygoid processes on the sphenoid bone and the pterygoid muscles

ptosis Drooping or sagging

pubic Relating to the pubis

pubis The pubic bone or the region over the pubic bone

pudendal Relating to the genital area

pudendum External genital organs, especially in the female; also called the *vulva*

pulmonary Relating to the lungs

Purkinje fibers Conduction myofibers of the heart; specialized cells that are part of the conduction system of the heart

pus The liquid product of inflammation that contains cellular debris, dead leukocytes, and dead bacteria

putamen The lateral portion of the lentiform nucleus, a region of gray matter in the cerebrum

pyloric Relating to the pylorus

pylorus The distal portion of the stomach; opening between the stomach and the duodenum

pyramidal Relating to or having the shape of a pyramid

quadrant One of four sections; used to designate regions of the abdomen

quadrate Having four sides, such as the quadrate lobe of the liver

quadratus lumborum One of the muscles of the posterior abdominal wall, lateral to the psoas muscles

quadriceps femoris Muscle mass of the anterior thigh; consists of four muscles

radial Relating to the radius, a bone in the forearm; diverging in various directions from a central point

radiograph The processed photographic film used in radiography

radius The lateral bone in the forearm

ramus (pl. rami) Branch; a branch of an artery, vein, or nerve

raphe A ridge or line that marks the union of two similar structures

receptor A sensory end-organ; it receives a stimulus and converts it into a nerve impulse

rectouterine pouch Peritoneal space between the rectum and uterus; also called the *cul-de-sac* or *pouch of Douglas*

rectovesical pouch Peritoneal space between the rectum and the urinary bladder

rectum Terminal portion of the intestinal tract; section of intestine that extends from the sigmoid colon to the anus

rectus Straight; used to describe some muscles that run a straight course, such as the rectus abdominis muscle and the rectus muscles of the eye

reflux Backward flow

renal Pertaining to the kidney

respiration The physical and chemical processes by which an individual acquires oxygen and releases carbon dioxide

respiratory Pertaining to respiration

retina The innermost layer of the eyeball; part of the eye that contains the visual receptors

retinaculum A bandlike ligament found in the wrist and in the ankle

retinal Relating to the retina

retromammary Located behind or deep to the mammary gland

retroperitoneal Located behind the peritoneum

retropharyngeal Located behind or dorsal to the pharynx

retroversion Backward tilt of an organ

rima A slitlike opening

rima glottidis The slitlike opening between the true vocal folds

rima vestibuli The slitlike opening between the vestibular or false vocal folds

rotation Circular motion around an axis

rotator A muscle that rotates a part

ruga (pl. rugae) A fold or wrinkle; gastric rugae are folds in the lining of the stomach

rupture To break or to tear apart; hernia

sac An anatomical structure that resembles a bag or pouch

saccule A small sac

sacral Relating to the sacrum

sacroiliac Relating to both the sacrum and the ilium, e.g., the sacroiliac joint

sacrum Curved, triangular bone made up of five fused vertebrae that are inferior to the lumbar vertebrae and are wedged between the two hip bones

sagittal plane A vertical plane that divides the body into right and left portions

salivary Relating to saliva; salivary glands produce saliva

saphenous Relating to either of two long, superficial veins in the leg, the great (long) saphenous vein and the small (short) saphenous vein; the great (long) saphenous vein is the longest vein in the body

sartorius A long, straplike muscle that courses obliquely across the anterior thigh and flexes the thigh and leg

scalene muscles A group of muscles associated with the first and second ribs

scalp The skin that covers the cranium

scapula (pl. **scapulae**) Part of the pectoral girdle that provides the attachment for the upper extremity; also called the *shoulder blade*

scapular Relating to the scapula

sciatic Relating to the hip or ischium, such as the sciatic nerve

sclera The outermost layer of the eyeball

scrotum The pouch or sac that encloses the testes and the lower part of the spermatic cord

sebaceous Relating to a fatty or oily substance called sebum

sella turcica A depression on the upper surface of the sphenoid bone that marks the location of the pituitary gland

semimembranosus One of the hamstring muscles located on the thigh

seminal Relating to the semen; seminal vesicles are paired glands, posterior and inferior to the bladder in the male, that secrete a component of semen into the ejaculatory duct

seminiferous tubules Tightly coiled ducts, located in the testes, where spermatozoa are produced

semitendinosus One of the hamstring muscles located on the thigh

septal Relating to a septum

septum (pl. **septa**) A wall or partition

septum pellucidum A thin partition between the two lateral ventricles in the brain

sequela (pl. **sequelae**) An abnormal condition that follows and is caused by another disease

sigmoid Crooked, or having the shape of the letter S; the sigmoid colon is the S-shaped portion of the colon, between the descending colon and the rectum

sinoatrial node The portion of the conduction system of the heart that initiates and establishes the rhythm of the heartbeat; also called the *pacemaker* or the *SA node*

sinus An air-filled cavity in a cranial bone; a dilated channel for the passage of blood or lymph

sinusoid Like a sinus; venous channels in some organs, such as the liver and spleen

skeletal Relating to the skeleton or bone

skullcap The top portion of the cranium; also called the *calvaria*

soleus Muscle in the calf of the leg, deep to the gastrocnemius muscle; plantar flexes of the foot

somatic Pertaining to the body or the soma

sperm Spermatozoa; mature male gametes or germ cells

spermatic cord Supporting structure of the male reproductive system that contains the vas deferens, the blood vessels, the lymphatics, the cremaster muscle, and the connective tissue

spermatogenesis The formation of spermatozoa

spermatozoon (pl. **spermatozoa**) Mature male gamete or germ cell; sperm

sphenoethmoidal Relating to both the sphenoid bone and the ethmoid bone

sphenoidal Relating to the sphenoid bone

sphincter A circular muscle that closes an opening when it contracts

spinal Relating to a spine; relating to the vertebral column

spine A short projection of bone, a spinous process; the vertebral column

splenic Relating to the spleen

squama (pl. **squamae**) Thin, flat portion of the temporal bone; squamous region of the temporal bone

squamous Flat or scaly

stapes One of three ear ossicles in the middle ear; attached to the oval window

stasis A stoppage or halt in the normal flow of fluids

Stensen's duct The duct from the parotid gland that empties into the oral cavity; also called the *parotid duct*

sternal Relating to the sternum

sternum A long, flat bone that forms the anterior portion of the thoracic cage; also called the *breast bone*

stratified Consisting of, or arranged in, many layers

stroma (pl. **stromata**) The supporting or connective tissue framework of an organ, as opposed to its functional part, the parenchyma

styloid process A long, pointed process on the temporal bone

substantia nigra A region of deeply pigmented cells in the cerebral peduncles

sulcus (pl. **sulci**) A groove or furrow

superficial On, or near, the surface; shallow, such as a superficial wound

superior Located higher, or toward the head; the upper surface of an organ

supination Act of lying on the back; rotation of the forearm so that the palm of the hand is forward or upward

supinator A muscle that supinates the forearm

supine Lying on the back

sura Calf of the leg

sutures Immovable joints that unite bones of the skull

sympathetic One of the two divisions of the autonomic nervous system

symphysis A slightly movable joint that has a pad of fibrocartilage between the opposing bones, such as the symphysis pubis

synapse The junction or region of communication between nerve cells

syndrome A set of signs and symptoms that are characteristic of a particular abnormal condition

synovial joints Freely movable articulations characterized by a membrane that secretes a fluid for lubrication of the joint

systemic Relating to, or affecting, the entire body

tailbone The coccyx

talus One of the tarsal bones that articulates with the tibia and fibula to form the ankle joint

tarsal Relating to the bones that form the heel, ankle, and instep of the foot

tarsus A collective term for the seven bones that form the heel, ankle, and instep of the foot

temporal Relating to the bone that forms the temple or side of the head

temporalis Muscle of mastication that extends from the temporal bone to the mandible

tendinous Having the nature of or relating to a tendon

tendon A cord of dense, fibrous connective tissue that attaches muscle to bone

tensor fasciae latae Superficial muscle of the lateral thigh; muscle that flexes and abducts the thigh

tentorium cerebelli An extension of dura mater that acts as a partition between the cerebrum and the cerebellum

teres major and minor Muscles associated with movement of the shoulder joint

tertiary Relating to the number three

testicular Relating to the testes

testis (pl. testes) Male gonad that produces spermatozoa and the male hormone testosterone; also called the *testicle*

thalamic Relating to the thalamus

thalamus (pl. thalami) An oval mass of gray matter, located on either side of the third ventricle in the cerebrum; primarily functions as a relay center for sensory impulses

thigh The proximal portion of the lower extremity, located between the hip and the knee

thoracic Relating to the thorax or chest

thorax The upper part of the body, between the neck and the diaphragm; the chest

thrombus A blood clot in an unbroken blood vessel, located at its point of formation, usually within a vein

thymus A lymphoid structure, located in the mediastinum posterior to the sternum; plays a role in the development of the immune system

thyroid A bilobed endocrine gland, located on either side of the trachea, that functions in the regulation of the body's metabolism

tibia Long bone in the thigh

tibial Relating to the tibia

tibialis anterior Muscle along the anterior surface of the tibia

tonsil A small mass of lymphoid tissue embedded in mucous membrane

tortuous Twisted

trabecula (pl. trabeculae) A supporting cord of connective tissue

trabeculae carneae Muscular bands or ridges of myocardium on the inner surface of the ventricles of the heart

trachea Passageway for air between the larynx and the bronchi, also called the *windpipe*

tracheal Relating to the trachea

transected Cut across

transverse Term indicating horizontal or crosswise direction

transversospinalis muscles Deep layer of intrinsic muscles associated with the vertebral column; includes the semispinalis, the multifidus, and the rotators

trapezius Superficial muscle of the upper back

trauma An injury

traverse To navigate, cross, bridge, or span

triceps brachii Large muscle with three heads, located on the posterior surface of the arm that functions to extend the arm at the elbow

tricuspid Having three cusps, the valve between the right atrium and the right ventricle

trigeminal Cranial nerve V

trigone Triangular area on the floor of the bladder marked by the openings for the two ureters and the urethra

trochanter One of two large prominences on the proximal femur

trochlea Any pulleylike structure or surface

trochlear Cranial nerve IV

tubercle A rounded elevation on a bone

tuberosity A rounded projection from a bone

tunic A layer or coating

turbinate Shaped like a scroll; a bone that is shaped like a scroll or conch shell; one of the nasal conchae

ulna The medial bone of the forearm

ulnar Relating to the ulna

umbilical Relating to the umbilicus or navel

umbilicus Region on the abdomen that marks the former attachment of the umbilical cord; also called the *navel*

uncinate Shaped like a hook; an extension or region of the pancreas

undifferentiated Not specialized, usually in reference to cells

uniaxial Allows movement along one axis, such as a hinge joint

unmyelinated Does not possess myelin, a fatty sheath; refers to nerve axons

ureter Tubular structure that conveys urine from the renal pelvis to the urinary bladder

urethra Tubular structure that conveys urine from the urinary bladder to the exterior

urogenital Relating to both the urinary (renal) system and the genital (reproductive) system; also called *genitourinary*

uterus The hollow, muscular organ in the female pelvis that is the site of menstruation, implantation of the fertilized egg, and the development of the embryo and fetus; also called the *womb*

utricle A part of the membranous labyrinth, located in the vestibule of the inner ear, that contains sense receptors for static equilibrium

uvula The fleshy projection at the posterior end of the soft palate

vagina The muscular tube that extends from the vestibule to the cervix of the uterus in the female

vaginal Relating to the vagina

vagus Cranial nerve X

vallecula A shallow groove; the groove between the epiglottis and the root of the tongue

vas (pl. vasa) A channel or duct, which conveys a liquid

vascular Pertaining to, or containing, vessels

vasculature The blood vessels of an organ

vastus muscles Part of the quadriceps femoris group of muscles on the anterior thigh: vastus lateralis, vastus intermedius, and vastus medialis

vein A vessel that carries blood toward the heart

vena (pl. **venae**) Latin for vein

venous Relating to veins

ventral Pertaining to the front or anterior side of the body; opposite of dorsal

ventricle A chamber or cavity, especially in the heart or brain

ventricular Pertaining to a ventricle

vermiform Shaped like a worm, such as the vermiform appendix

vermis Latin for worm; the central part of the cerebellum that connects the two cerebellar hemispheres

vertebra (pl. **vertebrae**) One of the bones that form the spinal column or backbone

vertebral Relating to the vertebrae

vesicle A small pouch or sac that contains liquid

vestibule A chamber or space, such as the vestibule of the larynx or vestibule of the inner ear

vestibulocochlear Cranial nerve VIII; functions in the sense of hearing and equilibrium

villus (pl. **villi**) A small, hairlike projection from the surface of a membrane

viscera The organs inside the ventral body cavity

visceral Relating to the viscera

vitreous body The soft, gelatinous substance that fills the posterior portion of the eyeball, between the lens and the retina

vomer Bone of the face that forms the lower portion of the nasal septum

vulva Collective term for the external genitalia of the female; also called the *pudendum*

Wharton's duct Duct of the submandibular salivary gland; also called *submandibular duct*

Wharton's jelly Homogeneous intercellular substance of the umbilical cord; also called *mucous connective tissue*

xiphoid Shaped like a sword; the distal portion of the sternum

zygomatic Relating to the cheekbone or the zygomatic bone, such as the zygomatic process or the zygomatic arch

zygomatic bone Cheekbone; also called *zygoma*

zygote Fertilized egg; single cell, resulting from the union of male and female gametes

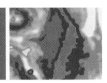

Many anatomical and medical terms are made up of combinations of word roots, or combining forms, together with prefixes or suffixes. Some of the more commonly used word roots and combining forms and their definitions are listed here, along with examples of their uses in a word and their definitions.

Ab– away from; *abduct*—to take away from

Abdomino– abdomen; *abdominopelvic cavity*—the portion of the ventral body cavity that includes the abdomen and the pelvis

Acro– extremity; *acromion process*—the extremity or extreme end of the spine of the scapula

Ad– toward; *adduct*—to move toward the axis of the body

Alb– white; *linea alba*—vertical white line in the center of the abdomen

Alveol– cavity, socket; *alveolus*—air cavity in the lung

Ante– before; *antecubital*—region in front of the elbow

Antero– in front, ventral; *anterolateral*—located in front and to one side

Atrio– relating to an atrium of the heart; *atrioventricular valve*—valve between an atrium and a ventricle

Bi– two; *biceps brachii*—muscle in the arm with two heads

Brachi– arm; *brachial artery*—the principal artery in the arm

Bronch– relating to the bronchi; *bronchoscopy*—direct visual examination of the bronchi

Capit– relating to the head; *capitulum*—a head-shaped eminence on a bone

Cardi– heart *cardiology*—study of the heart and its diseases

Cephal– head; *cephalad*—toward the head

Cerebello– relating to the cerebellum; *cerebellomedullary*—relating to the cerebellum and the medulla oblongata

Cerebro– brain; *cerebrospinal fluid*—fluid that circulates around the brain and spinal cord

Chondr– cartilage; *hypochondriac region*—abdominal region below the cartilage of the ribs

Coraco– relating to the coracoid process of the scapula; *coracoacromial ligament*—ligament between the coracoid process and the acromion process

Cor–, Coron– heart; *coronary arteries*—arteries that supply blood to the heart muscle

Cost– rib; *costal cartilage*—the cartilage that connects the ribs to the sternum

Crani– skull; *craniotomy*—surgical opening of the skull

Cysti– sac or bladder; *cystic duct*—duct from the gallbladder

Dorso–, Dorsi– denotes a relationship to the dorsal or the posterior surface; *dorsolateral*—on the posterior surface and to one side

Duodeno– denotes a relationship to the first part of the small intestine; *duodenojejunal flexure*—turn at the junction of the duodenum and the jejunum

Dura– hard or tough; *dura mater*—outer, tough membrane that covers the brain and the spinal cord

Ecto– outside; *ectopic pregnancy*—pregnancy or gestation outside the uterus

Endo– inside; *endocardium*—membrane that lines the inside of the heart wall

Epi– above or upon; *epidural*—above the dura mater

Ex–, Exo–, Extra– out or away from; *extrinsic muscles*—muscles outside the structure being acted upon

Fibro– denotes fibers; *fibrocartilage*—cartilage with an abundance of white fibers in the matrix

Gastr– stomach; *gastritis*—inflammation of the stomach

Gingiv– gum; *gingivitis*—inflammation of the gums

Glosso– tongue; *glossopharyngeal nerve*—nerve that provides innervation for the tongue

Hepato– liver; *hepatitis*—inflammation of the liver

Hyper– beyond or excessive; *hypertrophy*—excessive growth of a tissue

Hypo– under, below, deficient; *hypoglossal*—below the tongue

Hyster– uterus; *hysterectomy*—surgical removal of the uterus

Ileo– ileum; *ileocecal valve*—junction of the ileum and the cecum

Ilio– ilium; *iliosacral*—pertaining to both the ilium and the sacrum

Infra– beneath; *infraorbital foramen*—foramen below the orbit of the eye

Inter– among or between; *intercostal muscles*—the muscles between the ribs

Intra– within or inside; *intracranial pressure*—pressure inside the cranium

Labi– lip; *glenoid labrum*—rim or lip of fibrocartilage around the margin of the glenoid fossa

Laryngo– relates to the larynx; *laryngopharynx*—the portion of the pharynx in the region of the larynx

Lieno– relates to the spleen; *lienorenal ligament*—peritoneal ligament between the spleen and the kidney

Lingua– tongue; *lingual frenulum*—fold of tissue that anchors the tongue to the floor of the mouth

Lumbo– lower back, loin; *lumbar vertebrae*—vertebrae in the lower back region

Meningo–   membrane; *meningitis*—inflammation of the membranes around the brain and spinal cord

Meta–   after or beyond; *metacarpals*—bones of the hand, beyond the wrist

Metr–   uterus; *endometrium*—lining of the uterus

Mid–   located in the middle; *midsagittal*—sagittal section in the middle, divides into equal right and left portions

Musculo–   muscular system; *musculoskeletal*—pertains to both the muscular system and the skeletal system

Myo–   muscle; *myocardium*—muscle in the heart wall

Naso–   referring to the nose; *nasolacrimal duct*—duct that drains tears into the nasal cavity

Nephro–   kidney; *nephron*—basic functional unit of the kidney

Neuro–   nerve; *neuromuscular*—pertaining to both nerves and muscle

Oculo–   eye; *oculomotor*—nerve that transmits impulses to the muscles of the eye

Odont–   tooth; *odontoid process*—toothlike process on the second cervical vertebra

Oo–   egg; *oocyte*—egg cell

Ophthalm–   eye; *ophthalmology*—study of the eye and its diseases

Orchid–   testicle; *cryptorchidism*—failure of the testicle to descend into the scrotum

Oro–   mouth; *oropharynx*—region of the pharynx posterior to the cavity of the mouth

Oss–, osseo–, osteo–   bone; *osseous*—containing bone

Palpebr–   eyelid; *levator palpebrae superioris*—muscle that raises the upper eyelid

Para–   adjacent, alongside, or deviation from normal; *parasagittal section*—a sagittal section that is not in the midline

Parieto–   relates to the wall of a cavity; *parietal peritoneum*—layer of peritoneum that lines the wall of the abdominal cavity

Patho–   disease; *pathology*—study of disease mechanisms

Peri–   around; *pericardium*—membrane around the heart

Phon–   voice, sound; *phonation*—the production of sound

Phren–   diaphragm; *phrenic nerve*—nerve that stimulates the diaphragm

Postero–   a direction toward the back of the body; *posterolateral*—toward the sides on the back of the body

Pre–   before, either in time or in space; *prenatal*—before birth

Pulmon–   lung; *pulmonary*—relating to the lungs

Quadr–, quadri–   of or relating to the number four; *quadriceps femoris*—muscle group that contains four muscles

Radio–   relating to radiation; *radiograph*—picture formed by radiation

Radio–   relating to the radius; *radioulnar joint*—articulation between the radius and the ulna

Recto–   relating to the rectum; *rectouterine pouch*—pouch or cul-de-sac between the rectum and uterus

Retro–   situated behind or backward; *retroperitoneal*—located behind the peritoneum

Sacr–, sacri–   relating to the sacrum; *sacroiliac*—relating to both the sacrum and the ilium

Semi–   denoting half or partial; *semicircular canals*—canals that are shaped like half of a circle

Spheno–   relating to the sphenoid bone; *sphenoethmoidal*—relates to both the sphenoid bone and the ethmoid bone

Sterno–   relating to the sternum; *sternopericardial ligament*—membranous ligament located between the sternum and the pericardium

Stylo–   relating to the styloid process of the temporal bone; *stylomastoid foramen*—foramen located between the styloid process and the mastoid

Sub–   below or less than; *submandibular*—below the mandible

Supero–   relating to superior; *superomedial*—in a direction that is superior and medial to the reference

Super–, supra–   meaning above or too much; *supraspinatus muscle*—muscle above the spine of the scapula

Trans–   across, through, or beyond; *transected*—cut through

Tri–   three; *trigone*—a triangular region, marked by three openings, on the floor of the urinary bladder

Utero–   relating to the uterus; *uterovesical pouch*—peritoneal pouch between the uterus and the urinary bladder

Vas–   vessel or duct; *cerebrovascular*—pertaining to the blood vessels of the brain

Vertebro–   relating to the vertebrae; *vertebrosternal ribs*—ribs that are attached to the vertebrae and the sternum

Vesico–   relating to the urinary bladder; *vesicoprostatic*—relating to the urinary bladder and the prostate gland

Viscer–   organ; *visceral peritoneum*—peritoneum that covers the abdominal organs

EPONYMS

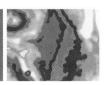

Eponyms are names of diseases, structures, or procedures that include the name of an individual. The current trend is to avoid, or at least to discourage, the use of eponyms because they are nondescriptive and often vague. Eponyms are still widely used, however, especially in clinical practice. This list has been prepared to help you relate common eponyms to the preferred terminology.

Eponym	Preferred Terminology
Achilles tendon	calcaneal tendon
Adam's apple	thyroid cartilage
ampulla of Vater	hepatopancreatic ampulla
antrum of Highmore	maxillary sinus
aqueduct of Sylvius	cerebral aqueduct
Bartholin's duct	major sublingual duct
Bartholin's gland	greater vestibular gland
Bundle of His	atrioventricular (AV) bundle
canal of Schlemm	scleral venous sinus
circle of Willis	cerebral arterial circle
Cooper's ligament	suspensory ligament of the breast
Cowper's gland	bulbourethral gland
crypt of Lieberkühn	intestinal gland
duct of Rivinus	lesser sublingual duct
duct of Wirsung	pancreatic duct
eustachian tube	auditory tube
fallopian tube	uterine tube

Eponym	Preferred Terminology
fissure of Rolando	central fissure (sulcus)
fissure of Sylvius	lateral cerebral fissure
foramen of Luschka	lateral aperture
foramen of Magendie	median aperture
foramen of Monro	interventricular foramen
foramen of Winslow	epiploic foramen
graafian follicle	vesicular ovarian follicle
island of Reil	insula
ligament of Treitz	suspensory muscle of the duodenum
organ of Corti	spiral organ
Peyer's patches	aggregated lymphatic follicles
pouch of Douglas	rectouterine pouch
Purkinje fibers	conduction myofibers
Skene's gland	paraurethral gland
Stensen's duct	parotid duct
Wharton's duct	submandibular duct
Wharton's jelly	mucous connective tissue

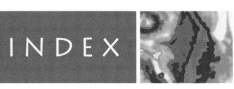
Page numbers followed by *f* indicate figures; *t*, tables.